Ruddy and McDaniel have the collective experience and persuasive examples to convince their readers why integrated care represents the best care available. Context matters. No matter whether joining people to guide their journey toward health or creating change in organizations, we need to understand the perspective of others and the forces that shape their choices. Whether new or experienced to a systems lens, this accessible text will transform your care of patients.

–**CATHERINE L. GILLISS, PhD,** RN, FAAN; DEAN AND STYLES PROFESSOR OF NURSING, UCSF, SAN FRANCISCO, CA

Complete with theory, policy, and practice evidence to manage the complexities of integrated behavioral health more effectively, Ruddy and McDaniel offer a comprehensive overview of behavioral healthcare integration. Regardless of readers' familiarity with integrated models of care at the clinical-, population-, and system-levels, this book will deepen practice knowledge and understanding.

–**LISA DE SAXE ZERDEN, MSW, PhD,** UNC CHAPEL HILL SCHOOL OF SOCIAL WORK, UNIVERSITY OF NORTH CAROLINA AT CHAPEL HILL, CHAPEL HILL, NC; & BRIANNA M. LOMBARDI, MSW, PHD, UNC CHAPEL HILL SCHOOL OF MEDICINE, UNIVERSITY OF NORTH CAROLINA AT CHAPEL HILL, CHAPEL HILL, NC

Written by two highly successful forerunners in the field of integrated healthcare, this book describes the challenges implementing integrated models of care and provides a pathway to addressing those barriers. The strong focus on navigating systems effectively makes it a unique resource. The collective wisdom of the authors shines through, making it a must-read for anyone who wants to thrive in integrated primary and specialty care settings.

–**BARBARA CUBIC, PhD,** PROFESSOR, DIRECTOR OF BEHAVIORAL HEALTH, WEST VIRGINIA UNIVERSITY SCHOOL OF MEDICINE, DEPARTMENT OF FAMILY MEDICINE, MORGANTOWN, WV

T0374844

Ruddy and McDaniel offer us a work that is encyclopedic in scope, balanced and authoritative in its content, and, finally ground-breaking for the field of integrated care. It serves as a manual for making integrated behavioral health the standard of care in medical settings, as relevant to clinicians entering the field as to policy makers and organizational leaders on the lead edges of innovation.

—ALEXANDER BLOUNT, EdD, PROFESSOR EMERITUS OF FAMILY MEDICINE AND COMMUNITY HEALTH, UMASS CHAN MEDICAL SCHOOL, WORCESTER, MA; PRESIDENT, INTEGRATED PRIMARY CARE, INC.

For the first time we have a clear and comprehensive account of the field of integrated clinical care—the elements from which it draws, the sociopolitical and economic crucible in which it is forged, the powerful tools that have emerged, and the most promising directions for the future. Drs. Ruddy and McDaniel are two distinguished clinician-scholars who have been there from the beginning, working in and shaping this field, and this volume is a brilliant culmination of decades of work. Well done!

—FRANK DEGRUY, MD, MSFM. PROFESSOR, DEPARTMENT OF FAMILY MEDICINE, UNIVERSITY OF COLORADO, BOULDER, CO

With a focus on systems, this text is a must-read for healthcare professionals who wish to have a sophisticated, yet practical understanding of current health conditions and why integrated care models are our best hope for achieving better health outcomes.

—TERRY STANCIN, PhD, ABPP, PEDIATRIC/CLINICAL CHILD & ADOLESCENT PSYCHOLOGIST, PROFESSOR, CASE WESTERN RESERVE UNIVERSITY, CLEVELAND, OH; FELLOW, AMERICAN PSYCHOLOGICAL ASSOCIATION

A SYSTEMIC APPROACH TO

BEHAVIORAL
HEALTHCARE INTEGRATION:

CONTEXT MATTERS

FUNDAMENTALS OF CLINICAL PRACTICE WITH COUPLES AND FAMILIES

*Best Clinical Practices for Treating Families in Juvenile
and Criminal Justice Systems*

CORINNE C. DATCHI

A SYSTEMIC APPROACH TO

BEHAVIORAL

HEALTHCARE INTEGRATION:

CONTEXT MATTERS

NANCY BREEN RUDDY AND SUSAN H. MCDANIEL

 AMERICAN PSYCHOLOGICAL ASSOCIATION

The opinions and statements published are the responsibility of the authors, and such opinions and statements do not necessarily represent the policies of the American Psychological Association.

Published by
American Psychological Association
750 First Street, NE
Washington, DC 20002
https://www.apa.org

Order Department
https://www.apa.org/pubs/books
order@apa.org

Typeset in Charter and Interstate by Circle Graphics, Inc., Reisterstown, MD

Printer: Gasch Printing, Odenton, MD
Cover Designer: Mark Karis

Library of Congress Cataloging-in-Publication Data

Names: Ruddy, Nancy Breen, author. | McDaniel, Susan H., author. | American
   Psychological Association, issuing body.
Title: A systemic approach to behavioral healthcare integration : context
   matters / Nancy Breen Ruddy and Susan H. McDaniel.
Other titles: Fundamentals of clinical practice with couples and families.
Description: Washington, DC : American Psychological Association, [2024] |
   Series: Fundamentals of clinical practice with couples and families |
   Includes bibliographical references and index.
Identifiers: LCCN 2023016630 (print) | LCCN 2023016631 (ebook) |
   ISBN 9781433835865 (paperback) | ISBN 9781433835872 (ebook)
Subjects: MESH: Mental Health Services | Patient-Centered Care | Delivery
   of Health Care, Integrated | Family Relation | United States | BISAC:
   PSYCHOLOGY / Clinical Psychology | MEDICAL / Public Health
Classification: LCC RA790.55 (print) | LCC RA790.55 (ebook) | NLM WM 30 AA1 |
   DDC 362.2--dc23/eng/20230602
LC record available at https://lccn.loc.gov/2023016630
LC ebook record available at https://lccn.loc.gov/2023016631

https://doi.org/10.1037/0000381-000

Printed in the United States of America

10 9 8 7 6 5 4 3 2 1

*For our mentors, whose work provides the foundation for ours,
and to our mentees who will expand this work in wonderful
and unimaginable ways.*

For our families, whose love and support makes our work possible.

For the families we serve, who seek resilience in the face of adversity.

Contents

Foreword

This book is a labor of love to all who would aspire to work in clinical settings on an integrated team of medical and behavioral health professionals. Its aim is to further a more effective and satisfying approach to understanding and intervening in matters of health, illness, and care. The authors have condensed two careers' worth of knowledge and wisdom into a succinct and coherent account of the history of the major concepts, professional issues, practical intervention strategies, research efforts, and policy enhancements and constraints that have led to our current state and next step challenges. The text is loaded with lists of resource material from governmental, professional, and academic sources for all who would delve further, depending upon personal interest and setting. Overall, the essentials are here for old hands and pilgrims alike.

Looking back roughly 50 years, we can identify three origin themes that shaped the development of integrated care. One is that primary care needed reforming. The doctor–patient relationship could benefit from input from behavioral scientists. A second is that many medical patients needed mental health services that were not being met within mental health settings. For various reasons, referrals weren't working, and things fell back on the primary care office to manage these needs. Surely behavioral health clinicians could team up to help with this. And third, focusing medical care on isolated parts does not always work. Our minds and our bodies function as wholes, and although we know there are significant psychological, familial, cultural, and community-based components to all medical problems and their treatment, not much was being done to address this reality. Again, behavioral health clinicians could help mend this rift and contribute to healing once they got their feet in the door. Their value would extend over time to far more than mental health care. A fourth, and more recent understanding, is that what has been good for primary care is also good for specialty care. It is unrealistic to think that we can train "superdocs" to deal effectively with the linchpins of patient and family behavior. But like-minded colleagues with a systems incli-nation from different professional disciplines, collaborating within integrated teams, have a much better chance. Drs. Ruddy and McDaniel consolidate these themes into a framework that could be constructed only by two authors who have spent their careers in multiple roles and settings where these issues were calling out to be addressed.

When I joined the Division of Ambulatory and Community Medicine at the University of California San Francisco (UCSF) School of Medicine in 1969, my role was to help develop a curriculum for a new pathway in family medicine for medical students and to teach "behavioral science" at a new residency program in family medicine at the Community Hospital of Sonoma County in Santa Rosa, California. The centerpiece was an introduction to family medicine course for first-year medical students that included a pre-ceptorship and a dinnertime home visit to a family chosen by the student's preceptor because of an interesting health reason. This occasion provided the opportunity to elicit a family health history, construct a basic genogram, and ask about the family members' experiences with their family doc, all to be written up in a family study.

The residency role involved adding one-way mirror observation rooms in the new family practice center, introducing video feedback, and providing con-sultation, including joining the residents in the exam room with whomever they wished, including their most difficult patients. I recruited several inter-ested psychologists and psychiatrists from the community to join the clinical faculty and be on hand for a couple of hours per week to help residents and patients in whatever way was needed.

One novel feature of this work, back in the day when time seemed less pressing, was for me to sit with an experienced family physician behind a one-way mirror and observe a resident for a full morning or afternoon patient care session, on occasion videotaping patient encounters, and then reviewing with the resident what went on, in a three-way conversation. One striking fact that inspired this two-on-one approach was my early discovery that it was possible for a future physician to go all the way through medical school and residency training without ever having been observed firsthand with a patient in an outpatient setting. (This was mind-boggling to someone who had been trained to do family therapy by being routinely observed through a one-way mirror.) With communication being the essence of the relationship between a patient and their doctor, that is where we started. The mental and eventual behavioral health dimensions of practice, patient care, and collaboration flowed from there.

Federal policymakers gave the effort covered in these pages an enormous boost when the federal Comprehensive Health Manpower Training Act of 1971 required all new family practice residencies seeking basic program support to include one full-time equivalent behavioral scientist for every 24 residents. This would ensure support for at least one faculty position in these new programs that most sponsoring hospitals would not see fit to fund. Fifty years later, providing much-needed wind for our sails, Larry Green and colleagues produced a manifesto, published in the January 2022 issue of *Family Medicine,* outlining a new "Decade of Family Medicine Residency Transformation" that calls out a central role for behavioral health professionals, teamwork, and integrated education and care. I would have thought, back in the mid-1970s when we launched the Task Force on Behavioral Science in Family Medicine and the Task Force on Family in Family Medicine, that near-universal integrated care within all contexts of primary care would be the norm by now, but it still is not. Now, as primary care continues its development, the benefits of integrated team care are being recognized by other medical specialties. The University of Rochester is leading the way with initiatives in 11 clinical departments. The book you are about to read gives a substantial lift to these ongoing efforts.

My first task at UCSF was a literature search on behavioral scientists and behavioral health clinicians working with medical students and residents. The most useful publications in those days described groundbreaking work in pediatrics on inclusion and collaboration that established the tradition embodied in the work of Nancy Ruddy, reflected throughout this book. That early work on training and the beginnings of team-based care inspired a cadre of like-minded colleagues to imagine what could be accomplished in family medicine.

I have known Susan McDaniel since she and Tom Campbell gave their first presentation at a Society of Teachers of Family Medicine conference in 1985. In the time since, no one has done more in more settings to advance the cause of systemic integrated care than has Dr. McDaniel. Her academic and professional leadership roles, her policy facilitation and contributions, and her body of conceptual and practical publications is unsurpassed. The core of that work runs through these pages.

In addition to covering the conceptual framework, research base, and clinical evolution of integrated care, the authors include three well-developed actual case studies illustrating how integrated team care can work over an extended period. Throughout the book the authors also interweave personal reflections on their successes and failures and identify the major obstacles blocking the path of progress today. Their comments resonate with my own experience entirely. Here are four observations.

First, the systems lens is essential. The family systems mindset informs team development and integration in ways well suited for healthcare settings of all kinds. Isolating the lens to the patient or thinking about team members as simply those multiple professionals identified in the electronic health record as having had contact with the patient ignores interconnectedness and forgoes an abundance of opportunities. The systems lens with its practical application is also crucial for organizational development. This is extremely difficult to achieve but essential if synergies are to replace internal competition and contradictions.

Second, the heavy lift in building teams is on the behavioral side. Therapists, whatever their professional degree, are primarily specialists by training and practice preference in that they offer a particular approach to change or prefer to see patients with only certain kinds of problems. There are few opportunities in training to be exposed to healthcare settings, and it is challenging to find true generalists who can work briefly, flexibly, and comfortably within free-flowing collaboration. I have been frustrated with this obstacle for 50 years. Fortunately, efforts to change this are picking up steam, and examples and opportunities are well-documented in this book.

Third, grant-funded demonstration projects, no matter how successful at achieving their goals, are almost always discontinued at the end of their extramural funding. There is a revealing explanation for this. Let's say that a demonstration grant provides funding for two behavioral health clinicians to provide on-site care for common problems and work collaboratively with medical clinicians. After 2 years, depending on the outcomes chosen to measure, the results may include reduced failures for mental health referrals, fewer visits to the emergency room, better preparation for major surgery leading to earlier discharge from the hospital and less use of postsurgical pain medication, fewer readmissions, overall higher satisfaction from patients and clinicians, and meaningful reduction in the overall cost of care. Why wouldn't the clinic administration celebrate these achievements and continue the employment of the behavioral health clinicians? It is because they do not benefit from the financial savings that accrue to these changes but only incur their costs. Clinic managers have budgets to which they are accountable. Their margins would be squeezed by two new employees that could not pay for themselves in the current reimbursement scheme, and the savings are not credited where they originated but roll up elsewhere to levels that do not have the behavioral clinicians on their immediate payrolls. The shibboleth, "No margin, no mission," needs to be revisited with the question "Whose margin and whose mission?" With federally qualified community health centers somewhat excepted because of their funding and salary mechanisms, the private and not-for-profit sectors are seldom structurally rationalized to make investments at the ground level that benefit the greater good.

Fourth, and connected to the issue above, the authors make a convincing case throughout the text for how the current predominant fee-for-service payment model, based on the resource-based relative value scale used by the Centers for Medicare and Medicaid Services and most other payers, undermines progress in primary care and undervalues what is needed to support integrated team care. They suggest some good-faith ways to work around this roadblock to adequate payment. Better for the integrated team enterprise by far would be national and state policy decisions to transform the whole system, but the very idea runs up against enormous resistance from entrenched interests that would have a lot to lose.

In their conclusion the authors note that the emergence of integrated care has served as a "systemic counterbalance" to the healthcare fragmentation of the last half century. Because primary care had to absorb many patients who could not or would not get their needs met in specialty mental health settings, this pressure led increasingly toward embedding mental health clinicians within the primary care setting. As time passed behavioral health clinicians demonstrated their value well beyond addressing mental health needs. As these participants joined their medical counterparts and worked together in teams, something special was added. The long-recognized reality that many of the problems of physical health, medical disease, and successful treatment are shaped by key psychological, social, and cultural determinants at last would have the right people in the right place to engage these issues. This emergence also led to something special for the new team members, something the authors identify as the "joy of practice." The promise of these new interprofessional teams is that providing health care can be more effective and personally rewarding when based in interprofessional relationships with a shared purpose and mission in a shared setting. What's better for the clinicians is better for patients and families, too.

What the future holds for these team-building health professionals depends not just on them but on many others who make decisions central to their fate.

Let's hope our healthcare leaders and policymakers have the good sense to support them. One thing I can assure everyone is that anyone interested in any aspect of the story of integrated team care will experience much joy in reading this superb book.

Donald C. Ransom, PhD
Senate Professor Emeritus
Department of Family and Community Medicine
University of California San Francisco

Preface

As we came to the end of writing this book, we turned our attention to placing our work in the context of our own journeys as clinicians, educators, and healthcare change agents. We contemplated, in the famous words of musician David Byrne, "How did we get here?"

Not surprisingly, our dialogue revealed patterns: some that we both had recognized for many years and some that emerged only as we each shared our version of the book's origin story. We anticipate the reader may recognize some of their own experiences in ours, reflective of a collective journey. We hope our transitions in viewpoint, focus, and values will reflect and illuminate the reader's own journey toward systemic integrated care.

TRANSITIONING FROM AN INDIVIDUAL LENS TO A SYSTEMIC LENS

We both were trained as clinical psychologists prior to our systemic training but felt something was missing. Susan discovered her interest in systemic work when she completed her internship at University of Texas Medical Branch in Galveston, working with Harry Goolishian and Harlene Anderson. Her internship and postdoctoral fellowship formed a systemic foundation she would later apply in her work in medical settings, as a clinician, educator, and delivery system architect.

Nancy first learned of family therapy as an undergraduate and was fascinated by a focus on relational patterns as she studied child psychology but had little opportunity to learn family therapy formally. She welcomed the opportunity to complete the postgraduate Family Therapy Training Program at the University of Rochester after finishing her internship in child psychology there. We both found systemic thought very natural and felt our training filled in the large missing puzzle piece in our approach to our work.

JOINING THE WORLD OF MEDICINE AND PRIMARY CARE—WITH A NOD TO THE POWER OF MENTORSHIP

Neither of us focused our training on medical issues. Relative to today, it was unusual for psychologists to work in medical settings and even more unusual to work in primary care. Susan was comfortable around medical clinicians as she came from a "medical family" in which her father was an obstetrician–gynecologist with a thriving practice in South Florida. She experienced significant illness as a small child so had firsthand experience regarding the impact of medical conditions on individual and family development, roles, and relationships. Her position in Family Medicine and Psychiatry was a natural fit, even if the role was not well-defined. She had mentorship from Lyman Wynne, MD, PhD, who helped her develop a keen understanding of the interplay of systems and health based in his lifelong work seeking to understand links between family relational patterns and somatic issues. George Engel, MD, also served as a mentor. The impact of his biopsychosocial model on the culture of the medical school created an environment ripe for integrated care.

In contrast, Nancy was not a fan of medical settings (especially hospitals) but accepted the opportunity to join the faculty in the Department of Family Medicine to maintain her connection to the university after internship. She was pleasantly surprised to find herself at home in the primary care setting and truly enjoyed working with the vulnerable families served by the residency practice. She appreciated that systemic thinking was normative. Over time she realized her luck—and it was luck—went far beyond finding a place that felt like home. She had somehow managed to land in a place with extraordinary colleagues like Tom Campbell, MD; Tillman Farley, MD; Barbara Gawinski, PhD; Dave Seaburn, PhD; Cleveland Shields, PhD; and of course, Susan.

Our gratitude to our mentors was a driving force in writing this book. The process expanded our appreciation and debt of gratitude to our professional colleagues and reminded us that both of our careers stand on the shoulders of George Engel, Lyman Wynne, and others. We both reflected on the way Lyman's and George's mentorship of Susan ultimately cascaded into more than 3 decades of mentorship from Susan to Nancy (and from Susan and Nancy to countless others). This book reflects what we have learned from our mentors and the power of mentorship to change lives and careers and perhaps spark a collective effort that improves our healthcare system.

LIFE GOALS: MAKING BIOPSYCHOSOCIAL SYSTEMIC INTEGRATED CARE NORMATIVE

In her early years in family medicine, Susan quickly recognized that primary care patients needed access to behavioral health. Initial attempts to garner assistance from the mental health community were largely unsuccessful. She and Tom Campbell realized that the volume and intensity of behavioral health need in family medicine could not be managed by referring people out to specialty mental health. They hired behavioral health clinicians to provide services in the residency practice, largely out of necessity. The evolution of integrated services took time. Initially, the services were primarily a colocated, in-house referral model with a great deal of collaboration and communication. However, they eventually morphed into a more integrated team-based approach.

Susan and Tom were two of a scattering of "pioneers" nationwide, as their work at Rochester paralleled that at several sites across the United States. These pioneers, their colleagues, and their trainees have worked tirelessly over the past 4 decades to create a new field. Their (and our) work defined integrated care, outlined integrated care competencies, developed educational programs, researched best clinical and implementation practices, and generated outcome data to facilitate integrated care advocacy.

Despite all of this incredible work, we share a concern that the centrality of a systemic lens is not well-established in the current dialogue about integrated care. To provide biopsychosocial systemic care with optimal impact, we must attend not only to the patterns of one level of life but also to multiple levels as well as the interaction of these levels. We felt writing a book that contextualizes the integrated care movement in its systemic origins and further development might bring these issues to the foreground, especially with the current focus on large systems and population health. We provide this perspective with clear recognition that there is no one "true narrative."

Another motivation was to further our shared goal of making integrated healthcare and the biopsychosocial systems model normative. Like many, we have come to believe that this model is both a foundational way to improve health care and an opportunity to advocate for social justice. But we also know from our decades of experience that as long as the reimbursement system and policies currently in place persist in the United States, establishing and maintaining truly integrated care will continue to be an uphill battle. We looked to the implementation literature and found excellent summaries of important potential issues and interventions that support integration (e.g., training, workflows). Our implementation part expands on these resources to focus on the leadership, team building, and change management processes that promote large-scale systemic change.

We base these beliefs in our shared experiences with integrated care implementation. Susan expanded the integrated model well beyond family medicine at University of Rochester Medical Center. To date, there are coaching and/or clinical roles for behavioral health clinicians in 12 University of Rochester Medical Center clinical departments. In so doing, she expanded access to behavioral health services for patients, families, and clinicians, managing a wide array of medical challenges. After leaving Rochester in 2000, Nancy served as a clinician and educator in three additional family medicine residency clinics and led multiple training programs that trained future psychologists to work in primary care. She worked with others to implement integrated care in dozens of community-based primary care practices. Both of us came to appreciate the hard work it takes to move from separate to colocated to fully integrated behavioral health. We also came to appreciate how rewarding this work can be and how integration efforts positively transform the experience of healthcare for patients and clinicians alike.

Each of us feels our systemic lens and process orientation were keys to success, helping us strategically assess system elements and intervene as needed. Therefore our implementation part focuses on how common patterns in various levels of the system in healthcare affect implementation processes. We look to the literature on leadership and systemic change management science to inform strategies to address behavioral and relational patterns that can impede integration efforts.

We strongly believe a relational, systemic approach to integrated clinical care facilitates successful patient outcomes and clinician satisfaction. Yet many integrated care behavioral strategies emphasize brevity and focus clinical assessment and intervention solely on the individual. We advocate a systemic approach to clinical care that recognizes the benefits of individual integrated care assessment and intervention approaches and places them—

along with relevant relational interventions—within a larger biopsychosocial treatment plan. Toward these ends, we apply medical family therapy strategies developed by Susan and others to the integrated care environment in the final part of the book.

Our ultimate motivation is a shared belief that our healthcare system is in dire need of disruption. Writing this book during the COVID-19 pandemic, we became all the more aware of the urgency of change. Integrated care can, and has, served as a disruptive factor. We hope that a biopsychosocial systemic lens for integrated care will catalyze and amplify change for you, your practice, your healthcare system, and our collective communities.

Acknowledgments

We want to acknowledge a number of people for their assistance in the writing of this book. Each helped to improve the final product. Some offered ideas and insights, some shared their experience of the evolution of integrated care, and some read portions of the text and offered feedback. We value these esteemed colleagues, from whom we have learned a great deal. We are exceedingly grateful for their help with this project. Thank you to the following people: Keisha Bell, Alexander Blount, Tom Campbell, Rebecca Copek, Barbara Cubic, Janette Dauenhauer, Lauren DeCaporale-Ryan, Frank deGruy, Ann Dobermeyer, Tillman Farley, Colleen Fogarty, Andrea Garroway, Barbara Gawinski, Catherine Gilliss, Jeffrey Goodie, William Gunn, Christine Henry, Julia Hill, Christopher Hunter, Lisa Kearney, Rodger Kessler, Parinda Khatri, Hochang Ben Lee, Larry Mauksch, Jessica Moore, Benjamin Miller, C. J. Peek, Carol Podgorski, Ellen Poleshuck, Donald Ransom, Donna Rasin-Waters, John Rolland, Tziporah Rosenberg, Julie Schirmer, David Seaburn, Cleveland Shields, Jenny Speice, Michelle Swanger-Gagne, Neftali Serrano, Terri Stancin, Kari Stephens, Lindsay Sycz, Traci Terrance, Douglas Tynan, Mark Vogel, Barbara Ward-Zimmerman, and Shanda Wells. We also want to thank the members of Dr. McDaniel's family medicine professional writing seminar. We also are grateful to Dr. Ruddy's teaching and research assistants: Lucas Brandt, Tenzin Dorjee, Shannon McCleery, Molly O'Reilly, Hannah Sokoloff-Rubin, and Joanna Sullivan.

We also appreciate our family psychology colleagues, Corinne Datchi, PhD, and Anthony Chambers, PhD, for encouraging us to write this book.

We are grateful to the American Psychological Association Publishing staff—Ida Audeh, Elizabeth Brace, Janette Lynn Neal, and Catherine Malo—as they have been invaluable partners in this process.

Finally, special thanks to our husbands, Tom Ruddy and David Siegel, who support us through thick and thin.

Prologue

The goal of integrated care is for physical and mental health professionals to work together to provide comprehensive patient care. The goal of integrated care sounds simple.

It is not.
It is powerful.
It is very effective.
It is deeply rewarding.
It is a prescription for medical and behavioral health clinician wellness.
It is often fun.

But it is not simple—it is multifaceted, reflecting the biopsychosocial complexity of the human experience. For that reason, it is important to use a systemic lens to understand the process and experience of integration at the clinical, educational, operational, policy, and larger system levels.

A SYSTEMIC APPROACH TO

BEHAVIORAL
HEALTHCARE INTEGRATION:

CONTEXT MATTERS

INTRODUCTION

Why a Systemic Lens Is Critical for Integrated Care

We have a neck for a reason. Common sense and decades' worth of data tell us that it is perilous to ignore the connection between our minds and bodies. Yet traditional clinical and training approaches segregate the biomedical and psychosocial aspects of the human experience. The U.S. healthcare system largely bifurcates care for our emotional, physical, and relational wellness. This dualistic, profit-driven structure impedes collaboration that can facilitate coordinated, comprehensive care to the people we serve. The status quo too often stymies service integration efforts aimed at bringing a team approach to necessary services and gathering expertise under one roof.

Despite these challenges, the advantages of integration have propelled expansion of interprofessional, team-based care in the latter part of the 20th century (Richman et al., 2020). The movement toward integration of behavioral health into medical care occurred in the context of larger system paradigm shifts over many decades. George Engel's (1977, 1980) description of the biopsychosocial approach in the 1970s spurred evolution in medical training, research, and standards of care. The biopsychosocial approach does

https://doi.org/10.1037/0000381-001
A Systemic Approach to Behavioral Healthcare Integration: Context Matters, by
N. B. Ruddy and S. H. McDaniel

not focus solely on the interplay of the mind and body. Rather, the approach acknowledges the impact of factors at every level—from the microscopic to the social stratosphere (see Figure 1). This expansion was prescient. In the years since publication of Engel's foundational article, research increasingly shows that social and behavioral factors are some of the most important aspects of health and wellness (Daniel et al., 2018).

Many healthcare professionals recognize and enjoy the benefits of multidisciplinary teams. However, integrated care has yet to become the agreed-upon standard of care. We believe it is critical to replace this parallel play between the medical and behavioral health systems with team-based, collaborative care

FIGURE 1. Hierarchy of Natural Systems

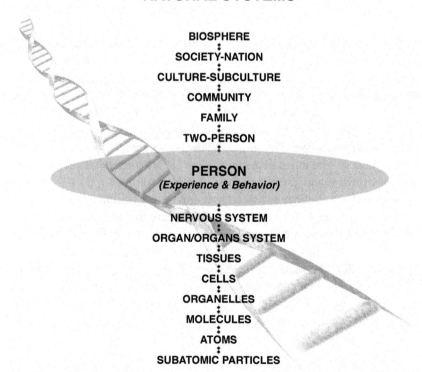

Reprinted from the "The Clinical Application of the Biopsychosocial Model," by G. L. Engel, 1980, *The American Journal of Psychiatry, 137*(5), p. 537. Copyright 1980 by the American Psychiatric Association. Background illustration printed with permission from Janette Dauenhauer.

that recognizes the patient and family as critical members of the team. We strive to make integrated care normative.

A central tenet of integrated care is to meet people where they are. Integrated care *literally* provides behavioral health services where the public seeks healthcare. Integrated family- and patient-centered care *figuratively* meets people where they are as well. The focus of care reflects the patient's, family's, and community's values and goals, recognizing that patients, families, and communities are more likely to engage when they feel they have a voice and a sense of agency in their own care (Baker, 2020).

Integrated care is part of a movement to care for the whole person. Whole-person healthcare focuses on the meaning of the healthcare experience, with a collaborative stance toward patients and families that emphasizes healing (Hutchinson, 2017). However, whole-person approaches still treat the individual as the unit of care. We advocate a systemic approach that not only recognizes the full spectrum of factors that influence an individual's health but also considers the relationships between these factors. Exploring these interactions enables a deeper reflection on the complexity of the human experience as it relates to our health and wellness.

Along these lines, one of our goals in writing this book is to highlight the importance of a *systemic lens*. A systemic lens recognizes nonlinear or circular/reciprocal causality, focuses on the relationships and patterns, anticipates unintended consequences, and emphasizes the role of the system in creating lasting, intentional change (Stroh, 2015). A systemic lens also enables us to integrate the influence of variables at each level of the system as well as the interplay among them. This interstitial space between our microbiology, organ systems, individual psychology and beliefs, family relationships, community, and culture is critical to improving the health of individuals, families, and communities. Finally, a systemic lens allows us to unravel the complexity of our fragmented healthcare system and revamp it to focus on effective, comprehensive care for patients and families.

This lens is particularly important when one seeks to influence systems in which

- a situation is chronic and defies attempted solutions;
- well-intended stakeholders struggle to align efforts despite shared goals;
- stakeholders tend to focus on optimization of their own part of the system, without consideration of the impact on the whole;
- efforts have, at times, actually undermined the stated goals;
- improvement efforts occur simultaneously with little to no coordination; and
- a focus on specific solutions (e.g., best practices) reduces engagement in continuous learning (Stroh, 2015).

Anyone familiar with our healthcare system will recognize these characteristics. Politicians, patients, and clinicians generally agree that the U.S. healthcare system functions poorly and is not financially sustainable. Ongoing reforms have yet to yield the needed transformative results. Too often, the system is stuck.

This book seeks to chart a path forward. Moving forward requires healthcare professionals to turn the mirror on ourselves and our system. We must create a road map for improving population health via integrating patient- and family-focused behavioral health into our healthcare structure and services. This road map, essentially a treatment plan for our healthcare system, must be evidence-based and cognizant of larger contexts. Therefore, we describe a path forward based on implementation science and clinical assessment, interventions, and outcomes research that recognizes how larger contexts facilitate and complicate efforts to integrate care.

SUCCESSFUL SYSTEMS CHANGE

As any experienced systems thinker appreciates, the foundations, history, systemic barriers and solutions, and clinical applications are intertwined like a bowl of spaghetti. We must be inclusive of the perspectives and expertise of all disciplines and roles because each serves different functions in our healthcare system. Yet each discipline and role ideally understand the larger context in which they function.

Clinicians and direct service staff can best facilitate reform when they understand the essential elements of integration, models of care, their genesis, and the systemic issues that affect care. Frontline clinicians can serve as the canary in the coal mine to inform implementation processes because they experience directly what is and is not working in their system. The more clinicians and staff understand and engage in the implementation process, the more likely the process will be successful. In parallel, administrators and systems architects need to understand and be able to explain exactly how these services look in the real world and how they will improve our healthcare system. They need to be able to highlight how clinicians' roles shift in integrated care while understanding the difficulty of changing clinical patterns. Ideally, their understanding of the end goal and the resources and processes needed to reach this goal can engender true practice transformation. Across the board, everyone needs motivation and a shared mental model of the desired end state, how to get there, why it matters, and how to measure and maintain progress.

Just as the biopsychosocial approach is foundational to integrated care, reflective practice and intentionality are foundational to practice transformation (Horton-Deutsch & Sherwood, 2017). We invite self-reflection regarding your readiness to change from a traditional, siloed approach to integrated, team-based care. Changing one's own behavior is challenging, particularly with regard to professional habits honed over years of training and practice. To successfully evolve toward integrated care, leaders, clinicians, and staff must believe that this shift will help them realize the shared "north star" to serve our communities via exceptional healthcare. To achieve this goal, health professionals must work collectively to alter daily routines and behaviors and adjust their interactions with each other and the patients and families they serve.

As family therapists ourselves, we assist families by helping them identify shared goals, make structural changes, and shift relational dynamics, communication, and behavioral patterns in service of the family's goals. Organizations and practice change efforts must engage in a parallel process to support systemic change toward integration. Successful integration implementation requires shifting healthcare structures, team dynamics, and communication and behavior patterns. As with families, the healthcare system has a strong pull to homeostasis that can derail change efforts (Selladurai et al., 2020). Such change is not simple, and it is not quick. Also as with families, integration implementation is most likely to be successful when stakeholders understand this new model of care and how it addresses some of the root causes of healthcare system pain points.

As change agents, we work with one hand tied behind our backs if we are unfamiliar with systemic concepts. Yet many healthcare professionals have not been trained in these concepts. The next part defines various systemic concepts and outlines how each concept is reflected in our review of systemic integrated care history, implementation, and clinical applications. We hope this helps readers less familiar with systemic thinking understand the meaning and application of these concepts. We encourage the reader to embrace a systemic spirit. As part of your self-reflection, notice any drift into thinking about these systems in a linear, cause-and-effect way and experiment with (or continue) to focus on the relational intertwining of elements and their function in the whole.

As you move forward, consider these wise words from Donella Meadows, an environmental scientist and writer who trained in system dynamics at the Massachusetts Institute of Technology and served as a professor of environmental sciences at Dartmouth. She wrote multiple bestselling books on systems thinking, as well as *The Global Citizen*, a well-regarded newspaper column that applied a systems perspective to global events.

> I don't think the systems way of seeing is better than the reductionist way of thinking. I think it's complementary and therefore revealing. You can see some things through the lens of the human eye, other things through the lens of the microscope and others through the lens of a telescope and still others through the lens of systems theory. Everything seen through each kind of lens is actually there. Each way of seeing allows our knowledge of the wondrous world in which we live to become a little complete. At a time when the world is more messy, more crowded, more interconnected, more interdependent, and more rapidly changing than ever before, the more ways of seeing, the better. The systems-thinking lens allows us to reclaim our intuition about whole systems and hone our abilities to understand parts, see interconnections, ask "what if" questions about possible future behaviors, and be creative and courageous about system redesign. Then we can use our insights to make a difference in ourselves and our world. (Meadows, 2008, p. 19)

APPLYING AND DEFINING A SYSTEMIC LENS

A systems lens serves as the foundational schema for how we understand integrated care. This lens informed our inclusion of the historical context of integrated care and serves as the underpinning of our approach to integrated care implementation and clinical services.

Part I of the book focuses on the *historical context* of integrated healthcare because the developmental context of any system is critical to understanding a system's current state and future direction. Therefore, we review the emergence and evolution of integrated care as well as the systemic underpinnings of our current healthcare state.

Part II of the book focuses on our belief that a systems lens underlies successful integration *implementation*. A systemic approach to healthcare reform and transformation is based on understanding the structure and regulation processes of the healthcare system. Therefore, in the implementation part of the book we discuss healthcare system structure, organization, subsystems, and interactional patterns.

Part III of the book shifts to address systemically oriented *direct clinical service*. Systemically focused clinical assessment and intervention require a specific mindset and set of competencies that transcend any one discipline. We review key concepts of medical family therapy, its evidence base, and its application in various healthcare settings and populations.

Table 1 describes how these particular concepts are relevant in the three parts of the book: historical context, implementation, and clinical application. These concepts can be difficult to understand based on verbal descriptions; for visual learners we suggest "Habits of a Systems Thinker" from Thinking Tools Studio, available at https://thinkingtoolsstudio.waterscenterst.org/cards. Below are definitions of systems concepts:

- **General systems theory:** A paradigm that recognizes that (a) the whole is greater than the sum of its parts (nonsummativity); (b) systems have hierarchies, executive organization, and subsystems; and (c) systems self-regulate and strive toward self-preservation (Gerhardt, 2019).

- **System:** A coherently organized set of elements interconnected in a pattern or structure that serves a specific purpose or set of purposes (Meadows, 2008).

- **Family system:** The family is an organism in which no one person orchestrates interactional patterns, so no one person can be to blame for issues. In a family systems perspective, all behavior makes sense in context. The patterns of interactions between family members and their context reflect mutually negotiated, often implicit, system rules and norms (Gerhardt, 2019).

- **Complex adaptive system:** A system made up of semiautonomous units that evolve over time, based on schemas or shared mental templates that inform this evolution. Multiple systems and schemas exchange information and/or resources. Understanding a complex adaptive system requires consideration of the way many elements interact with many other elements. This interlocking web of relationships among elements sets the stage for exponential "tipping point" change, depending on levels and natures of interconnection in the system (Dooley, 1997). Complex adaptive systems in healthcare are made up of diverse agents who can learn and adapt or coevolve with their environment, whose relationships are highly interconnected or interdependent, and who self-organize to complete tasks (Noël et al., 2013; Sturmberg, 2018).

- **Systems thinking (or systems lens):** An approach that recognizes nonlinear or circular/reciprocal causality, focuses on the interrelationship and patterns of behavior of system elements, anticipates unintended consequences, and emphasizes the role of the system in creating lasting change (Stroh, 2015).

- **Hierarchy:** An aspect of system structure related to the level of power in different parts of the system, or subsystems (Meadows, 2008).

TABLE 1. How Systems Concepts Can Inform Integrated Care

Concept	Part I: Historical Context	Part II: Implementation	Part III: Clinical Application
General systems theory	Context matters—the healthcare system cannot be well-understood outside of its historical evolution.	Implementation efforts are affected by the interrelation of healthcare system elements and its structure and the system's natural tendency to support the status quo.	The interplay of families, communities, health, and the healthcare system all affect and should be considered in clinical work.
System	A description of how healthcare system elements and their relationships evolved over time	How multiple systems (e.g., education, healthcare, government) can spur and deter implementation of systemic integrated care	How systemic elements in the family affect healthcare management and vice versa
Family systems	Healthcare expanded its purview to include the family system and other social factors in health.	Description of the parallels between family dynamics and healthcare system and clinical team dynamics in healthcare provision	A focus on the assessment and interventions strategies based in family systems theory.
Complex adaptive system	Healthcare increasingly recognizes the complexity inherent in its mission. This recognition has had broad implications for its evolution.	The barriers and facilitators of integrated healthcare are based in and reflect the complexity of our contextual system, practice organizations, and even the interplay of professionals, patients, and families in the provision of clinical care.	A systemic approach to clinical care requires consideration of how multiple systems interact with and around the patient and family.
Systems thinking (or systems lens)	The emergence of systemic thinking, including how this paradigm shift affected healthcare and the evolution of systemic integrated care	A description of how a systemic lens is critical to successful systemic integrated care implementation and practice transformation, including the application of organizational change theory	A description of how health conditions stress family systems, including systemic assessment, intervention strategies, and the interplay of family and clinical team dynamics

Hierarchy	How power hierarchies in the healthcare system have shifted over time	How power differentials across the systems of interest affect implementation and how the various subsystems within the healthcare system relate to one another	How health conditions can affect family structures and hierarchies and the impact of power differentials on team function and care provision
Nonsummativity	How shifting paradigms and mental models of health and healthcare have far-reaching effects on the healthcare system	The import of recognizing nonsummativity in implementation efforts, focusing on potential unanticipated consequences	A means of understanding and addressing challenging patient, family, and care team interconnections and their potential parallel processes
First-order and second-order change	How second-order changes in healthcare contexts related to the evolution of systemic integrated care, and how second-order change in one element (e.g., education system) may facilitate second-order change in other elements	How second-order change, or practice transformation, is the ultimate goal of implementation, requiring development and assessment of system and implementation strategies to foment second-order change	How health conditions can set the stage for second-order changes in families, who often benefit from strategies to manage problematic shifts and seek meaning in the experience by shifting the mental model and interactions in a positive way
Homeostasis	The patterns of recursive change in our healthcare system illustrate the push-pull of change and homeostasis.	Relevant strategies to deal with the inevitable counterweight of homeostasis that must be overcome to achieve practice transformation	How health conditions can disrupt family development and homeostasis and also how some health conditions can actually serve to maintain a homeostasis that is problematic in the long run for the family or clinical team

- **Nonsummativity:** A full understanding of a system requires attention to elements' interrelatedness and organization, particularly in complex adaptive systems. A system's interconnected elements cannot be understood fully in isolation from one another (Goldenberg et al., 2017).

- **First-order and second-order change:** First-order change reflects surface changes that do not fundamentally alter the structure of the system (like rearranging the furniture in a living room). First-order change tends to be transient, as the system self-regulates back to its original state. In contrast, second-order change reflects a shift in the structure and/or rules of the system such that the system itself fundamentally changes (like building a new house with an entirely different living room). Second-order change tends to be more lasting (Gerhardt, 2019).

- **Homeostasis:** The tendency of systems to maintain the status quo and the dynamic process by which a system maintains this equilibrium (Gerhardt, 2019).

ORGANIZATION OF THIS BOOK

Part I of this book focuses on foundational elements of integrated care. In Chapter 1, we outline levels of integration that are common in our healthcare system, ranging from completely separate to fully integrated services. We illustrate each level via a case-based care narrative that contrasts patient encounter experiences to highlight the benefits and challenges of each. We then describe elements that define fully integrated care as well as how these elements are operationalized in different models of integrated care. Additionally, we present a brief, high-level overview of outcomes research on the two established integrated care models. The intent is to ensure that readers recognize key elements of integrated care, the similarities and differences of the models, and their implications for the patient, family, and clinician experience.

In Chapters 2 and 3, we turn to the historical context of systemic integrated behavioral health. We start with historical context to help us chart the path forward, mindful of lessons learned from history. We outline how healthcare is shifting, in parallel with other sciences, from a mechanistic, linear model to a broader, biopsychosocial systemic approach. Our underlying schemas, or mental models, reflect this shift toward contextualization and increased focus on interrelationships and complexity in how we understand and define healthcare. These mental models are foundational, as they reflect "concentrated, personally constructed, internal conceptions of external phenomena (historical, existing or projected), or experience, that affect how a person acts" (Rook, 2013, p. 11).

The shift toward a biopsychosocial systems mental model of healthcare set the stage for the growth of integrated behavioral health. As we embraced this broader, relational approach to healthcare, our standards shifted. The pursuit of these new standards required evolution in care provision, research, and policy reform. Our historical review specifically outlines the emergence of integrated behavioral health. We describe how this new approach required professionals to develop novel concepts and competencies to meet new bio-psychosocial relational standards of care. We also describe how these shifts influenced researchers. Researchers began to recognize the need to adjust their mental models and research methodologies to better understand complexity and systems of care. The goal of these evolving research models is to provide more usable guidance to clinicians, policy makers, and healthcare system architects to facilitate evidence-based care and needed process and infrastructure changes. Across the board, our historical review illustrates how healthcare stakeholders slowly realized progress comes only when we recognize the need for a systemic lens and acknowledge the inevitable messy complexity of healthcare.

Part II of the book focuses on the implementation of integrated care. We describe and utilize Lau and colleagues' (2016) conceptual framework regarding elements that influence implementation efforts. They highlight four levels of analysis:

- external contexts, including policy, incentives and funding, dominant paradigm, and infrastructure;
- organizational, including culture, resources, skill mix, and relationships;
- professional, including philosophy of care (which we term *mental model of care*), competencies, professional role, and relationships; and
- intervention, including implementation challenges related to clinical intervention content and modality.

Chapters 4, 5, and 6 parallel the first three levels of analysis: external contexts, the organizational level, and the professional level. (Intervention, the fourth level of analysis in the conceptual model, is the focus of Part III of the book.) Chapter 4 focuses on the interplay of external contexts in healthcare and the movement toward reform and integration. These external contexts include multiple sociocultural systems, such as the health professional education and training system, government healthcare policy, reimbursement systems, and systemic racism and other social issues that affect health. With regard to these sociocultural issues, we argue that change occurs only when we name facilitators and barriers to change, engage in community-based advocacy, and adopt reflective practices to identify opportunities for change. Furthermore, we emphasize the social justice mission inherent in healthcare reform toward integration. We argue that systemic integrated care can improve inequities, recognizing that the most vulnerable among us often receive subpar care and suffer negative outcomes (Baciu et al., 2017; O'Loughlin et al., 2019).

Chapter 5 shifts to systemic factors at the level of regional and community healthcare organizations and practices. We review how organizational factors such as leadership engagement, culture, and resources affect the implementation process. For example, a practice's culture can influence whether it embraces or rejects change processes. The degree to which the practice has resources to support practice shifts has a significant impact on the implementation process and its outcome (Kyle et al., 2021).

In Chapter 6, we attend to how professionals within the organization approach integration, reflecting both individual and team practice patterns. We review the importance of shared mental models of care, clinician and staff attitudes toward change and collaboration, and professional role definitions. Understanding these elements and associated patterns is crucial to integrated care efforts because a shift toward integration requires clinicians and staff to interact with their community, families, patients, and each other differently than is done in standard care (Blount, 2019a, 2019b).

For each level of analysis, we discuss specific facilitators and barriers to care. Implementation research informs strategies to assess, address, and mitigate or capitalize on these factors. We advocate a measurement-based process in which ongoing assessment informs the need for changes in strategy and approach and provides stakeholders with information regarding their own and their team's performance. In addition, we describe and apply an evidence-based, systemic change management approach that recognizes the need for a strategic process to motivate healthcare organizations and professionals to make necessary changes. We specifically review how leadership and team functioning influence the implementation process. Vignettes illustrate these external large-system, organizational, and professional characteristics as well as the suggested implementation strategies.

Part III of the book illustrates the application of the systemic approach to integrated clinical services, with a specific focus on evidence-based family interventions and the interface of families and health. It is critically important to expand our healthcare purview to engage families, communities, and social structures as allies and partners to achieve optimal care. One of our goals of writing this book is to highlight how clinicians and other healthcare leaders can broaden their lens to include the family and other social systems to improve their effectiveness, even in the fast-paced healthcare environment.

Toward this end, we describe strategies to include family and social issues in clinical care (Chapter 7) and provide a high-level overview of the evidence base for the family's influence on health and the utility of family systems approaches to care (Chapter 8). We apply a relational, systemic lens to adult (Chapter 9), children's (Chapter 10), and women's (Chapter 11) primary care by outlining the application of these concepts to common presentations, illustrating them using clinical descriptions and examples.

HOW TO USE THE BOOK

We examine integrated care from three perspectives: a foundational, historical context; implementation and dissemination; and clinical applications. Parallel to the way a systemic clinician seeks to understand and approach a clinical issue from multiple biopsychosocial perspectives, we seek to explore issues that facilitate and impede the development of integrated care in their contexts.

Just as healthcare is intended to serve the needs of patients, this book is intended to serve the needs of the reader. We hope that reading the book cover to cover builds knowledge from one level of a system to the next. We believe that every chapter in this book instills a deeper understanding of systemic, family-oriented integrated care. At the same time, we recognize that some readers might be primarily interested in specific parts of the book, so we encourage readers to ask themselves, Why did I pick up this book?

Do you have an incomplete understanding of the various levels and approaches of integrated care? Do you need to understand the real-world applications of integrated care models better before you move forward? Chapter 1 describes essential elements of integrated care and clinical models of integration from the patients' and family's experience.

Do you want to understand the historical context of integrated care to inform the process of moving forward from the current state? Chapters 2 and 3 describe the U.S. healthcare system's development with regard to integrated care. We then offer possible pathways to the future.

Do you need to understand the root, systemic issues that complicate and facilitate integration implementation? In Chapter 4, we review external contextual factors that promote or impede integration efforts. We highlight strategies to address these challenges, recognizing that only through individual and collective action will we successfully change the system.

Are you working to begin or enhance integration in a practice or multiple practices in a given healthcare system? In Chapter 5, we offer a review of healthcare organizational barriers and facilitators as well as organizational change strategies. We draw from numerous existing integrated care implementation guides and offer resources and tips to serve as key elements for successful integrated care implementation. We also outline how to develop a systemic change roadmap based on organizational change principles. The goal is to chart a course forward that aligns with local system values and goals by curating key ingredients and applying them strategically.

Have you struggled to engage various practice members in an integration process? Successful integration requires engagement across functions in the practice team, with ongoing support from key practice team members. In Chapter 6, we review professional practice patterns as they relate to integration efforts as well as strategies to motivate administrators, clinicians, and staff to adopt integrated, team-based care. We also leverage existing training resources and other change-incubation methods as part of an overall, strategic change management process. Our goal is to help the reader motivate and prepare professionals to engage in integrated team-based care.

Are you a clinician working in a healthcare setting, seeking new approaches to meet patients' and family's needs? Perhaps your training did not prepare you for an integrated setting. Perhaps you are finding that siloed, individually oriented assessment and intervention strategies are not optimally effective in a healthcare environment. Part III of the book focuses on direct service, outlining clinical applications of systemic and relational approaches to expand clinical assessment and intervention options. Chapter 7 offers a general overview of medical family therapy, a family-oriented, relational, systemic approach that serves as a helpful mental model to guide clinical practice shifts that support integrated care. Chapter 8 reviews the evidence regarding the interface of health and social connection with a specific focus on family relationships and health. In addition, we review the evidence for family-oriented healthcare assessment and intervention, summarizing large-scale systematic and strategic literature reviews. Chapters 9, 10, and 11 highlight clinical approaches that are useful in adult primary care, pediatrics, and women's health. In each chapter, we outline common presenting concerns, medical family therapy strategies to address these common issues, and collaboration and integrated care strategies that align with the setting's culture and population served. We illustrate these strategies via case vignettes.

In general, each part and chapter of the book can stand alone. We recognize each reader brings contextual knowledge and experience and seeks to apply this information to a specific system in a specific community, time, and place. Because of the dynamic nature of integrated team-based care implementation and provision, the reader may find different parts of the book useful at different times.

PART I

OVERVIEW: THE SYSTEMIC EVOLUTION OF INTEGRATED CARE

Part 1 lays the groundwork for subsequent parts of the book that focus on implementation of integrated care models and systemically based clinical strategies. We begin in Chapter 1 by describing how medical and behavioral health services can interface in different practice models. These configurations range from completely separate services to different integrated service models. We define *integrated behavioral healthcare* and describe current thinking regarding its essential elements and the need to move beyond specific models. Because model-driven integrated care is still common, we describe the two foremost models of integrated behavioral healthcare and the evidence base for each. We differentiate these models of care by the patient experience, highlighting the benefits and challenges of each approach. In so doing, we hope to preserve a focus on the most important team members: the patient and their family.

The next two chapters in this part describe the evolution of integrated care in the U.S. health system, with a focus on critical incidents. We begin this narrative in Chapter 2 with the evolution of mental models used in healthcare and how these models influenced, and were influenced by, the emerging fields of primary care, family therapy, and integrated healthcare. In Chapter 3, we focus on how the definition and application of integrated care evolved in different settings, bringing us to where we are today. This chapter also outlines the interplay of healthcare reform and integration efforts, with a focus on how research models shifted to explore and understand the complexity inherent in how patients with multiple, ambiguous, biopsychosocial problems often present in healthcare, especially primary care.

Our goal is to help the reader think about the larger systemic factors that influenced—and continue to influence—the evolution of this field. Integrated healthcare did not evolve in a vacuum. Understanding the historic influence of these larger systems informs our understanding and our path forward.

Different professions and perspectives form multiple interwoven branches of the integrated care origin story. Each branch evolved during similar time periods but in different contexts. Each was informed by the progress of the others and adapted to many of the same challenges and facilitators over time that occurred in pediatric primary care, family medicine, and various specialties such as genetics, cancer, and geriatrics as well as health systems such as community-based federally qualified health centers, TRICARE (the healthcare system for the U.S. Department of Defense), and the Department of Veterans Affairs (VA). Each of these systems was integral to the development of integrated care in the public and private primary healthcare sector.

We do not review the development and evolution of "reverse integration," in which primary care is embedded into the system of care for people with serious and persistent mental illness. We instead refer the reader to McGinty and colleagues' (2021) excellent review of these models and the evidence that supports them.

1 MODELS OF INTEGRATED CARE AND BEYOND

Before reviewing the evolution of the integrated care movement, we review various levels and models of integrated behavioral health and consider how these models affect care in actual practice. What is the experience of a given patient at different levels of integration? How do these experiences facilitate or impede provision of behavioral health services?

Rampant fragmentation and a lack of patient-centeredness are oft-cited factors for U.S. healthcare systems failure. The lived experience of those who seek care often reflects these realities, with too many patients experiencing substandard care secondary to fragmentation, frustration, and confusion. Healthcare economists liken the challenges associated with obtaining services to an ordeal that patients must endure to receive care. They posit that these ordeals serve as a naturalistic sorting process in which only those patients who are willing and able to navigate barriers ultimately obtain treatment. This sorting process may be a major factor in health disparities because vulnerable populations face significant barriers and often do not have the resources to overcome them (Zeckhauser, 2021).

Poor access to care and poor coordination across medical and behavioral healthcare is common, particularly for people experiencing severe mental

https://doi.org/10.1037/0000381-002
A Systemic Approach to Behavioral Healthcare Integration: Context Matters, by
N. B. Ruddy and S. H. McDaniel

health issues (Goetter et al., 2020). Ultimately, only half of patients with diagnosable behavioral health issues seek care from physical or mental health professionals. For those who do, patient follow-up to initiate behavioral health services is poor (Mojtabai et al., 2011). If the patient is able to initiate service, the subsequent time and money necessary to engage in traditional psychotherapy can be insurmountable. Insurance plans often limit access to care or require complicated administrative oversight.

In addition, although stigma regarding mental and behavioral health issues is easing, many experience ambivalence as they consider seeking care (Arnaez et al., 2020; Clement et al., 2015). Patients often do not know what to expect from psychotherapy or may have mixed feelings about discussing emotionally difficult topics. These factors can derail even determined patients and may deter those whose symptoms limit their perseverance and function, as can occur with depression or anxiety.

Segregated behavioral health services typically require patients to seek a therapist independently, with an extended waiting period prior to initial contact. Even when the patient manages to initiate services, little to no communication may occur between behavioral health and medical clinicians. Pence and colleagues (2012) described a depression treatment attrition pattern in which only 24% of patients who present to primary care with symptoms meeting criteria for a diagnosis of depression receive any treatment at all, with 9% receiving treatment that aligns with guidelines and only 6% achieving remission.

As the treatment pattern suggests, recognizing a behavioral health issue is but the first step. How treatment proceeds or stalls from that point can depend on the model of care delivery (Haack et al., 2020). In this chapter, we use Amber's story to describe a patient's experience of different models of care.[1] The first narrative describes traditional segregated care, followed by Amber's story if she was to experience the earliest level of integrated care, now called *colocated care*. Some models of colocated care meet the definition by Peek (2019; Peek & National Integration Academy Council, 2013) described later; others do not.

Before presenting narratives that outline Amber's experiences in more fully developed integrated care models, we define *integrated behavioral healthcare*. We present a detailed historical narrative of the field in subsequent chapters; in this chapter we present some context to understand how the field continues to evolve. Of great import more recently is a movement

---

[1]The case description aligns with common presentations in healthcare but does not reflect a real person or specific situation.

to understand the critical elements of integrated care. Toward this end, we present the work of integrated care proponents who outline a Cross Model Framework. A Cross Model Framework is a blend of the elements of the two prominent approaches to integration: the Primary Care Behavioral Health (PCBH) model and the Collaborative Care Model (CoCM). In addition, we describe the evidence base for these models and research efforts underway to ground our understanding of integrated care's key elements.

To understand the elements each approach brings, we then describe PCBH and CoCM in more detail. We present the evidence base of each model as well as the limitations of this research. We return to Amber's story to illustrate how these approaches shape the patient's experience. Reviewing care from the patient's perspective in each of these approaches highlights how practice workflows and larger system processes inhibit or facilitate access to care.

After sharing Amber's story, we present examples of how Amber might experience four different approaches to care. With the first three examples, we include a figure that represents graphically what is explained in the text. We describe Amber's experience, highlighting the benefits and challenges of each model of care.

AMBER'S STORY

Amber is a 54-year-old woman who lives alone. She is divorced and has one adult child who lives out of state. Amber and her daughter have a close but conflictual relationship, which bothers Amber a great deal. Amber was diagnosed with diabetes 6 years ago and has never really been successful in managing the illness. She struggles to lose weight, falling into the severely obese category. Amber acknowledges that difficult interactions with her daughter are a trigger for her own binge eating. Until recently, Amber felt content with her life, aside from her relationship with her daughter. She enjoyed her job and had a small circle of friends that kept her busy and engaged. About 8 months ago, she had a falling out with several friends. Amber also has a new boss whom she does not like. She has started to feel like she can't seem to get along with anyone, as evidenced by her divorce and the relationship difficulties with her daughter, friends, and boss.

Over the past few months, Amber has been feeling down. She has difficulty concentrating and doesn't enjoy things the way she used to. She has been isolating from her family and friends so that recently her daughter expressed concern about her. Amber's sister convinced her that she needs to seek help. Amber does attend appointments regularly with her endocrinologist, who works in a multidisciplinary diabetes center. Amber would not describe herself as depressed—she describes herself as "out of sorts." Furthermore, she is ambivalent about sharing her struggles, especially in a medical context. Prior to the appointment, Amber obtained routine diabetes blood work. Her hemoglobin A1c, which indicates her blood sugar levels over the past 3 months, rose from 8 to 10.5, revealing that her diabetes is even less controlled than it was previously.

AMBER GETS STANDARD CARE

Standard care, like that in specialty mental health, involves separate behavioral health and medical services with behavioral health and medical clinicians linked only through referrals and shared patients. Regular communication is rare, and segregated behavioral health clinicians may not provide information that is practical for use in a healthcare setting. Access to mental health services is cited as a major problem in care by primary care and other medical clinicians.

Amber attends her appointment for a regular diabetes checkup with a medical clinician in the diabetes center. She is not screened for mental health or relational issues, but the medical clinician does ask about stress. Because of Amber's high blood glucose level, the medical clinician orders bloodwork and asks Amber to return. The visit likely has a biomedical focus. For example, Amber's report that she has been feeling out of sorts may be attributed to her high blood glucose levels and poor diabetes management. The discussion might focus on how she needs to do a better job of managing her diabetes. The medical clinician may not ask about Amber's social supports or learn about her difficult relationship with her daughter and its connection to Amber's weight issues. Involving family members in her management plan often is not considered. During the follow-up appointment, the focus shifts to psychoeducation about how her blood glucose levels, stress, and emotional distress may underlie Amber's concerns. Amber sees a diabetes educator to learn more about diabetes management. The diabetes educator may assess how relational issues are relevant but does not have relational training to address these issues. Family members may not be invited to participate.

If Amber's mood becomes a focus, the medical clinician may turn to psychotropic medication. Prescribing medication is a relative comfort zone for the medical clinician, and behavioral health services may be hard to come by. Amber may receive a prescription for an antidepressant but may not adhere to the prescribed regimen due to side effects, medication costs, or conflicting beliefs. Amber may not receive appropriate counseling from the clinician about these medications or adequate follow-up to monitor effectiveness and side effects. Only occasionally do patients like Amber receive a psychotherapy referral.

If Amber does receive a psychotherapy referral, the likelihood of Amber successfully following up to initiate treatment depends greatly on the medical clinician's support and Amber's perseverance, organization, and motivation to seek therapy. Qualitative research indicates that some people who seek psychotherapy do so only after feeling medications were not helpful or they hit "rock bottom" (Wells et al., 2020). If Amber decides to seek therapy, the medical clinician may offer a referral. However, it is up to Amber to determine which clinicians are in-network with her insurance company. She likely would have little information to guide her choice of a behavioral health clinician, remaining unaware of the different approaches and skill sets of the various behavioral health disciplines. Amber also must determine which behavioral health clinicians are taking new patients and wait for an opening. And she must be willing and able to pay significant copay costs.

All the tasks involved in finding a therapist can be particularly challenging for people who are suffering impairments in concentration and motivation or who have lost a sense of hopefulness for the future (e.g., people who are depressed). People are often fearful and ambivalent about seeking therapy. Qualitative research indicates that some patients have misgivings about attending psychotherapy and may not understand the process, even after completing initial sessions (MacFarlane et al., 2015). If family members are not aware of the referral, they cannot help the patient navigate the system or support the patient in seeking and continuing treatment. Even when people successfully initiate treatment, the opportunity cost (e.g., financial transportation, time) may be prohibitive.

For the sake of argument, we'll assume that Amber overcomes all of these barriers and schedules an initial appointment. She likely will have to wait weeks for a first session. Protracted wait times for a first session have been associated with poor follow-through and poor outcomes, particularly for underserved families (Ofonedu et al., 2017). Approaches to the initial session vary; her first sessions may focus on information gathering rather than symptom-mitigation strategies. Clearly, a single session with a support person focused on the patient's story may bring some relief (Hymmen et al., 2013; Talmon, 2012). However, other studies indicate that initial sessions that did not meet expectations for symptom relief and/or practical strategies predict early termination (Ofonedu et al., 2017). In addition, research shows that professional context factors such as payment, limited session time, and the spacing of sessions can make patients like Amber doubt the therapist's genuine care and commitment (Levitt et al., 2016). These issues, in combination with the ordeals associated with seeking therapy, likely derail many patients.

Even if Amber continues with therapy, a behavioral health clinician working outside a medical context may not collaborate with the diabetes center clinicians or include her family members (Durbin et al., 2012). Many specialty behavioral health clinicians prioritize confidentiality over collaboration even when the patient has a chronic illness and prefer a more collaborative model of care along with family involvement. Ultimately, insufficient communication between healthcare professionals negatively impacts care, particularly for patients like Amber who have a chronic health condition. In addition, the medical clinician and family often do not know if a patient terminates behavioral health treatment prematurely, as is common. This outcome reflects another missed opportunity to offer support from both professional and personal support systems.

Figure 1.1 illustrates the struggles Amber likely would face in a standard, segregated care model. To summarize, too often behavioral health issues may not be detected, and relational and family elements are not considered during medical care. Behavioral health services can be expensive and difficult to access, and the selection of a behavioral health clinician too often borders on random selection. Sometimes initial services do not impart confidence or comfort or access important social supports. Behavioral health clinicians may not close the loop with medical clinicians or themselves include family members, potentially hampering optimal care.

AMBER GETS COLOCATED BEHAVIORAL HEALTH SERVICES

In response to the challenges involved in standard care, the first level of integration is colocated care. Practices with colocated care typically contract with a behavioral health clinician or practice to provide services to patients and families of the medical practice. The behavioral health clinician may be a partner in the practice or rent space, and contractual variables differ depending on their state's regulations and the preferences of both the practice and the behavioral health clinician (Coons & Gabis, 2010).

Colocation generally improves access to care and can be described along a continuum such that some have none to few elements of integration, whereas others have many. The behavioral health clinician is located in the healthcare setting and typically tries to accept common insurance plans, potentially

FIGURE 1.1. Amber Experiences Standard Care

Amber attends appointment	Focus on diabetes	Blood work, return for follow up
Return appointment	Elicit stress as issue	Prescribe antidepressants	Psychotherapy referral?
Amber seeks psychotherapy	Call insurance to find clinicians	Call BH clinicians	Find BH clinician taking new patients
Amber attends first appointment	"Blind date" of talking to new person	May not focus on symptom relief	Likely interplay of chronic illness and mood is not a focus
Follow up to psychotherapy initiation	BH clinician communicate w/ PCP?	Amber attend more than one session?	Amber follow through with antidepressants?

BH = behavioral healthcare; PCP = primary care provider.

reducing some of the financial and other barriers to care. Engagement in collaboration ranges. Some colocated behavioral health clinicians offer siloed care, seeing patients in traditional psychotherapy within the medical clinic without sharing clinical information or initiating shared problem solving with the referring clinician. Others meet patients at the time of the referral (also known as a *warm handoff*); attend joint appointments with the patient, family, and medical clinicians; run groups that meet specific practice needs; and have more interaction with their medical colleagues about patient care because of their common location. However, because these behavioral health clinicians are typically a separate business entity from the medical practice, they must focus time on reimbursable activities, primarily psychotherapy. Some clinicians also bill for encounters that focus on health behavior change for patients with a chronic illness. Reimbursement for these services can fall under health and behavior Current Procedural Terminology® (CPT) codes (B. F. Miller et al., 2014).

In this model, illustrated in Figure 1.2, Amber makes an appointment at the diabetes center for her regular check-in. With behavioral health services available on-site, the center may (or may not) routinely screen for emotional distress. When Amber screens positive for depression, it can trigger a consultation with the behavioral health clinician during Amber's visit. However, some behavioral health clinicians who are colocated may not see patients in real time because they are scheduled with existing patients. This lack of availability can hamper connection and referral because the clinician and Amber must connect another time, so Amber's concerns are not addressed during the present encounter. To address these access issues, some colocated practices provide a very brief, real-time introduction to the behavioral health clinician to facilitate follow-up for behavioral health services. In some cases, the behavioral health clinician provides a very brief consultation as well.

With the support of the on-site behavioral health clinician, the medical clinician may be more likely to explore stress, emotional, and relational issues. This discussion may, in and of itself, help Amber recognize how stress and relational issues are a source of her disease from the beginning. Furthermore, if the medical clinician suggests psychotherapy, Amber may be more likely to meet the on-site behavioral health clinician that day, increasing the likelihood she will follow up on the referral (Mullin & Funderburk, 2013). If a positive connection occurs or Amber experiences relief from even this brief encounter, the real-time connection may motivate Amber to return to care. If the on-site therapist is able to take Amber's insurance, then Amber returns at some later time to begin therapy. However, the initial appointment may take weeks to months to occur because the service demand usually exceeds capacity, particularly if the behavioral health clinician is available only a few days a week.

FIGURE 1.2. Amber Experiences Colocated Care

Amber attends appointment	Amber's depression screen positive	Amber meets on-site clinician	Blood work, return for follow up
Return appointment	Amber must schedule separately with medical and MH clinicians	Medical clinicians may prescribe antidepressants	Amber must wait to see MH clinician check with insurance
Amber sees MH clinician	Focus on depression and social factors	Follow up discussion on antidepressant medication	Communication with PC medical clinician?
Follow up to psychotherapy initiation	Biopsychosocial management of diabetes and depression?	Focus on chronic disease management and health behaviors?	Amber follow through with antidepressants?

MH = mental health; PC = primary care.

As Amber engages in therapy, her behavioral health clinician may speak directly with the medical clinician with Amber's consent, or there may be little to no communication. Amber's clinical notes may go into a shared medical record that all clinicians in the practice can access. If the clinician is not an employee of the practice or a common healthcare system, her records may be kept completely separate to comply with Health Insurance Portability and Accountability Act of 1996 (HIPAA) regulations.

Colocation offers improvements over standard care, with Amber's concerns detected and managed more quickly, and makes access to behavioral healthcare easier. Patients in need of behavioral health referral may meet the behavioral health clinician in a warm handoff, but that is less likely to lead to a full assessment or intervention than in more integrated settings. The behavioral health clinician's schedule typically is structured around 50-minute hour psychotherapy, such that they cannot spend more than a few minutes with the patient during the warm handoff. More thorough assessment and intervention are more likely to occur in the intake appointment. If, as with segregated care, the first encounter with the behavioral health clinician is delayed or relatively brief, Amber may be less likely to follow through and engage further (Mautone et al., 2020). When the behavioral health clinician is not an employee of the practice, their income depends on fee-for-service (FFS) income, limiting their options regarding intervention modalities. Obtaining reimbursement for time spent communicating with families and other clinicians can be complicated in FFS reimbursement.

These complications may contribute to suboptimal communication between the behavioral health clinician, Amber's medical clinician, and her family. So, although Amber does not have to run the gauntlet to seek outside services, she may not get real-time, highly coordinated care. In addition, she may not have the substantial financial resources, time, and transportation to attend separate appointments with the mental health clinician.

In the next part, we shift to a discussion of care that aligns with definitions of integrated behavioral healthcare. In reality, the line between colocated and integrated services is not so stark. Colocating care often serves as a precursor to integrating services, a way-stop on the way to more full integration, so to speak. Second, many practices offer enhanced colocation that borrows workflows and strategies for integrated care. For example, the behavioral health and medical clinicians may have regular meetings to discuss shared patients and communicate regularly during happenstance contacts that occur in a shared clinical space. Some practices prioritize a more robust warm handoff in which the behavioral health clinician engages in a first encounter, more akin to the PCBH encounter we describe shortly.

THE DEVELOPMENT OF MORE FULLY INTEGRATED MODELS OF CARE

Integrating behavioral health more fully into medical settings reflected a larger paradigm shift in healthcare toward systemic, biopsychosocial team-based care. Chapters 2 and 3 present a historical narrative that contextualizes the emergence and current state of integrated care. Here in Chapter 1, our purpose is to define integrated care and illustrate common models. Toward this end, we focus on how the challenges patients and medical clinicians faced (and continue to face) in separate—and colocated—behavioral healthcare set the stage for the emergence of new, integrated, behavioral healthcare models.

For example, research conducted in the early 1980s showed that only a third of patients experiencing significant depressive symptoms received medication management that aligned with treatment guidelines (Keller et al., 1982). Subsequent research revealed only 10% of depressed patients received behavioral interventions (Katon et al., 1995). Furthermore, medical clinicians, particularly those in primary care, noted concerns and abject frustration with the barriers to care inherent in bifurcated medical and mental healthcare systems (Vickers et al., 2013). Clearly, bifurcated care did not meet patient or medical clinician needs.

To address these issues, many healthcare systems explored integrating behavioral health clinicians into medical settings, starting with colocation, and moving to models involving even more collaboration. The emergence of the new field of integrated behavioral health was not linear, with different solutions and models developing in parallel processes (D. J. Cohen, Davis, Hall, et al., 2015). As often occurs in the emergence of a new discipline (Kuhn, 2012), confusion ensued regarding the very definition of integrated care and its elements. Subject matter experts convened to create a definition of this new field. The generally accepted definition of integrated primary care that emerged from this process is as follows:

> A practice team of primary care and behavioral health clinicians working together with patients and families, using a systematic and cost-effective approach to provide patient-centered care for a defined population. This care may address mental health and substance abuse conditions, health behaviors (including their contribution to chronic medical illnesses), life stressors and crises, stress-related physical symptoms, and ineffective patterns of health care utilization. (Peek & National Integration Academy Council, 2013)

This definition set the stage for subsequent research that sought to reveal and define the essential elements of integrated care. In a subsequent publication, Peek (2019) drilled down into the elements of this definition, differentiating the clinical aspects of care provision and the organizational support necessary to sustain integrated care clinical care. We delve into organizational support as part of implementation in Part II of this book. In this chapter, we focus on clinical services. For the integrated care team to address the needs of the population served, Peek noted they must

- have team members with the necessary relevant behavioral health expertise and role functions;

- ensure clinicians understand team clinical roles and relationship, culture, and team-building; and

- share operations in the same space, workflows that promote collaboration, and a practice culture that does not bifurcate medical and mental healthcare.

Peek further clarified that integrated care teams share a patient population and ascribe to a mission of whole-person care that does not separate medical and mental healthcare. Toward this end, integrated care also requires systematic processes to

- identify patients who need behavioral health assistance,
- engage patients and families in identifying and defining their care needs and shared decision making,
- utilize explicit shared care plans that unify care goals and processes, and
- follow up and adjust the shared care plan if improvement is not as expected.

This shared definition of integrated care facilitated research and implementation. However, there was great variability in *how* systems implemented these elements, resulting in different models of integrated care. Later in this chapter, we describe in detail the two most referenced and studied models of integrated behavioral health services: CoCM and PCBH. Both models were developed to embed behavioral healthcare into primary care, improve access to care, and support primary care medical clinicians in quality care provision. However, they emerged from very divergent missions and cultures. CoCM was developed at the University of Washington, guided over time by a research program in an academic health center. CoCM sought to manage depression by applying Wagner and colleagues' (1996) chronic care model, a framework that, to this day, guides management of chronic medical conditions (Berwick, 2019). In contrast, PCBH evolved in numerous types of primary care clinical settings serving a broad array of patient populations with a wide variety of presenting concerns (Freeman, 2011; Funderburk et al., 2012; C. L. Hunter et al., 2014; McDaniel, Doherty, & Hepworth, 2014; Ogbeide et al., 2014; Reiter et al., 2018). It evolved in response to direct clinical care needs of patients and primary care medical clinicians, reflecting more of a clinical than a research culture (Peek, 2019). One mantra of the PCBH approach is to "meet patients where they are," reflecting a strong emphasis on patient-centricity and addressing patient and medical clinician needs in real time (Funderburk et al., 2021).

Of note, both of these models of care were developed in the context of primary care. Behavioral health services are now often part of specialty medical settings, and the models of care offered in these settings can parallel the models we describe shortly. Throughout this text, we advocate for integrated behavioral health services across the spectrum of healthcare. Our goal is to facilitate adoption of the elements of integrated care described above such that they become normative. This approach enables customization of the services to meet patients' and families' needs across specific healthcare settings. Increasingly, healthcare settings committed to integrating behavioral healthcare recognize that PCBH and CoCM complement each other (Raney, 2017; Unützer, 2016). CoCM helps to identify patients who are struggling with serious or intransigent behavioral health issues, following their progress as they receive care management and optimized psychotropic medication therapy. PCBH addresses a broader range of patient and family presentations and offers real-time patient assessment and intervention (meeting patients where they are) and real-time consultation to medical clinicians (directly addressing practice pain points). Blending elements of both models in a Cross Model Framework can help patients get the care they need, when they need it, and ensure that their care uses a track-to-goal process that aligns with practice guidelines.

In addition, as the field of integrated behavioral health has evolved, these models have become more aligned to share common essential elements. PCBH and CoCM have served as guideposts in the movement. However, we are shifting away from comparing these two models toward seeking to understand integrated care as a collection of elements (Buchanan et al., 2022; Coates et al., 2020; Funderburk et al., 2021; Giese & Waugh, 2017; Stephens et al., 2020). We appear to be on the cusp of a new stage in the development of integrated care, one that will identify the best of both models and apply them to the local context, using measurement against key benchmarks to optimize quality outcomes.

BEYOND MODELS—MOVING TOWARD A CROSS-MODEL FRAMEWORK

After the development of colocated, CoCM, and PCBH models, D. J. Cohen and colleagues set out to understand the reality of integrated care practices on the ground (D. J. Cohen, Balasubramanian, et al., 2015). Their observations of real-world practices revealed patterns and practices that did not fit neatly into the well-described models of care. Although these models are recognized to be on continua, the results of this study indicate that integrated behavioral health takes myriad forms that defy this type of "pure" categorization. They stated:

> As more practices move towards integrating care, there is likely to be an increasing need to migrate away from some existing heuristics (e.g., levels, models) and sharpen the focus on the particulars in practices' approaches to integration. Models have tremendous relevance in identifying common conceptual elements or behaviors, and these have led to standardizations critical for unifying the field of integration. Yet, these conceptual and definitional frameworks . . . cannot be expected to mirror the many nuances emerging among practices integrating care in real-world settings. (D. J. Cohen, Balasubramanian, et al., 2015, p. 8)

In short, research indicates that many healthcare settings integrate behavioral health in ways that do not align with either model (D. J. Cohen, Davis, et al., 2015).

The movement to transcend models—to focus on the *what* as well as the *how*—moved forward in Stephens and colleagues' (2020) development of a Cross-Model Framework based on research and expert opinion. The model paralleled Peek's themes, outlining five core principles, 25 key processes, and nine clinic structures (Stephens et al., 2020). Stephens and colleagues (2020) described these principles as follows:

- patient-centric care—"Ensure the patient is well engaged with the entire care team, understands the various roles for themselves and their providers, and is supported and guided to manage their lives, health, and treatment."

- treat to target—"Ensure clear goals and measures are defined to guide and track care."

- use evidence-based behavioral treatments—"Ensure the best evidence-based care is used across medical and mental/behavioral care."

- conduct efficient team care—"Ensure integrated behavioral healthcare is efficient and comprehensive, supported by appropriate policies and procedures."

- population-based care—"Ensure limited services reach the most patients while targeting the patients most in need." (p. 530)

A survey of experts showed broad agreements on importance and feasibility of these identified elements (Stephens et al., 2020). Stephens and colleagues also noted that these elements map onto existing measures of integrated care, reflecting construct validity.

Subsequent research has found identifiable patterns of these elements across practices with some form of integrated care. Of interest, the data suggest that team-based care appears to be associated with higher levels of integration and serves as a key factor in differentiating practices with high versus low levels of integration (Buchanan et al., 2022). The authors emphasized that the integration elements occur along continua and that these elements come together to enhance or stall integration. In their conclusion, they stated, "Findings indicated that IBH [integrated behavioral healthcare] implementation was not globally 'complete,' but benefitted from being assessed multidimensionally" (Buchanan et al., 2022, p. 323). Aligning models to local needs requires flexibility in application, such that our focus must shift toward understanding how to customize integrated care to specific contexts.

Although much of the field is shifting away from pure models, the PCBH and CoCM models of care and related research do form important underpinnings to the provision of integrated care to this day. As such, we present these models in their pure form to illustrate the common elements and differences. We again use Amber's experience of care to highlight how care unfolds as a patient and clinician experience.

PRIMARY CARE BEHAVIORAL HEALTHCARE

The PCBH model evolved in numerous types of clinical settings serving a broad array of patient populations with a wide variety of presenting concerns (Freeman, 2011; Funderburk et al., 2012; C. L. Hunter et al., 2014; McDaniel, Doherty, & Hepworth, 2014; Ogbeide et al., 2014; Reiter et al., 2018). The organic growth of the model resulted in an initial lack of clarity regarding its definition (C. L. Hunter, Funderburk, et al., 2018). However, over time, patterns and key elements emerged (Peek & National Integration Academy Council, 2013). P. J. Robinson and Reiter (2016) captured these elements with the acronym GATHER:

- G: Generalist approach
- A: Accessible
- T: Team-based
- H: High volume
- E: Educational
- R: Routine

This acronym was further fleshed out by Reiter and colleagues (2018), who provided the following definition of the PCBH model:

> The PCBH model is a team-based primary care approach to managing behavioral health problems and biopsychosocially-influenced healthcare conditions.

The model's main goal is to enhance the primary care team's ability to manage and treat such problems/conditions, with resulting improvement in primary care services for the entire clinic population. The model incorporates into the primary care team a behavioral health consultant (BHC), sometimes referred to as a behavioral health clinician, to support the primary care provider (PCP) and team. The BHC works as a generalist and an educator who provides high volume services that are accessible, team-based, and a routine part of primary care. Specifically the BHC assists in the care of patients of any age and with any health condition (Generalist); strives to intervene with all patients on the day they are referred (Accessible); shares clinical space and resources and assists the team in various ways (Team-Based); engages with a large percentage of the clinic population (High Volume); helps improve the team's biopsychosocial assessment and intervention skills and processes (Educator); and is a routine part of biopsychosocial care (Routine). (p. 112)

Operationally, PCBH behavioral health clinicians function as part of the medical team, enhancing care via a longitudinal, shared treatment plan. PCBH clinicians are often employed by the primary care practice and must meet productivity requirements, as do medical clinicians and other team members. However, these requirements typically build in time for collaboration and nonbillable services, recognizing the value of these services to the practice.

Behavioral health clinicians engage in proactive case-finding, seeking patients who will benefit from behavioral health consultation. They examine the medical charts of patients with scheduled appointments to determine which patients may have issues with chronic disease management, health behavior targets, and/or emotional and relational issues. The behavioral health clinician also meets with other team members, ideally in a team huddle that occurs prior to patient care (H. P. Rodriguez et al., 2015), seeking to identify patients who might benefit from consultation. Medical clinicians also can request behavioral health consultation for myriad patient care issues or because they are struggling with some aspect of patient care and desire assistance (Reiter et al., 2018). Screening also plays a role in identifying patients in need. Upon arrival, patients complete screening instruments such as the Patient Health Questionnaire-9 (PHQ-9; C. L. Hunter et al., 2009; Kroenke et al., 2001). The intent is to identify people in distress in real time, so that patients receive care when they need it (Pomerantz et al., 2008). Not infrequently, patient concerns that arise during a medical visit will spur a warm handoff to a behavioral health clinician, who then meets with the patient for a brief consultation (Reiter et al., 2018).

A key component of the PCBH model is team-based care planning prior to, sometimes during, and/or after clinical encounters. In PCBH practices the behavioral health clinician is accessible to the rest of the team for real-time consultation and collaboration. The behavioral health clinician maintains availability by building in breaks between scheduled patient encounters. They also emphasize that team members can interrupt them during patient care, if needed. Because the behavioral health clinician shares workspace with other team members, there is ongoing collaboration throughout the day. These conversations can focus on the clinical care of shared patients, debriefing challenging encounters, brief coaching, or information sharing to enhance patient care. These elements of collaboration are reflected in the consultant and educator roles of the behavioral health clinician as they help team members provide optimal care (Kearney et al., 2014).

Behavioral health consultations with patients are brief, typically less than 30 minutes. First contacts usually occur as part of the patient's office visit for medical care. The focus of the behavioral health patient encounter can relate to a broad array of patient and medical clinician concerns (Reiter et al., 2018). PCBH consultation might help patients cope with or manage a health condition. They might work on health behavior change, such as smoking cessation. They might address difficult clinician–patient interaction patterns and communication issues or utilization-of-care issues such as frequent emergency department visits. They might help patients navigate the healthcare system or connect to community resources. And, of course, they often work with patients who are struggling to manage stress, relationship problems, a mental health issue, or a substance use issue. The goal of the encounter is to identify a target change that is important to the patient and offer systemic and/or behavioral management strategies to facilitate that change (Davis et al., 2019). In addition, behavioral health consultants assess motivation and readiness to change. Motivational interviewing, behavioral activation, psychoeducation, cognitive behavior therapy, problem-solving therapy (C. L. Hunter et al., 2009), and brief relational or family systems therapy (McDaniel, Doherty, & Hepworth, 2014) are common interventions.

Behavioral health clinicians do not automatically assume that patients will initiate a series of consultations or a course of psychotherapy. Follow-up care varies based on patient need, motivation, and interest in engaging with the behavioral health clinician. The behavioral health clinician's role in PCBH often is episodic. In other words, patients can return to care with a behavioral health clinician at any time they feel it would be beneficial. Barry and colleagues (2020) noted that termination in primary care behavioral health reflects a decision to end an episode of care, rather than necessarily to end a treatment relationship. This soft termination enables the behavioral health clinician to be available on an as-needed basis and to meet with patients when they are in the practice for medical care, rather than necessarily scheduling separate subsequent visits. The PCBH model emphasizes continuity of care with the entire team, rather than with just one clinician. The goal is for the behavioral health clinician to provide low-intensity interventions to a high volume of patients (Peek, 2019). Toward this end, behavioral health clinicians may augment consultations and brief psychotherapy with ancillary services to extend reach, including group medical appointments, call-in hours, telehealth, and preventive services (Reiter et al., 2018).

The broad array of PCBH services is well-suited to including family members and focusing on relational issues. Research suggests that adults are accompanied to healthcare visits in one third to one half of routine encounters (Wolff & Roter, 2011). Obviously, a family member is present even more frequently in pediatric medical visits. However, much of what has been written about the PCBH model has been focused on the individual patient, with a few exceptions (Hodgson et al., 2014; McDaniel, Doherty, & Hepworth, 2014; Mendenhall et al., 2018).

Amber Gets Primary Care Behavioral Healthcare

As we recognize that PCBH can vary greatly in its execution, the following description of Amber's care in the PCBH model exemplifies how care might unfold. As we advocate for a systemic approach that values families' and significant others' involvement in care, we highlight the BHC's and team's opportunities to engage the family. In the PCBH model, Amber's care might occur as illustrated in Figure 1.3.

Amber is flagged by the behavioral health clinician prior to her appointment via chart review based on her diabetes lab results. During their huddle, the team discusses whether a brief behavioral health consult for Amber could be helpful.

Amber is screened upon arrival, typically with the PHQ-9. Any screening outside normal limits is shared with the behavioral health clinician. The results of Amber's screening spur the behavioral health clinician to briefly consult with the medical clinician to determine next steps. PCBH workflow and roles are negotiated between clinicians based on who can best meet the patient's needs.

In this scenario, the team agrees that the behavioral health clinician should initiate Amber's appointment. Amber's behavioral health clinical encounter is very different from a typical intake in specialty behavioral health. The behavioral health clinician begins by introducing the team model and their role. This description clarifies information sharing in a team-based care environment, highlighting the benefits of a shared plan. The level of information sharing among the team is another departure from specialty behavioral healthcare. Although some behavioral health clinicians balk at

FIGURE 1.3. Amber Experiences the Primary Care Behavioral Health Model

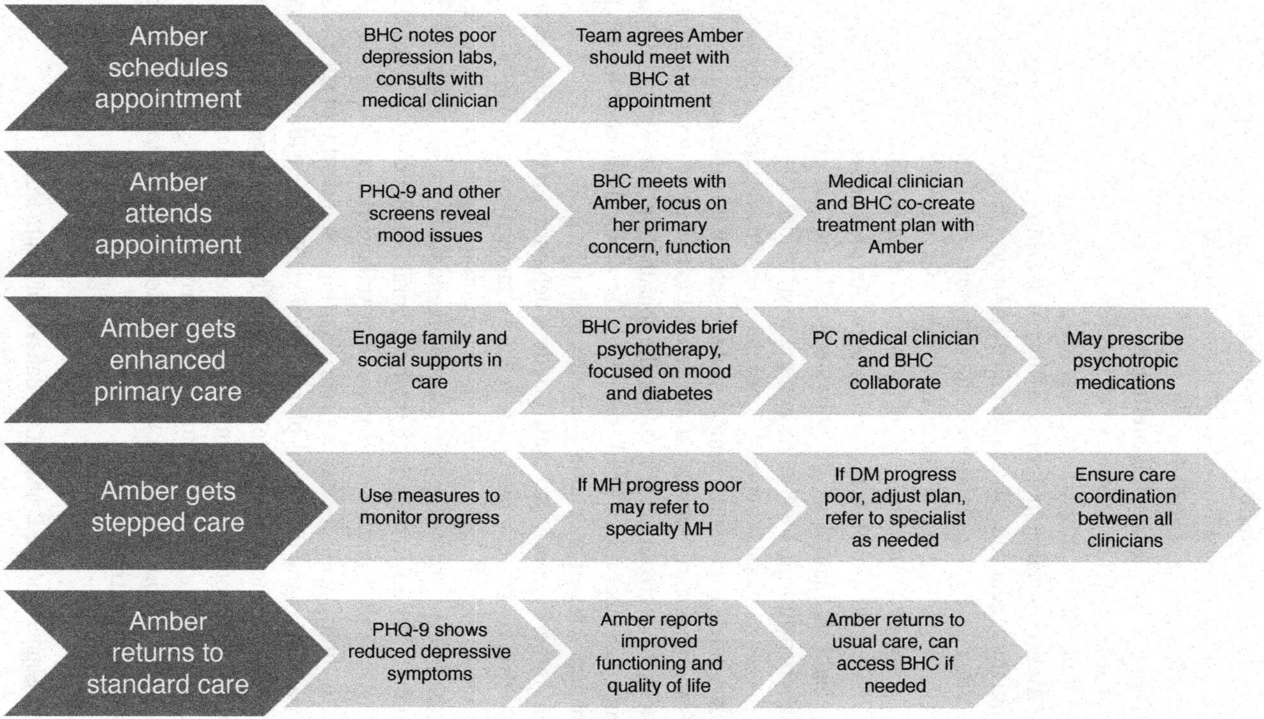

Amber schedules appointment	BHC notes poor depression labs, consults with medical clinician	Team agrees Amber should meet with BHC at appointment	
Amber attends appointment	PHQ-9 and other screens reveal mood issues	BHC meets with Amber, focus on her primary concern, function	Medical clinician and BHC co-create treatment plan with Amber
Amber gets enhanced primary care	Engage family and social supports in care	BHC provides brief psychotherapy, focused on mood and diabetes	PC medical clinician and BHC collaborate. May prescribe psychotropic medications
Amber gets stepped care	Use measures to monitor progress	If MH progress poor may refer to specialty MH	If DM progress poor, adjust plan, refer to specialist as needed. Ensure care coordination between all clinicians
Amber returns to standard care	PHQ-9 shows reduced depressive symptoms	Amber reports improved functioning and quality of life	Amber returns to usual care, can access BHC if needed

BHC = behavioral health clinician; DM = diabetes mellitus; MH = mental health; PC = primary care; PHQ-9 = Patient Health Questionnaire-9.

the confidentiality parameters that emphasize collaboration among the integrated care team members, research indicates that patients respond positively to this level of collaboration and communication, feeling they benefit from the teamwork and usually assume it is part of good care (Balasubramanian et al., 2017; Davis et al., 2018).

The behavioral health clinician then assesses Amber's mood, stress level, degree of insight, and motivation for change, as well as the impact of her symptoms on daily functioning. In systemic integrated care, the assessment also reviews Amber's social supports and family relationships, seeking opportunities to expand the system and garner assistance for Amber (Zubatsky & Mendenhall, 2018). The clinicians collaborate to identify one or two specific behavioral goals with Amber and explore behavioral strategies and tools to help her meet her goals. For example, Amber might want to follow through on appropriate limit-setting with her daughter and engage in brief problem-solving therapy. Or Amber might be focused on remembering to take her diabetes medication so she might benefit from medication adherence strategies. Often, the behavioral goal reflects a functional improvement related to activities that are important to Amber and sometimes her family. Amber's session is active and pragmatic. The session ends with a review of a cocreated follow-up plan to be discussed with the diabetes treatment team. After the consultation, the behavioral health clinician and Amber might briefly meet with the medical clinician prior to her medical appointment encounter to discuss their joint goals.

With Amber's consent, a family-oriented behavioral health clinician may seek to involve Amber's daughter in future medical or behavioral health appointments. A joint telehealth or phone conversation can help the care team understand her perspective, concerns, and potential role in Amber's treatment.

If Amber chooses to meet with the behavioral health clinician repeatedly, the team actively communicates regarding Amber's progress. In many systems, the clinical team measures progress using a standard tool such as the PHQ-9, adjusting the treatment plan as needed. This measurement process is not built into the PCBH model, and some research suggests that robust measurement is not normative in real-world settings (Beehler et al., 2017). If Amber does not improve, she might be referred to specialty mental health services, with supportive care from the behavioral health clinician while she awaits this appointment.

Research Support for the Primary Care Behavioral Health Model

As we noted earlier, the PCBH model arose organically out of many clinical settings. Peek (2019) noted that the model reflects a clinical culture that may prioritize clinical care and access over rigorous measurement. Given the great deal of variability in its execution, PCBH has been likened to more of a platform for care as opposed to a specific intervention (Pomerantz et al., 2010). This heterogeneity complicates evaluating PCBH model efficacy.

In this context, the research data, as described in two reviews, are in a developmental phase (C. L. Hunter et al., 2018; Possemato et al., 2018). C. L. Hunter and colleagues (2018) noted most studies used a pre–post design, with no comparison group, limiting interpretation. In their meta-analysis of the data, Possemato and colleagues (2018) concluded that

> This review finds that PCBH services improve access to and utilization of behavioral healthcare along with positive preliminary evidence of improved patient health outcomes and satisfaction. However, the great variability in methodological rigor of the reviewed studies minimizes the meaningful conclusions that can be drawn. . . . In conclusion, the implementation of PCBH services is ahead of the science supporting the usefulness of these services. (pp. 9–10)

There is more robust evidence that PCBH is associated with patient satisfaction (Angantyr et al., 2015; Funderburk et al., 2012) and with high medical clinician satisfaction (Hill, 2015), improved clinician efficiency (Torrence et al., 2014), and recognition of behavioral health issues (Sandoval et al., 2018). Funderburk et al. (2012) tied these improvements to behavioral health clinician accessibility.

C. L. Hunter and colleagues (2018) concluded their literature review by acknowledging the developmental nature of the research but also stating that the PCBH model

> has great face validity, makes sense to patients and providers, and has been disseminated, implemented, and sustained in large healthcare systems. The growth and sustained uptake of the model is encouraging and suggests that the model is liked and perceived by these systems as beneficial. (p. 141)

In short, the data supporting the efficacy of this model to improve patient outcomes over usual care are slim. Proponents argue this reflects the difficulties inherent in studying a heterogeneous set of practice patterns (Funderburk & Shepardson, 2017). Others argue that the "dosage" of behavioral health services in PCBH is inadequate to create lasting change for patients (Unützer, 2014). However, subsequent PCBH research with a pre–post design again evidenced significant functional improvement for patients with functional impairment secondary to mental health concerns, particularly for those with severe impairment at baseline. Of interest, research that specifically examined number of encounters and outcomes indicated that most of the benefit was in patients with fewer than four visits (Wilfong et al., 2019), hypothesizing that those patients who needed more encounters reflected presentations that likely needed a specialty-care level of intervention (Wilfong et al., 2019). Again, this study was a pre–post design, limiting interpretation. However, proponents of PCBH point to its potential utility for a large group of patients who seek care in medical settings and for engaging patients in some form of behavioral healthcare to enhance care. In Chapter 4, we discuss the interface of healthcare research and clinically focused models such as PCBH.

COLLABORATIVE CARE MODEL

CoCM applies Wagner and colleagues' (1996) chronic care model to address research indicating primary care management of depression and anxiety did not align with practice guidelines (Wang et al., 2005). In the early versions of CoCM, patients' service needs were identified via screening with the PHQ-9. Patients with elevated PHQ-9 scores were approached by the care manager and invited to become part of a programmatic intervention. The program offered ongoing outreach and support from a care manager. In addition, the patient's primary care medical clinician received ongoing psychiatric consultation to optimize diagnostic clarity, application of treatment guidelines, and psychotropic medication management (Raney, 2017). Most diagnostic consultations relate to patient mood, anxiety, or substance use disorders (Norfleet et al., 2016). Patients complete the PHQ-9 over time to monitor progress. The care team of a consulting psychiatrist, a care manager, and a primary care medical clinician collaborate to adjust treatment as needed. Patients return to usual care when the PHQ-9 indicates resolution of depression symptoms and improved functioning.

The psychiatrist's role primarily was, and largely continues to be, indirect consultation via the care manager (Norfleet et al., 2016). Early research indicated only 5% to 7% of patients required direct contact with the psychiatrist (Unützer et al., 2002). The use of indirect consultation is intended to maximize a psychiatrist's reach and efficiency (Raney, 2015).

Over time, the model expanded to new populations, settings, and presenting concerns (Katon et al., 2010). Research outcomes informed assessment and intervention strategies as well as team workflows and roles. Dissemination and implementation efforts were supported by the University of Washington Advancing Integrated Mental Health Solutions (AIMS) Center. Extensive implementation guidance and training disseminated CoCM best practices, supporting model fidelity and customization across settings. The ability to adapt the model to the local circumstances was reported to be a key theme of implementation success and medical clinician satisfaction with the model (Holmes & Chang, 2022).

Tracking patient progress to their goal is a foundational element of CoCM. As the model expanded to numerous types of patient presentations, outcome tracking expanded beyond the PHQ-9 to assess progress in other areas, such as anxiety, and to track mental health and medical symptom severity. CoCM emphasizes the use of patient registries to track all patients "to make sure no one falls through the cracks" (Unützer, 2014). The AIMS Center offers a registry tool that helps behavioral healthcare managers track care, with a specific focus on identifying those patients who are not improving to adjust treatments or stimulate psychiatric review (AIMS Center, 2023c).

The role of the behavioral healthcare manager (formerly, care manager) has evolved over time. Behavioral healthcare managers typically manage a case load of between 60 and 120 patients, depending on the population served and program scope (AIMS Center, 2020). The behavioral healthcare manager role encompasses the following tasks (Chwastiak et al., 2017):

- comprehensive health assessment to guide an individualized health plan with specific and measurable targets;
- psychoeducation regarding chronic illness self-management;
- brief, evidence-based behavioral interventions such as motivational interviewing and behavioral activation;
- care coordination among clinicians and outside professional supports such as social service agencies; and
- consistent case review with medical clinicians and psychiatric consultants for all patients who are not improving on their current care plan.

The AIMS Center additionally noted the key role of the behavioral healthcare manager in notifying the primary care medical clinician if the patient is not progressing. The behavioral healthcare manager also works directly with the patient to support implementation of the medical plan and to offer brief problem-solving therapy (AIMS Center, 2023a).

Behavioral interventions that align with a chronic care model were foundational to early studies that sought to improve care for people with depression and poorly controlled diabetes or cardiac problems (e.g., Katon et al., 2010). A 2014 meta-analysis of 74 CoCM studies that examined the efficacy of specific model elements found that the behavioral interventions, as opposed to the psychiatric medication management, are the key factors in much of the clinical improvement (Coventry et al., 2014). In this regard, behavioral healthcare managers offer a variety of behavioral interventions that parallel those used by behavioral health clinicians in the PCBH model, such as motivational interviewing, psychoeducation, behavioral activation, relapse prevention, and brief problem-solving therapy (AIMS Center, 2023a).

As part of a systematic review of CoCM implementation, Whitfield et al. (2022) highlighted the following programmatic key performance indicators. These reflect foundational elements of the CoCM program and its emphasis on measurement:

- patient engagement, defined as frequency of contact between the behavioral healthcare manager and medical clinician;

- pharmacotherapy adherence/prescription tracking;

- counseling delivery and tracking patient adherence to counseling;

- monitoring measurement-based care, which is defined as completion of behavioral health symptom measures during clinical encounters;

- CoCM team collaboration, defined as communication among CoCM clinical team members;

- stepped-care fidelity, defined as adjustments to treatment based on patient improvement; and

- when needed, facilitating direct mental health specialist care, defined as direct contact between the patient and a behavioral healthcare specialist, such as psychologist or psychiatrist, if patient improvement stalls.

CoCM does not offer the immediate access to behavioral health consultation for patients and medical clinicians that is the hallmark of the PCBH model. However, it does systematically apply treatment guidelines and measurement-based care processes to ensure that the care plan shifts if a patient is not improving (Raney, 2017). CoCM requires a change in the treatment plan every 2 to 3 months if validated measures indicate the patient has not experienced at least a 50% reduction in symptoms (AIMS Center, 2023b). For patients with depression and dysthymia (PHQ-9 score > 10 at time of program enrollment), the remission rate for depressive symptoms was approximately 3 months, as compared to over 20 months in usual care (Garrison et al., 2016).

Amber Gets Collaborative Care

The following description of the patient experience of CoCM describes how this model uses care management, behavioral interventions, and remote psychiatric consultation to enhance care for patients with moderate to serious mental health problems and health issues.

As illustrated in Figure 1.4, in a practice with CoCM, Amber seeks care because she is feeling out of sorts. Prior to her appointment with the medical clinician, she is screened for depression using the PHQ-9. Because she scores above the threshold for depression, a CoCM behavioral healthcare manager approaches Amber to further assess her concerns. During this conversation, Amber learns about the CoCM program, including the opportunity for ongoing support and access to psychotropic medication consultation.

Amber agrees to enroll in the program, and her care is monitored by the behavioral healthcare manager via a patient registry. As described previously, the registry tracks the services she accesses and her progress over time using instruments like the PHQ-9 and other measures of psychiatric symptomatology and functioning.

Amber's behavioral healthcare manager engages with her when she attends medical appointments and reaches out to her in between appointments. The program is designed to reduce treatment burden to the patient, so Amber can access support via phone or telehealth visits and receive outreach when she does not attend scheduled appointments. During visits, the behavioral healthcare manager provides psychoeducation designed to empower Amber by enhancing her understanding of her conditions and how they interface. They discuss treatment adherence strategies and target her symptoms of depression via behavioral activation and problem-solving therapy. As Amber improves, they shift to developing a collaborative relapse-prevention plan to help her maintain her gains by developing a sensitivity to signs of relapse (Raney, 2015, 2017).

Throughout the time Amber is in the CoCM program, the behavioral healthcare manager also works collaboratively with a consulting psychiatrist or other prescribing medical clinician to manage her psychotropic medication. Amber does not meet with the prescriber directly. Rather, the behavioral healthcare manager and prescriber review Amber's care plan if measurement indicates she is not improving significantly after 2 to 3 months (Bao et al., 2016; Raney, 2015). Recommendations from this consultation are shared with the direct care clinical team during a team case conference focused on care plan revision. Although Amber never met the consulting psychiatrist, her care is enhanced with this expert consultation and the support of the behavioral healthcare manager.

After the care team meeting, Amber and the behavioral healthcare manager review the new plan. If the plan includes a change in her psychotropic medication, Amber meets with her on-site medical clinician to complete this change. The behavioral healthcare manager continues regular contact with Amber to monitor her progress, address any psychotropic medication

FIGURE 1.4. Amber Experiences the Collaborative Care Model

Amber attends appointment
- Amber's depression screen positive
- Amber meets CoCM behavioral health care manager (BHCM)
- Amber agrees to join CoCM care management program

Prior to return appointment
- BHCM consults w/ psychiatrist to optimize medication management
- Primary care medical clinician prescribes psychotropics based on recommendation
- BHCM provides psychoeducation, care coordination, brief interventions

Amber engages in CoCM
- Completes PHQ-9 regularly to track progress, if poor adjust care plan
- Consistent connection to BHCM for resources & support
- PC medical clinician manages diabetes and depression w/ input from psychiatry

Amber completes CoCM program
- PHQ-9 shows reduced depressive symptoms
- May have improved diabetes management with support from BHCM
- Amber returns to usual care, screened at each appointment

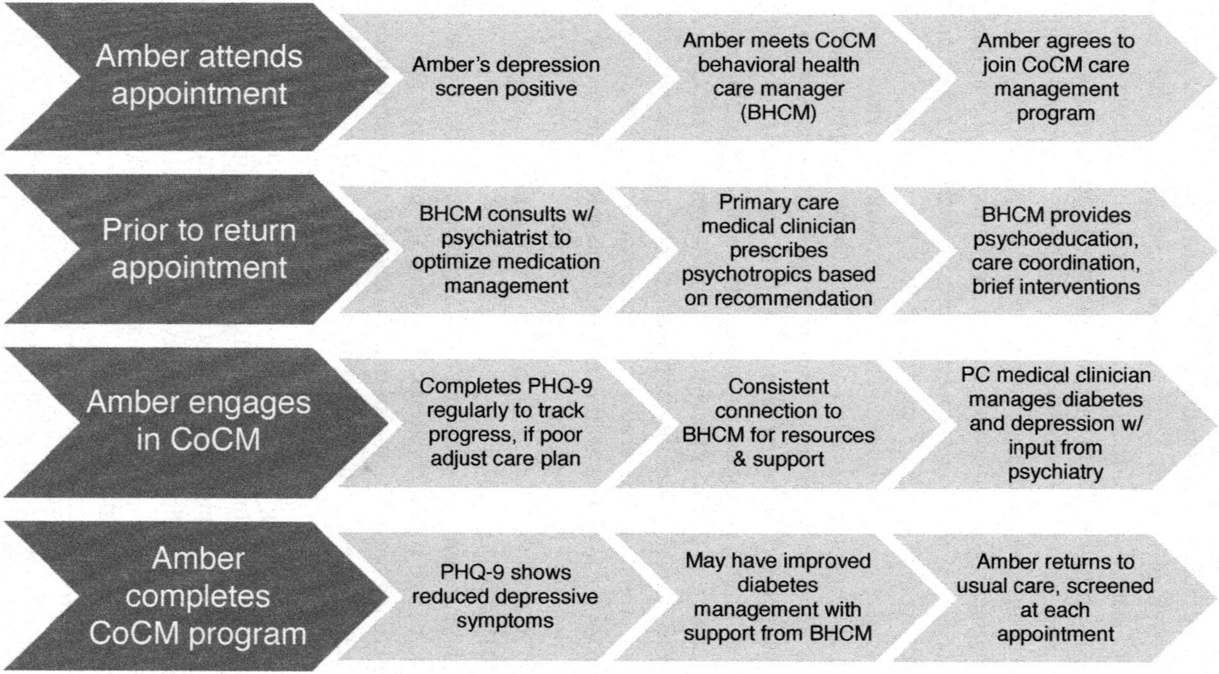

BHCM = behavioral healthcare manager; CoCM = collaborative care model; PC = primary care; PHQ-9 = Patient Health Questionnaire-9.

side effects, and continue behavioral interventions to target symptoms and improve functioning. Across time, Amber's team collaborates closely, meeting regularly to track Amber's progress, adjusting her treatment plan as needed, and connecting directly with the consulting psychiatrist when necessary. As long as she continues to make progress, Amber remains in the CoCM program until she is ready to return to routine care. Amber is referred to specialty behavioral health resources if her needs are not met by CoCM.

Amber and her behavioral healthcare manager work together to plan discharge from the program, based on measures of her symptoms and functioning, her relapse-prevention plan, and her own readiness to move forward. The focus on relapse prevention becomes more central, preparing Amber to self-monitor and recognize signs of trouble early; coping strategies to prevent relapse are reviewed as well. The behavioral healthcare manager emphasizes to Amber that she can reenroll in the program should she begin to experience problems again.

Although the model's primary assessments and interventions do not specifically address relational issues, behavioral healthcare managers can focus on enhancing social support, connecting with community resources, and engaging family members. Both PCBH and CoCM emphasize addressing social determinants of health and healthcare system issues. Behavioral healthcare managers often specifically address the patient's experiences related to healthcare system access and management challenges (Reising et al., 2022). For example, if Amber struggled to obtain subspecialist care to manage diabetes symptoms, she might receive help navigating the healthcare system or accessing social services to address financial and other resource-related barriers to care.

Reimbursement for CoCM includes both FFS and value-based elements (Carlo et al., 2018). During the time that Amber is enrolled in the program, the practice bills for visits and uses a programmatic billing code that pays the practice a monthly fee. The programmatic fees augment FFS billing to cover behavioral healthcare manager time engaged in nondirect clinical service. Typically, the psychiatrist is an independent contractor or employed by the larger healthcare system that owns the medical practice, so the psychiatrist bills separately. The behavioral healthcare manager and other members of the direct care team are employees of the practice.

Research Support for the Collaborative Care Model

Extensive evidence supports the efficacy of CoCM in reducing anxiety and depressive symptomology and improving chronic disease outcomes in multiple conditions, including diabetes and cardiac disease (Katon, 2012; Muntingh et al., 2016; Thota et al., 2012). A 2012 Cochrane review determined that

CoCM offered improved outcomes over standard care in both the short and long term for adult patients struggling with depression and anxiety (Archer et al., 2012). Multiple systematic reviews and meta-analyses indicated that patients enrolled in CoCM achieved higher levels of remission, better psychotropic medication adherence, improved symptoms, and higher satisfaction over usual care (J. M. Baker et al., 2018; Coventry et al., 2014; Thota et al., 2012). However, a review of data regarding patient-reported quality of life was inconclusive (Thota et al., 2012).

CoCM has been implemented in many different types of healthcare systems across the globe with strong results (Ali et al., 2020). Researchers now are exploring enhanced technological advances to maximize the scalability of the model (Carleton et al., 2020). Workforce issues have been a challenge for CoCM implementation because many areas of the country do not have sufficient behavioral health professionals, particularly psychiatrists (Andrilla et al., 2018). In this context, a systematic review examined the impact of having both the behavioral healthcare manager and consulting psychiatrist work remotely from the integrated medical setting (Whitfield et al., 2022). The results indicated that remote administration of the CoCM model garnered results similar to those found with on-site administration, potentially increasing the flexibility of the model and somewhat addressing identified workforce barriers to implementation.

A systematic review of 15 studies examined the experiences of primary care medical clinicians with CoCM. Primary care medical clinicians reported that CoCM improved their knowledge of chronic care management and management of mental health issues. They also reported high levels of satisfaction with the program and an enhanced sense of efficacy in patient care (Holmes & Chang, 2022).

SUMMARY

The paradigm shift toward integrated behavioral healthcare is ongoing. In this chapter, we presented the key models as a point of education and context. PCBH and CoCM have served as guideposts in the movement, but we appear to be on the cusp of another paradigm shift in that many clinics and practices now take the best of both and apply them to the local context, utilizing measurement against key benchmarks to ensure quality outcomes.

In the next chapters, we shift to the process of implementing integration models into healthcare systems and medical practices. The Cross Model Framework, based on real-world practices, reflects the complexity of this process and is but one reason that a systemic lens is critical to success in integration efforts. Practices and healthcare systems have complex inter-acting elements. Like families (or any other system), they tend to resist major changes secondary to homeostatic processes. Like families, they are made up of individuals who may or may not share the same goals, behaviors, and values. Recognizing these challenges while also valuing the many significant advantages of integration, practices and healthcare systems benefit from embracing strategies and processes that enhance outcomes and address barriers at various systemic levels to facilitate integration efforts.

TAKEAWAY POINTS

- Patients face many barriers in accessing specialty behavioral healthcare, including poor communication with other healthcare clinicians that contribute to care fragmentation.

- Integrated care models improve access to behavioral health services, communication among clinicians, and care quality.

- Several models of integrated care approach issues of access, communication, and quality of care differently.

- CoCM is a programmatic intervention that focuses on detecting behavioral health concerns via depression screening, then provides care management and medication consultation to enhance care.

- PCBH uses multiple strategies to identify patients in need of behavioral health and health behavior issues. PCBH addresses a broad array of presenting concerns, focusing on real-time services to address emotional and relational concerns, chronic disease management, healthcare utilization, and other issues.

- Many systems have moved to the Cross-Model Framework, an integrated care service that blends these models to leverage their different advantages.

- Each model has different applications, benefits, and challenges. All require practices that currently engage in traditional separate services or colocated services to engage in substantial practice transformation.

2 THE RISE OF INTEGRATED CLINICAL APPROACHES

In this chapter, we present a narrative that describes the evolution of integrated care in the U.S. health system, with a focus on critical incidents. Our systemic assessment includes reflecting on how larger systems factors influenced the field's evolution. It also includes historical influences, recognizing that integrated healthcare did not evolve in a vacuum. All these factors inform our path forward.

We begin the narrative with the evolution of mental models used to understand health and healthcare and how these models influenced and were influenced by the emerging fields of primary care, family therapy, and integrated healthcare. We then review the evolution of integrated care itself, focused on how different definitions, settings, and implementation processes evolved. This version of history is formed, in part, from first-person accounts. We compared and compiled narratives to acknowledge different perspectives. This history is not intended to be exhaustive but rather one contextualized, systemically focused review.[1]

---

[1] Others who experienced the evolution of integrated care from 1985 to 2023 might select different critical incidents or tie them together in a different way.

https://doi.org/10.1037/0000381-003
A Systemic Approach to Behavioral Healthcare Integration: Context Matters, by
N. B. Ruddy and S. H. McDaniel

Perspectives from different professions and their cultures form multiple interwoven branches of the integrated care origin story. An integrated care narrative is incomplete without acknowledging parallel processes, or evolutionary branches, that occurred in different healthcare systems for children and families. The branches evolved during similar time periods but in different contexts such as academic medicine, public health, and large-scale health systems such as the Department of Veterans Affairs (VA). Each was informed by growth in other branches as integrated primary care professionals collaborated with one another. Each evolved in adaptation to many of the same facilitators and challenges. Integrated care evolved somewhat differently across systems, in part reflecting the needs of specific patient populations such as those served in federally qualified healthcare centers, TRICARE (the healthcare system for the Department of Defense), and the VA.

EVOLVING MENTAL MODELS OF HEALTHCARE: TOWARD A MORE WHOLISTIC SYSTEMIC APPROACH

The practice of healthcare is based on a mental model of care, reflecting myriad assumptions and heuristics that facilitate our management and understanding of complexity. Our mental model reflects how we understand what makes healthcare work and what we view as the definition of "good" or "normative" healthcare over time. Mental models regarding clinical care evolve, reflecting new evidence and shifting standards of care. This section reviews this evolution of mental models—how we think about and prioritize variables in the complex work of healthcare—and how this evolution has influenced the ongoing shift toward integrating behavioral health into medical settings.

We focus on four major mental models in healthcare that represent shifts that set the stage for integrated care:

- the biopsychosocial approach,
- application of a systemic lens,
- the patient-centered home and interdisciplinary team-based care, and
- the chronic care model.

Mental Model Shift #1: Expanding the Purview of Healthcare With a Biopsychosocial Approach

George Engel's seminal article titled "The Need for a New Medical Model: A Challenge for Biomedicine" (G. L. Engel, 1977) signaled a new healthcare paradigm. Engel (1977) argued that medical care must expand its purview beyond biomedicine to recognize and intervene with psychological, relational, and social factors that influence health and wellness. This perspective challenged medical professionals to include nonbiomedical issues in their assessment and management of health issues. The expanded purview required a shift in medical training toward this biopsychosocial approach (Waldstein et al., 2001). It also set the stage for eventual greater collaboration and integration with behavioral health clinicians.

Regier and colleagues' seminal 1978 article recognized this interplay. They argued that most behavioral health issues present and are managed in primary care, referring to primary care as the "de facto mental health system." In this context, Regier and others emphasized that primary care teams need specific expertise in assessing and managing behavioral and social components of health to provide optimal care. The issues with access to behavioral health services persist to this day, as evidenced in a 2022 U.S. government report calling for increased coordination and integration of care (U.S. Senate Committee on Finance, 2022). Public health experts also note that the disease burden of neurological, mental health, and substance abuse issues has risen precipitously over the past 2 decades and emphasize the importance of a primary-care-based care delivery system for these clinical presentations.

Time restrictions and limits on the competencies of any one discipline may be factors underlying the struggle to provide care to the whole person. In the late 1980s Donald Bloch took the position that comprehensive, systemic healthcare requires at least two health professionals: a clinician focused on physical health and one focused on emotional–relational health (Bloch, 1988). He called this approach the "Dual Optic." At the time, many felt that physicians, with appropriate training, could meet a wide variety of patient needs by practicing biopsychosocial medicine, with occasional consultations from specialists. However, it became clear that Bloch was correct: This feat is unrealistic and rare in fast-paced healthcare settings. Despite general agreement that the expanded purview of care ultimately requires an expanded team-based approach, research still seeks to discern the best team-based care structures, elements, and strategies (Shekelle & Begashaw, 2021).

Mental Model Shift #2: Family Therapy and Family Medicine Come Together and Demonstrate Systemic Thinking in Healthcare

General systems theory swept through the basic sciences in the first half of the 20th century (Hammond, 2002). The application of general systems theory to health, mental health, and behavior change occurred in the second half of the 20th century and affected medicine, nursing, and family therapy.

Even so, the disciplines then—and sometimes now—paid little attention to each other's literature.

During the 1960s and 1970s, a handful of psychiatrists (Bowen, Minuchin, Whitaker, Wynne), psychologists (Anderson, Goolishian, Watzlawick), and research social scientists (Bateson, Haley, Weakland) experimented with direct involvement of family or other significant others in the treatment of people with a broad array of vexing issues. These efforts to apply systems theory to human relationships were especially influenced by ongoing discoveries based on systems theory in physics. Second-order cybernetics (Mead, 1968; von Foerster, 2003) especially focused on how parts of a system influence the behaviors of each other and how the observer is necessarily a part of—not outside—the system. Although generally focused on all relevant relationships, this clinical approach came to be called *family therapy*. Early family therapy pioneers, most of them psychiatrists, believed the application of general systems theory to human experience, what is now called a *biopsychosocial systems approach* (McDaniel, Doherty, & Hepworth, 2014), would be a unifying theory that recognizes that mind and body are inextricably intertwined and influenced by the social environment.

This perspective was also influential in nursing. A popular textbook, *Distributive Nursing Practice: A Systems Approach to Community Health* (J. E. Hall & Weaver, 1977), proposed that context matters—"the experience of illness was framed by social, psychiatric, and behavioral forces" (C. Gilliss, personal communication, August 12, 2022). Catherine Gilliss (1991) eventually helped to describe the field of family nursing research, theory, and practice. In a seminal paper titled "There Is Science, and There Is Life" (Gilliss, 2002), she described theory and research supporting the application of family interventions to chronic disease management.

In parallel, family medicine emerged as a new medical discipline in the late 1960s, in part a reaction to the increased focus on specialization in medicine throughout the 20th century (Gibson et al., 2016). Family medicine embraced a collaborative, systemic, biopsychosocial approach to medical care. In the United States, family therapist Bill Doherty, PhD, and family physician Mac Baird, MD, modeled this collaboration and wrote the first book that focused on a truly family approach to primary care, *Family Therapy and Family Medicine* (1983). They were followed by Canadian family physician Janet Christie-Seely, who wrote *Working With the Family in Primary Care: A Systems Approach to Health and Illness* (1984).

Family medicine educators emphasized interprofessional collaboration, requiring all residency training programs to have a "behavioral health" faculty member (Accreditation Council for Graduate Medical Education, 1989). This requirement was central in development of the field of integrated primary care as it set the stage for behavioral health clinicians and researchers to serve a central role in primary care education. It facilitated real-time collaboration, integration, and easy communication between professionals across medical and behavioral health fields (Blount, 1998; McDaniel et al., 1992). Increasingly, medical and behavioral health trainees worked together, altering practice patterns for both. Recently, the field has further embraced integration of behavioral health by considering requirements that all residency training practices offer integrated behavioral health services (deGruy & McDaniel, 2021).

Similarly, behavioral health clinicians (psychologists, psychiatrists, psychiatric nurse practitioners, social workers, counselors, and marriage and family therapists) broadened their purview to focus beyond emotional and relational health to include the impact of health concerns on individuals and families. As in medicine, a systemic lens facilitated embracing this complexity. In 1992, McDaniel, Hepworth, and Doherty wrote *Medical Family Therapy: A Biopsychosocial Approach to Families With Health Problems,* updated in 2014 as *Medical Family Therapy and Integrated Care* (McDaniel, Doherty, & Hepworth, 2014). *Medical Family Therapy* is a guide to help behavioral health clinicians move toward a systemic, biopsychosocial framework for helping families cope with health issues. The approach delineates assessment and therapeutic strategies to help families cope with and successfully manage the challenges of medical illness. Of note, all three authors of *Medical Family Therapy* served as faculty in family medicine residencies. To this day, integrated care and medical family therapy thought leaders often share this history of learning and working in family medicine residencies (Hodgson et al., 2014).

Mental Model Shift #3: The Transition to the Patient-Centered Medical Home and Team-Based Care

As with family medicine, pediatrics played a key role in the story of integrated behavioral health and team-based care. As early as the mid-1960s, the president of the Academy of Pediatrics James Wilson (1964) stated:

> The need for pediatricians, for persons skilled in organic disease, to give comfort to the parents who turn to them for advice, is clear, but their ability, their desire, and their willingness to meet this need are far less clear. I feel very strongly that one of the things I would do if I could control the practice of pediatrics would be to encourage groups of pediatricians to employ their own clinical psychologists. . . . I will grant you that there is some aversion by some psychologists to working "under" pediatricians, but better cooperative effort between these two groups would be greatly appreciated by our public and would do an immense amount of good. Such an approach, it seems to me, is

the only practical step to aid us in solving many of the problems in childhood and adolescence which are associated with organic disease or the question of it. (p. 988)

Dr. Wilson's vision may not align with today's more collaborative, egalitarian, team-based model. Yet it is clear that his statement reflects a recognition of the need for physical and mental health clinicians to collaborate, an early recognition that no one discipline can address the broad needs of children.

This recognition set the stage for the development of the patient-centered medical home (PCMH) concept. The PCMH is defined as

a model of care in which patients are engaged in a direct relationship with a chosen provider who coordinates a cooperative team of healthcare professionals, takes collective responsibility for the comprehensive integrated care provided to the patients, and advocates and arranges appropriate care with other qualified providers and community resources as needed. . . . PCMH practices develop transdisciplinary care teams to improve care coordination and care management of patient populations aiming to improve safety, efficiency and quality in patient care. (Primary Care Collaborative, 2015)

This definition of the PCMH reflects a long evolutionary process. Early conceptualizations of the PCMH focused on reducing fragmentation of care for seriously ill or disabled children and children with special needs (American Academy of Pediatrics Council on Pediatric Practice, 1967). The concept expanded over time to highlight the importance of continuity of care and ongoing collaboration between families and medical professionals (Sia et al., 2004). It set the stage for the inclusion of behavioral health clinicians in the pediatric practice team. In 1967, E. E. Smith and colleagues published an article advocating for and outlining the role of the clinical psychologist in pediatric practice, touting the benefits to patients and clinicians alike (E. E. Smith et al., 1967). Carolyn Schroeder, PhD, helped define the role of a behavioral health clinician in a pediatric primary care practice (Schroeder, 1979, 2004), highlighting new ways of interacting with patients and families such as improving access to care via call-in hours and very brief assessment and intervention strategies. Current integrated care strategies still reflect Dr. Schroeder's early work.

Although the pediatric community continued to advocate for these practice shifts throughout the late 20th and early 21st centuries, widespread integration of behavioral health professionals into pediatric practice has lagged. Fifteen years after advocating for team-based care focused on psychosocial issues, Terry Stancin, PhD, a leading pediatric psychologist, and James Perrin, MD, a former president of the American Academy of Pediatrics and an early proponent of integrated care, stated: "Despite the early interest of psychologists and a natural partnership between psychology and pediatrics, psychologists' impact on the range of services for children in *primary care* [emphasis added] settings has not maximized its potential" (Stancin & Perrin, 2014, p. 332). Systemic approaches to pediatric care continue to develop.

Over time, the structure and focus of PCMH concepts and operational elements evolved with healthcare reimbursement systems. Primary care practices were incentivized to become certified as a PCMH, with the practice elements necessary to achieve certification increasing over time. These PCMH elements supported value-based care, that is, payment for quality of care and outcomes rather than for frequency of procedures or visits (Conrad et al., 2014). PCMH certification initially focused on a rubric of practice elements to determine the level of PCMH alignment (Kellerman & Kirk, 2007; Kilo & Wasson, 2010). Over time, the definition of PCMH became more conceptual, encompassing a mental model (Cronholm et al., 2013) with five core elements:

- comprehensive care, requiring a team of clinicians;
- patient-centered care, focused on the relationship between clinicians and the patient;
- coordinated care, ensuring clear communication between clinicians;
- accessible care, in real time whenever possible; and
- safe, quality care, using evidence-based practices that engage in quality improvement. (Agency for Healthcare Research and Quality, n.d.).

In the early 21st century, integrated primary care was not foundational in the PCMH rubric, as the focus was primarily on electronic health records, transitions of care, and care coordination (Ader et al., 2015). However, the requirements eventually shifted to team-based care and colocated behavioral health clinicians. The research and policy worlds began to pay greater attention to new integrated models of care such as the collaborative care model (CoCM) and the Primary Care Behavioral Health (PCBH) model (Crowley & Kirschner, 2015).

Mental Model Shift #4: The Chronic Care Model Supports Patient-Centered, Team-Based Care

Late in the 20th century, Edward Wagner et al. (1996) argued that people with chronic conditions need a reorganized system of care that is proactive and planned rather than reactive to issues as they arise. In this model, clinicians focus on enhancing patient engagement, offering a cadre of resources and outreach strategies based on patient goals and values. Most important for our discussion, Wagner and colleagues noted that chronic care management must focus on behavior change and actively engage patients and families in self-management. They described this model as delivered best by a team of clinicians who can provide "ready access to relevant expertise" (p. 518). Substantial research supports the efficacy of this model (Kastner et al. 2018) and serves as the foundation of CoCM (Katon, 1995). CoCM specifically focuses on the interplay of behavior, mental health, and chronic disease management. Exhibit 2.1 outlines the ethos underlying this approach, in the form of "mottos" selected by C. J. Peek (2006).

Impact of Mental Models

Shifting mental models of healthcare toward a biopsychosocial systemic approach revealed a need for an integrated team of clinicians. Each of these paradigm shifts raised expectations for the quality and scope of healthcare such that no one clinician could meet these expectations. Addressing complex care needs, some rooted in relational and social determinants of health, supported a move toward a more integrative, systemic lens. Embedding behavioral health, other clinicians, and ancillary supports into healthcare settings facilitated an expanded focus on the whole person, family, and social context. As an outgrowth of the healthcare system's increasing focus on quality of care,

EXHIBIT 2.1. Mottos for Chronic Care Management

1. When it comes to chronic care, no one has all the marbles.
2. The general ability to work well across disciplines on behalf of patients is good clinicianship.
3. Preventing the classic and predictable fragmentations and misunderstandings in care may be the most important part of your job.
4. Hold the baton until you are sure that the next person has it and knows he or she has it.
5. The right kind of time at the front of a case saves time over the life of the case.
6. Most difficult patients started out merely as complex.
7. Evaluation of the patient's case goes along with evaluation of the patient.
8. Healthcare relationship problems can complicate health problems.
9. Patients can't participate effectively in care plans that they don't understand and embrace.
10. Clinicians must be able to show how every move and technique serve the care plan.
11. Disability management is often bigger than symptom management.
12. Be sure the treatment doesn't increase the disability.
13. Groom patients for referral—make sure patients can verbalize why they are going to the next clinician.
14. Patient resistance is usually a sign of a problem in approach, negotiation or timing.

BH = behavioral health; PC = primary care. From "Appealing to What Matters in Chronic Care," by C. J. Peek, 2006, *Biofeedback*, 34(4), p. 142. Copyright 2006 by *Biofeedback*.

access, and coordination, the PCMH and aligned models of care (such as the chronic care model) and propelled interprofessional team-based care. Some disciplines within medical and mental health embraced these values, setting the stage for collaborations and the emergence of new approaches, such as medical family therapy. Next, we outline how these initial attempts at team-based care ultimately evolved into a new field—integrated behavioral health.

EVOLVING CLINICAL MODELS: THE RISE OF INTEGRATED APPROACHES

In this section, we review how and why medical practices sought to integrate behavioral health services into daily practice. Our review focuses on a relatively narrow time period from the 1980s to the present.[2]

The Emergence of Integrated Primary Care

Many early pioneers in integrated primary and specialty care worked to adapt family therapy concepts and strategies to these settings. Donald Bloch, MD, was a psychiatrist who served as the director of the Ackerman Institute for the Family and the second editor of the premier family therapy journal, *Family Process*. His work focused on the application of systems theory to health and healthcare, developing the field of *family systems medicine*. In 1983, he used private funding to establish the journal *Family Systems Medicine* (now *Families, Systems, & Health*) with colleagues Barry Dym, Michael Glenn, and Donald Ransom (Bloch, 1983). A clinical psychologist, Ransom wrote an influential column, *Random Notes*, that focused on applying systemic principles of healthcare delivery (e.g., Ransom, 1984). Like other early integration proponents, Ransom served as a family medicine faculty member in the Department of Family and Community Medicine at the University of California San Francisco (UCSF). In 2003, he retired from UCSF and shifted his focus to establishing the value of these systemic ideas within the Sutter Pacific Medical Foundation. This jump from the academic world into leadership in healthcare practice was another watershed moment in the development of this nascent field as Ransom and colleagues sought to shift healthcare provision. They, along with Nicholas Cummings at Kaiser Permanente,[3] created a real-world test of these concepts, with outsize effects on the healthcare system.

During the 1980s, other pockets of professionals in family medicine, psychiatry, internal medicine, and pediatrics focused on behavioral and

---

[2]The interested reader can find a more detailed description of the evolution of models of mental healthcare, the disciplines of primary care, and their eventual shifts toward collaboration and integration in B. F. Miller and Hubley (2017).

relational health issues in primary care, working to heal the mind–body split in our medical system. Systems thinkers recognized that a patient is to a family as a clinician is to a healthcare team, noting that healthcare teams had their own group dynamics that often parallel those of the family. Ultimately, the treatment system was defined collectively as the patient and relevant members of their family and the clinician and relevant members of the healthcare team (McDaniel, Doherty, & Hepworth, 2014).

In 1994, Bloch organized a small, seminal conference of systems-oriented innovators at the Wingspread Conference Center in Racine, Wisconsin. The Wingspread Conference launched the Collaborative Family Healthcare Coalition, now the Collaborative Family Healthcare Association (https://www.cfha.net), which continues to serve as the professional home for many healthcare professionals working in integrated care to this day.

Pragmatic issues in healthcare provision also supported integrating behavioral health into healthcare. Medical clinicians, on a daily basis, confronted the reality that effective collaboration was difficult to establish with external, community-based mental health clinicians. Beyond access-to-care issues, healthcare clinicians were challenged by patients unwilling or unable to seek specialty mental healthcare and poor communication among healthcare colleagues. Recognition of the interplay of mental health issues and chronic disease outcomes was but one factor that spurred development of the CoCM model (Katon et al., 2010).

Eventually, some healthcare systems began to experiment with having behavioral health clinicians on-site in primary care (Dym & Berman, 1986). For example, at the University of Rochester, Drs. McDaniel and Campbell brought a family therapist (Dave Seaburn, PhD) to work on-site in the residency practice. Vexing problems of access and communication evaporated almost immediately. Within a year, they hired two more family therapists, who functioned as embedded therapists and researchers. They engaged in systemic conceptualization, significant collaboration, and occasional "cotherapy" with their medical colleagues. Thirty-eight years later, in 2023, this same clinic has evolved to employ four master's-level clinicians, three PhDs, a consulting adult psychiatrist, and a child and adolescent psychiatrist. The clinic trains family medicine residents alongside psychology fellows and interns, and several marriage and family therapy graduate students.

---

[3]Nicholas Cummings, PhD, was a visionary psychologist who served as chief of mental health at Kaiser Permanente from 1959 to 1979 then left to develop the first successful behavioral health managed care organization. It was a service delivery and treatment model that focused on patient-driven, whole-person healthcare in collaboration with medical professionals, with more than 25 million covered lives. Cummings was a strong supporter (and funder) of integrated care, developing the Cummings Graduate Institute for Behavioral Health Studies to educate and train professionals in a doctorate of behavioral health program.

All are embedded into integrated healthcare teams. This process occurred almost simultaneously in other family medicine residency programs (e.g., UCSF, University of Minnesota, University of Oklahoma, University of Washington), incubating this new model of care.

These shifts were not just in academic health centers. In the mid to late 1980s and 1990s, prior to large-scale adoption of PCMH tenets, healthcare systems began embedding behavioral health clinicians to facilitate real-time collaboration, integration, and easy communication. Cherokee Health Systems started a community-based, integrated, primary care service in 1984, the beginnings of a health system that served as a national model for integrated care (Khatri, Perry, & deGruy, 2017). Although this process occurred largely independently across geographically dispersed health systems and sites, practice approaches and structures aligned in many ways. These similarities may reflect how various places ultimately settled on a similar set of solutions to many healthcare pain points such as the interplay of mental health and general health and mental health access issues. Alexander Blount (1998) documented the growth of this embedded mental health model in his book *Integrated Primary Care: The Future of Medical and Mental Health Collaboration* (1998). Blount provided a blueprint to advance integration, describing how behavioral health and medical clinicians collaboratively can address clinical issues created by the schism between the medical and behavioral healthcare systems. Blount's book emphasized the importance of not bifurcating medical and behavioral issues. Whereas the biopsychosocial systems approach described a clinical framework, integrated behavioral health described a service delivery model based on the biopsychosocial approach. Blount presented the case for this approach, reviewed implementation strategies, and illustrated the concepts by describing exemplar programs.

Over the next decade, growing pains emerged. The similar approaches developed by early adopters began to diverge. In addition, the language used to describe various elements was poorly defined, causing confusion and complicating outcome research efforts. C. J. Peek and colleagues worked with the Agency for Healthcare Research and Quality to precisely define and measure these integrated care concepts to facilitate practice-level outcome research (Peek & National Integration Academy Council, 2013). The Substance Abuse and Mental Health Services Administration also sought definitions of integrated primary care (e.g., Doherty et al., 1996) that linked to behavioral and structural anchors. Just as the PCMH rubric set benchmarks and measured progress toward PCMH designation, these efforts to define the continuum of integration helped identify a baseline and a course for a desired state. Clarifying and defining roles and processes continues to this day, as research shows that the clinical strategies of behavioral health clinicians in primary care continue to be variable (Beehler et al., 2017). Exhibit 2.2 outlines the six levels of

EXHIBIT 2.2. Substance Abuse and Mental Health Services Administration Levels of Integrated Care

Integration Categories	Integration Levels	Description
Coordinated Care	**Level 1**–Minimal Collaboration	BH and PC providers work at separate facilities and have separate systems. Providers communicate rarely about cases. When communication occurs, it is usually based on a particular provider's need for specific information about a mutual consumer.
	Level 2–Basic Collaboration at a Distance	BH and PC providers maintain separate facilities and separate systems. Providers view each other as resources and communicate periodically about shared consumers. These communications are typically driven by specific issues. For example, a PC physician may request a copy of a psychiatric evaluation to know if there is a confirmed psychiatric diagnosis. BH is most often viewed as specialty care.
Colocated Care	**Level 3**–Basic Collaboration On-site	BH and PC providers are colocated in the same facility but may or may not share the same practice space. Providers still use separate systems, but communication becomes more regular due to close proximity, especially by phone or email, with an occasional meeting to discuss shared consumers. Movement of consumers between practices is most often through a referral process that has a higher likelihood of success because the practices are in the same location. Providers may feel like they are part of a larger team, but the team and how it operates are not clearly defined, leaving most decisions about consumer care to be made independently by individual providers.
	Level 4–Close Collaboration with Some System Integration	There is closer collaboration between PC and BH providers due to co-location in the same practice space, and there is the beginning of integration through some shared systems. A typical model may involve a PC setting embedding a BH provider. In an embedded practice, the PC front desk schedules all appointments and the BH provider has access and enters notes in the medical record. Often, complex consumers with multiple health care issues drive the need for consultation, which is done through personal communication. As processionals have more opportunity to share consumers, they have a better basic understanding of each other's roles.

EXHIBIT 2.2. Substance Abuse and Mental Health Services Administration Levels of Integrated Care (*Continued*)

Integration Categories	Integration Levels	Description
Integrated Care	**Level 5**–Close Collaboration Approaching an Integrated Practice	There are high levels of collaboration and integration between BH and PC providers. The providers begin to function as a true team, with frequent personal communication. The team actively seeks system solutions, as it recognizes barriers to care integration for a broader range of consumers. However, some issues, like the availability of an integrated medical record, may not be readily resolved. Providers understand the different roles team members need to play and they have started to change their practice and the structure of care to achieve consumer goals.
	Level 6–Full Collaboration in a Transformed/ Merged Practice	The highest level of integration involves the greatest amount of practice change. Fuller collaboration between providers has allowed antecedent system cultures (whether from two separate systems or from one evolving system) to blur into a single transformed or merged practice. Providers and consumers view the operation as a single health system treating the whole person. The principle of treating the whole person is applied to all consumers, not lust targeted groups.

From *Evaluation of the SAMHSA Primary and Behavioral Health Care Integration (PBHCI) Grant Program: Final Report (Task 13)*, by D. M. Scharf, N. K. Eberhart, N. S. Hackbarth, M. Horvitz-Lennon, R. Beckman, B. Han, S. L. Lovejoy, H. A. Pincus, & M. A. Burnam, 2014, p. 25. Copyright 2014 by RAND Corporation.

integrated care, a rubric commonly used to describe practices and guide shifts toward integration (Scharf et al., 2014).

The Emergence of Integrated Care Training Models

Eventually it became clear that integrated healthcare clinicians need distinct team-based care and behavioral health competencies. The requisite brief interventions and models of care (e.g., the stepped-care model, family and systemic approaches to health issues) were not taught in many educational programs for mental health clinicians. Similarly, medical professionals were often trained to work as individual contributors will little interprofessional team-based experience. Ultimately, educators in medicine and various health and mental health disciplines recognized the need to prepare our workforce differently.

One of the major educational shifts came with the recognition that developing intentional teamwork competencies requires self-reflection, collaboration, systemic thinking, and other distinct knowledge, skills, and attitudes. The science of teamwork revealed that comprehensive healthcare is most effectively delivered by a team that is intentional about its complementary roles, relationships, and processes (Salas et al., 2018). Yet, these skills typically were not explicitly developed or defined in healthcare education. In 1992, the Interprofessional Education Collaborative convened an expert panel that sought to define team-based care competencies. Notably, no behavioral health professionals were included in the team that created the core competencies for Interprofessional Collaborative Practice (Interprofessional Education Collaborative Expert Panel, 2011). However, behavioral health educators were at the table in 2001 when a National Academies of Practice expert panel report built on these competencies by describing best training practices to instill interprofessional healthcare competencies (Brashers et al., 2001). In 2014, an Institute of Medicine report described educational programs for establishing transdisciplinary professionalism for improving health outcomes (McDaniel, Campbell, et al., 2014). As the ongoing reports suggest, education about team-based care has evolved—and continues to evolve.

In addition to instilling teamwork competencies, the education system recognized the need to instill distinct direct clinical service competencies based in a proactive, systemic, population health-focused integrated care model. In the 1980s and 1990s, prior to these educational innovations, integrated behavioral health clinicians adapted their clinical approach "on the job." These early behavioral health clinicians realized that many specialty mental health assessment and intervention strategies were ill-suited to the culture, pace, and volume in healthcare settings and began to experiment with new ways of providing behavioral health services that did align with these contextual factors (Pomerantz et al., 2009).

Much as with team-based competency skills, the healthcare education community worked to define and instill these new behavioral health competencies. Initially, most of the training was experiential; clinical supervisors passed down these new adapted strategies to students in practica, internships, and fellowships. As integrated-care-based experiential learning sites proliferated, educators sought to define critical PCBH competencies across multiple domains (clinical, consultation, collaboration, quality improvement, population health and research, to name a few). Some of these efforts were discipline-specific, some interdisciplinary. Exhibit 2.3 lists some of the various competencies that have been identified by disciplines involved in integrated behavioral health.

To this day, few future clinicians are exposed to these interprofessional and integrated care behavioral health competencies during typical discipline-based training. Trainees who complete experiential training in the VA, some academic health centers, and federally qualified health centers are more likely to be exposed to integrated care model, but many trainees do not train in these settings.

EXHIBIT 2.3. Categories of Integrated Primary Care Competencies

Selected Clinical Competencies

Appropriately document consultation and clinical services.

Engage patients and families in care.

Exhibit knowledge of common medical conditions, effects on psychological and relational health.

Provide psychoeducation.

Understand and provide psychopharmacology and pharmacology consistent with scope of practice.

Use standardized outcome measures, measurement-based care.

Selected Leadership Practice Management Competencies

Create and implement discipline-based and interprofessional curriculum.

Engage in advocacy for integrated care.

Engage in health management practice.

Engage in practice-based learning and quality improvement.

Provide discipline-based and interprofessional clinical supervision.

Understand role of informatics in integrated team-based care.

Selected Professionalism Competencies

Engage in self-assessment and reflective practice.

Engage in self-care.

Exhibit professional values and attitudes.

Selected Interprofessional Teamwork Competencies

Engage in interprofessional collaboration.

Engage in team-based care planning and care management.

Exhibit knowledge of discipline-based competencies, roles, and responsibilities.

Promote and engage in a shared mental model based in the biopsychosocial systems approach.

Selected Diversity, Inclusion, and Equity Competencies

Attend to cultural elements in health and healthcare.

Exhibit cultural humility.

Support efforts to reduce health disparities.

Selected Ethics Competencies

Balance patient confidentiality with team-based care communication.

Engage in interdisciplinary ethical practice.

Selected Scholarship Competencies

Consume and contribute to health-focused research and evaluation.

Consume and contribute to interdisciplinary scholarship.

Note. These competencies are specific to interprofessional team-based care and augment discipline-specific competencies. They are compiled from integrated primary care competency lists for educators from various disciplines in the following documents: American Association for Marriage and Family Therapy (2018); American Psychological Association: McDaniel, Grus, et al. (2014); Farley Center for Primary Care: B. F. Miller, Gilchrist, et al. (2016); Interprofessional Education Collaborative: Interprofessional Education Collaborative Expert Panel (2011); National Association of Social Workers: Horevitz & Manoleas (2013), Raney (2013), Ratzliff et al. (2014); Substance Abuse and Mental Health Services Administration: Hoge et al. (2014); and Sunderji et al. (2016).

Integrated care's rapid growth and the relative lack of focus and exposure during behavioral health training have resulted in a workforce challenge such that too few practicing behavioral health clinicians have the necessary knowledge, skills, and attitudes to work successfully in integrated care (Serrano et al., 2018). It has been difficult to address these training gaps, in part because there are few faculty, especially at the graduate level, with integrated care experience to champion, develop, and teach coursework and establish experiential training. To fill this gap, integrated behavioral health experts developed didactic training resources to complement experiential training. Resources were developed to meet accreditation requirements of a specific discipline or geared to a specific training audience (Horevitz & Manoleas, 2013; McDaniel et al., 2002; Speice & McDaniel, 2015). We review training resources in Chapter 4, focusing on programs designed to instill these competencies with behavioral health and medical clinicians.

These educational innovations occurred in the context of healthcare reform focused on team-based care. As it became clear that workforce issues were a major barrier to successful implementation of integrated models (Serrano et al., 2018), the government increasingly supported integrated care training efforts. Support included the development of grant programs that provided training stipends, faculty support, and technical support (e.g., Behavioral Health Workforce Education and Training Program, Graduate Psychology Education Program). These grants facilitate the development of both didactic and experiential training experiences for behavioral health clinicians that, at a minimum, introduce trainees to integrated care and, ideally, create a workforce pipeline.

Because so few practicing clinicians had access to this type of training, many integrated care settings developed postgraduate training opportunities. Exhibit 2.4 lists a number of such programs, which offer both in-person and remote training for behavioral health clinicians from various disciplines and at different levels of training. The government also supported integrated care via the VA and U.S. military healthcare systems (TRICARE). These programs served important roles in the development and definition of integrated care models, research on the impact of integrated care, and workforce preparation. Next we review how these healthcare systems play an integral role in our integrated care historical narrative.

The Role of the Department of Veterans Affairs and TRICARE in Integrated Primary Care

The Department of Defense (DOD) and the VA operate two of the largest healthcare systems in the United States. Both systems made significant

EXHIBIT 2.4. Integrated Behavioral Healthcare Clinical Training Resources

Institution	Website	Modality
Agency for Healthcare Research and Quality Integration Academy	https://integrationacademy.ahrq.gov	Online
AIMS Behavioral Healthcare Manager Training	https://aims.uw.edu/online-bhcm-modules	Online
American Association for Marriage and Family Therapy	https://www.aamft.org/Courses/Courses.aspx	Online
American Psychiatric Association	https://education.psychiatry.org	Online continuing medical education
American Psychological Association	https://www.apa.org/education-career/ce	Online continuing education
American Psychological Association	https://www.apa.org/ed/graduate/primary-care-psychology	Directory of psychology training programs with IPC elements
Arizona State University DBH	https://chs.asu.edu/programs/behavioral-health-clinical-dbh	Online, also offer DBH in IPC management
Cherokee Health Systems Integrated Care Training Academy	https://www.cherokeehealth.com/professional-training/integrated-care-training-academy	In person
Collaborative Family Healthcare Association	https://www.cfha.net/your-career/early-career-mentorship	Early career mentorship
Medical Family Therapy	https://www.medicalfamilytherapy.org/education-opportunities-1	Directory of family therapy training programs with medical family therapy focus
National Council for Mental Wellbeing Center of Excellence for Integrated Health Solutions	https://www.thenationalcouncil.org/integrated-health-coe/learn-with-us	Online training and learning collaboratives
University of Massachusetts Medical School Center for Integrated Primary Care	https://www.umassmed.edu/cipc	Online courses
University of Michigan Online Certificate in Integrated Behavioral Health and Primary Care	https://ssw.umich.edu/offices/continuing-education/certificate-courses/integrated-behavioral-health-and-primary-care	Online courses, with pediatric and adult tracks
University of Rochester School of Medicine and Dentistry	https://www.urmc.rochester.edu/psychiatry/institute-for-the-family/family-therapy/mfti.aspx	In person and online course on integrated health care and medical family therapy
Department of Veterans Affairs Center for Integrated Healthcare	https://www.mirecc.va.gov/cih-visn2/clinical_resources.asp	Online training

AIMS = Advancing Integrated Mental Health Solutions; DBH = doctorate in behavioral health; IPC = integrated primary care; SAMHSA = Substance Abuse and Mental Health Services Administration.

commitments to integrated primary care in the late 20th century and early 21st century, well ahead of most healthcare systems in the private sector.

The DOD Military Health System initially implemented somewhat different models of integration in the various branches of the military as part of their shift toward the PCMH model. Each had a strong focus on and prioritization of behavioral health services (C. L. Hunter & Goodie, 2012). Integration of behavioral health clinicians into primary care started as early as 1997, when the Air Force launched the Tinker Project as a pilot (P. G. Wilson, 2004); the Behavioral Health Optimization Program began in 2000. Despite the development of a training program for primary-care-based social workers and psychologists in the Air Force (C. L. Hunter, Goodie, et al., 2014), it soon became clear that systemic factors stymied integration efforts. In 2006, the DOD formed a work group to standardize implementation and enhance training regarding the integrated model. By 2012, the Air Force had systematically trained behavioral health clinicians in 88% of their primary care sites (C. L. Hunter, Goodie, et al., 2014). The Army implemented a collaborative care and case management effort in 2004, focused on improving the identification and management of depression and posttraumatic stress disorder (C. L. Hunter & Goodie, 2012). This program, called RESPECT-MIL, was also very successful, providing screening at more than a half million visits and subsequent behavioral healthcare coordination to more than 10,000 soldiers as of 2012 (C. C. Engel et al., 2008; Wong et al., 2015). In 2013, DOD policy guided all branches to adopt a model similar to that developed in the Air Force (C. L. Hunter, Goodie, et al., 2014).

Another output of this work was a seminal book that facilitated workforce training and integrated primary care implementation in the private sector as well. In 2009, some of the architects of the DOD's integrated care model published *Integrated Behavioral Health in Primary Care: Step-by-Step Guidance for Assessment and Intervention* (C. L. Hunter, Goodie, et al., 2014). This practical guide for assessment and intervention in common primary care presentations outlined shifts behavioral health clinicians can make to be successful in primary care. In 2016, the authors updated the text, with a broadened focus on the implementation of integrated behavioral health (C. L. Hunter et al., 2017). The work that emanated from the DOD's journey to integration has facilitated progress throughout healthcare, particularly in training and implementation processes.

The VA also played a major role in furthering integrated primary care. The shift started with interprofessional care teams focused on improving care for geriatric populations. The Geriatric Interdisciplinary Team Training Program was implemented throughout the 1970s and 1980s and ultimately served as a precursor to integration efforts throughout the VA (Rasin-Waters et al., 2018).

The White River Junction VA Center in Vermont was a pioneer in integrated behavioral healthcare (Pomerantz & The Primary Mental Health Care Clinic at the White River Junction VA Medical Center, 2005). In the early 1990s these shifts were reflecting in the VA's training efforts via the Interdisciplinary Team Training Program. By the late 1990s, all VA-funded training was required to have an interprofessional element (Rasin-Waters et al., 2018). More specific to behavioral health, the Primary Care–Mental Health Integration Program aligned with CoCM, helping veterans who were struggling with both chronic illness and serious mental health issues. Increasingly, all VA centers were required to offer a full spectrum of behavioral health services, with larger sites mandated to integrate these services into primary care (Kearney et al., 2014).

These innovations and the lessons learned had a large impact on workforce development. The VA highlighted that staff training and practice transformation consultation were key to facilitate movement toward truly integrated services. For example, from 2007 to 2011, the VA offered didactic trainings on foundations of practice in integrated primary care. In 2009, Pomerantz, Corson, and Detzer published an article titled "The Challenge of Integrated Care for Mental Health: Leaving the 50 Minute Hour and Other Sacred Things." They noted that many traditional mental health clinicians struggled to transition to primary care and that these clinician adaptation issues hampered consistent implementation.

These and many other lessons learned from the VA implementation process inform our guidance on implementation, outlined in Part II of this book. The VA shared these lessons learned via training and consultation to outside health systems. Internally, they developed a fidelity measure to measure the extent to which the behavioral health clinician is embedded, part of the primary care team, as opposed to a colocated clinician providing more traditional psychotherapy (Beehler et al., 2013, 2020). This measure focuses on the behavioral health clinician's role to differentiate between fully integrated services and enhanced colocation services as described in Chapter 1 (Oxman et al., 2006). This measure guided a hub-and-spoke model of training to help behavioral health clinicians develop clinical competencies that align with fully integrated services. The training also addressed systemic barriers to integration. The training model was largely successful. The specifics are outlined in Kearney and colleagues' 2020 article "Creation and Implementation of a National Interprofessional Integrated Primary Care Competency Training Program: Preliminary Findings and Lessons Learned."

The contributions of the DOD and VA went beyond training. These organizations also contributed to research on the impact of integrated care models. In particular, the research evaluated the clinical effectiveness of different implementation models. They also described and evaluated training processes. These projects now guide implementation and clinician training across many healthcare settings.

SUMMARY

Fifty years ago, integrated healthcare largely did not exist. In a relatively brief time, this field has become more clearly defined and disseminated, especially in primary care. Yet there is still a great deal of work to be done to make these models of care normative and available to all.

Some of the challenges that have impeded progress toward the goal of making integrated healthcare normative are embedded in large system factors. In the next chapter, we review how shifts in healthcare policy have both supported and stymied these efforts. Because policy often follows from evidence, we also describe the ongoing evolution of research methodologies to better study complex models of care such as behavioral health integration. To set the context of how and why some of these challenges persist, we review the intertwining evolution of healthcare system research on models of care as well as healthcare reform as it relates to systemic integrated care.

TAKEAWAY POINTS

- Our paradigm for healthcare has changed over time to embrace a systemic approach in recognition of health and healthcare complexity. Significant contributors to the development of integrated care in this regard include
  - family therapy and family medicine focused on the family and significant others as partners in care;
  - pediatrics focused early on coordinating care for high-needs children; and
  - internist Edward Wagner's development of the chronic disease model bringing an evidence-based population health lens to prevention and chronic care.
- Systemic integrated care and team-based care are foundational to reaching the Quadruple Aim of improving healthcare outcomes, improving patient and provider satisfaction, and lowering healthcare costs.
- The DOD and VA were early innovators in the training and implementation of integrated care models.
  - Many practicing clinicians still have not had access to training on integrated care models.
- Interprofessional teams that leverage the differential expertise of various healthcare disciplines facilitate care for chronic conditions and may play a role in reducing health disparities.

3 HEALTHCARE REFORM AND EMERGING MODELS OF RESEARCH

In this chapter, we review the intersecting narratives of healthcare reform and research. Over the past 50 years, a variety of stakeholders have sought evidence-based improvements in the healthcare system. Healthcare reform has facilitated the development and dissemination of integrated team-based care, in part because these shifts have been viewed as an opportunity to improve care and potentially decrease costs. A significant policy push from the U.S. government supported integrated care implementation, training, and research. These efforts included changes to reimbursement strategies and accreditation and certification requirements that incentivized implementation of integrated care models. In addition, the government offered grant programs to incentivize system change directly as well as address barriers such as workforce readiness. Grant support for integrated care research also increased significantly. Here we describe how shifts in the research agenda helped to define integrated care best practices. In addition, we review how research methods are evolving to better capture and understand the complexity inherent in healthcare provision. These shifts include a movement toward investigating models of care rather than specific treatment strategies

https://doi.org/10.1037/0000381-004
A Systemic Approach to Behavioral Healthcare Integration: Context Matters, by
N. B. Ruddy and S. H. McDaniel

and prioritizing research methods that emphasize real-world applicability to guide practice standards.

HEALTHCARE REFORM AND SYSTEMIC INTEGRATED CARE

The relatively fast adoption and evolution of integrated care did not happen in a vacuum. These new models of care emerged as the United States and other healthcare systems turned a mirror on themselves and began to recognize and seek to rectify their flaws. In particular, it became clear that systemic weaknesses such as fragmented care and access issues contributed to suboptimal clinical outcomes and challenging experiences for patients (Institute of Medicine Committee on Quality of Health Care in America, 2001). These issues were also associated with increased costs and reduced patient and professional satisfaction (Ede et al., 2015). As a result, healthcare leaders and policymakers began to focus on major problems in need of solutions.

In the 1990s, the Institute of Medicine (IOM), now the National Academy of Medicine, examined ways our healthcare system was coming up short. The 1999 IOM report, *To Err is Human*, revealed a troubling truth: Patient safety in the U.S. medical system was far from secure (Kohn et al., 1999). In a follow-up report 18 months later, *Crossing the Quality Chasm* (IOM Committee on Quality of Healthcare in America, 2001), the IOM strongly stated the need for reform:

> In its current form, habits, and environment, American healthcare is incapable of providing the public with the quality healthcare it expects and deserves. (p. 45)

Crossing the Quality Chasm redefined the goals of healthcare reform toward the "Triple Aim" (Berwick, 2002). The Triple Aim goals are to improve the patient's experience of care (patient satisfaction), improve the health of populations (quality outcomes of care), and reduce per capita costs of healthcare (improving efficiency and reducing waste). The report then outlined a pathway to achieve these goals, with a focus on changing systems of care as well as moving toward systems-minded care. In 2014, Bodenheimer and Sinsky noted that high rates of burnout among healthcare professionals are a significant threat to the system's ability to reach the Triple Aim. They suggested a shift to the "Quadruple Aim," expanding the focus to encompass needed improvements in the work life of healthcare professionals, both staff and clinicians.

In a "user's manual" for the *Quality Chasm* report, Berwick called on the healthcare education community to instill systemic thinking in future healthcare professionals, noting the need for a new breed of citizenship in the system of work. He designated cooperation as a premier professional value, encouraging the healthcare education system to shift its focus. Furthermore,

> The overall strengths of the Quality Chasm report lie foremost in its *systems view* [italics added]. Rooted in the experiences of patients as the fundamental source of the definition of quality, the report shows clearly that we should judge the quality of professional work, delivery systems, organizations, and policies first and only by the cascade of effects back to the individual patient and to the relief of suffering, the reduction of disability, and the maintenance of health. (Berwick, 2002, p. 89)

Researchers focused on achieving the Triple Aim for decades to come. This is still a work in progress, and success has been elusive. Regarding the goal of reducing costs, between 1996 and 2016 healthcare costs in the United States rose from $1.4 trillion to $3.1 trillion, accounting for 18% of the nation's economy (Dieleman et al., 2020). The Patient Protection and Affordable Care Act (ACA) enabled major strides forward in quality outcomes, as data show that the improved access to care facilitated by the ACA improved healthcare outcomes (Sommers et al., 2017). Yet, healthcare outcomes in the United States continue to lag behind other wealthy nations while our costs far exceed theirs (Schneider et al., 2017).

Integrated care has been touted as a key element in improving these outcomes. For example, integrated primary care has been shown to reduce preventable inpatient hospitalization (Lanoye et al., 2017), a major driver of healthcare costs. It has also been associated with improved patient outcomes (Archer et al., 2012; Possemato et al., 2018).

INTEGRATED CARE AND THE QUADRUPLE AIM

Rates of clinician burnout and dissatisfaction with the healthcare system continue to be significant issues, highlighting the need for renewed focus on the Quadruple Aim (Shanafelt et al., 2019). These issues were exacerbated by the stress of the COVID-19 pandemic (Restauri & Sheridan, 2020). Within primary care, surveys conducted by the Larry A. Green Center and the Primary Care Collaborative revealed unsustainable levels of burnout, turnover, stress, and uncertainty (Larry A. Green Center, 2021). Integrated team-based care may be part of the solution to this complex problem. Integrated care has not yet been shown to be a causal force in reducing burnout directly but has been linked to reduced stress for medical clinicians. In addition, medical clinicians report benefits for both patients and themselves when integrated services are implemented. This link has been found in academic health centers (Funderburk et al., 2012), and federally qualified health centers (Torrence et al., 2014). Integrated primary care enhances medical professionals' perceptions of the availability and quality of mental health services available to their patients, as well as their own perceived ability to manage behavioral health issues (Zallman et al., 2017). Summarizing their research on physicians' perceptions of integrated care, Miller-Matero and colleagues (2016) stated,

> The overwhelming majority of physicians were satisfied with having access to an integrated psychologist (97.4%). Physicians believed that integrated care directly improves patient care (93.8%), is a needed service (90.3%), and helps provide better care to patients (80.9%). In addition, physicians reported that having an integrated psychologist reduces their personal stress level (90.1%). (p. 51)

HEALTHCARE REFORM AND BARRIERS TO INTEGRATED CARE

Despite these benefits, integrated care is not normative. Multiple characteristics of the healthcare system impeded integration efforts. One of the key barriers, if not the key barrier, to integration in the U.S. healthcare system is our reimbursement system (Kathol et al., 2010). We go into more depth about reimbursement issues in Chapter 4, which focuses on external contextual factors affecting integration implementation. In short, problems include significantly lower reimbursement for behavioral health and primary care and a fee-for-service (FFS) reimbursement structure that pays individually for specific services (B. F. Miller, Ross, et al., 2017). Although integrated care is recognized as an important tool to improve our system, reformers have not addressed key reimbursement issues that hamper team-based care. For example, many services foundational to integrated care (e.g., collaboration, care coordination) typically are not reimbursed activities in FFS systems. In addition, many payers do not allow reimbursement for services rendered by different health professionals on the same day (Marlowe et al., 2014). Despite many efforts to address these issues, the lack of consistent reimbursement for important elements of integrated care has made comprehensive implementation challenging.

Reimbursement issues are not the only barrier to integrated care. Our patchwork of local, state, and federal healthcare policies both support and complicate integrated care adoption (Lewis et al., 2014). On the one hand, the federal government supports integration training and research initiatives and provides a resource clearinghouse and other services through the Substance Abuse and Mental Health Services Administration's Center of

Excellence for Integrated Healthcare Solutions. On the other hand, state-level policies can inhibit the success of integrated care. Some states, for example, fund mental health and medical services from separate offices with separate budgets, disincentivizing collaboration between the two systems. To the frustration of integrated care clinicians, some states even have regulations that preclude shared waiting rooms or shared clinical spaces for mental health and medical care (Budde et al., 2017).

Consequently, the uptake of integrated models varies greatly across states. National clinician data from 2010 revealed that the volume of healthcare sites with primary care and behavioral health colocated was highly variable across states, ranging from 27% in New Jersey to 65% in Massachusetts. The study found lower rates of colocation in rural areas, despite government efforts to support rural integrated care (B. F. Miller, Petterson, et al., 2014). B. F. Miller and colleagues (2014) noted that state-level policies and workforce initiatives were correlated with the concentration of integrated services. In 2020, similar methodology revealed that colocation rates had increased slightly since the 2014 study but still lagged in rural areas and in small practices (Richman et al., 2020). Richman and colleagues (2020) also found variation by state, with 2018 colocation rates ranging from 23% in Nevada to 69% in Massachusetts. Both studies emphasize the importance of targeting state-level policies that impede integrated care.

A 2021 report by the National Academies of Sciences, Engineering, and Medicine made the following recommendations to ensure that high-quality primary care is implemented in the United States:

- Pay for primary care teams to care for people, not just for doctors to deliver services;
- Ensure that high-quality primary care is available to every individual and family in every community;
- Train primary care teams where people live and work; and
- Design information technology that serves the patient, family, and interprofessional care team (Phillips et al., 2021).

Recommendations to increase access and pay for team-based care are not new. Repeated calls for these changes have not resulted in sufficient recalibration of the U.S. healthcare system reimbursement structure and policies to support integrated team-based care.

Why has change been so slow? Healthcare policy and reimbursement systems reflect a complex system that does not change quickly. When one looks with a very long lens, the development of integrated care and its popularity in the past 50 years is remarkable. But its full implementation will take longer. At least in theory, healthcare reformers look to the academic literature to guide and define best practices. In the next section, we discuss how the interface between healthcare research and delivery systems may have impeded our ability to understand the impact of integrated care and how recent shifts set the stage to enhance progress.

THE EVOLUTION OF RESEARCH IN PRIMARY CARE AND INTEGRATED PRIMARY CARE

The story of healthcare policy and reimbursement is intertwined with that of healthcare research. Policy and reimbursement are, to some extent, driven by data and outcome research. Just as research and data revealed the problems to be solved in our healthcare system, reformers seeking improvement looked to the research community to guide healthcare policy shifts.

These shifts in the research community form an important undercurrent to the integration evolution story. Emerging questions about established models and processes for empirical inquiry have impacted the research on integrated care itself. This story is still unfolding as our research approaches continue to evolve to meet the need for evidence to guide clinical practice.

Some researchers in academic health centers began to question the ways their work did and did not adequately inform clinical practice, notably in primary care. The gold-standard research model was (and to many, still is) the randomized controlled trial (RCT). This research model informs clinical guidelines and has facilitated the development of myriad medical interventions. RCTs, by definition, require researchers to study a very specific population, using specific procedures, with focused outcome measures that assess only one aspect of an individual's health. Because of the methodological specificity and reductionistic strategy, many began to question the utility of RCTs for guiding the complexity of human health and clinical practice (Bothwell et al., 2016). In short, RCTs did not yield the data many clinicians saw as useful because clinical plans often encompass myriad issues, including social factors and comorbidities that were often excluded from prior studies.

Some scholars and many clinicians believe that RCTs do not reflect how healthcare, particularly primary care, is practiced in the real world (Peek et al., 2014). Common concerns include the following:

- RCTs typically study people with only one diagnosis, ruling out those with comorbidities. This reduces generalizability to complex clinical populations with multiple diagnoses, comorbidities, and/or social issues affecting health.

- Many reductionistic intervention protocols and specific outcome measures based in RCTs cannot be implemented or tracked in the real world.

- Research populations have tended to overrepresent White middle-class men who do not face many of the social struggles of women, people of color, or the poor. Thus, these studies do not capture fully the impact of social factors, particularly systemic racism and the social determinants of health.

Lawrence W. Green (2008), a public health researcher, wrote a seminal paper entitled "Making Research Relevant: If It Is an Evidence-Based Practice, Where's the Practice-Based Evidence?" Green argued that traditional research and research dissemination models suffer from two fallacies. The "fallacy of the pipeline" reflects that research and clinical guidelines tend to be disseminated in one direction: from the researcher to the clinician, with little input from clinicians to ensure generalizability and real-world application. The second, the "fallacy of the empty vessel," refers to assumptions that the clinician is an "empty vessel," thereby responding to new evidence without reference to the individual's prior knowledge or experience. This "empty vessel" assumption is clearly not based in reality; clinicians have enormous reserves of information based on daily practice, not to mention education. In fact, research has revealed that most physicians' clinical practices are relatively fixed over time and do not evolve in step with clinical guidelines, related to a variety of factors such as established routines and preferences as well as difficulty interpreting and applying the academic literature (Launer, 2015). Consequently, Green recommended more collaborative, participatory models of research that consider context and emphasize generalizability.

Others have called for the research community to develop and prioritize methodologies that can expand knowledge in more generalizable ways (Frieden, 2017). Kessler and Glasgow (2011) even suggested a decade-long moratorium on RCTs to make way for "pragmatic, transparent, contextual, and multilevel designs that include replication, rapid learning systems and networks, mixed methods, and simulation and economic analyses to produce actionable, generalizable findings that can be implemented in real-world settings" (p. 637). Public health experts and primary care clinicians still look to RCT results and clinical guidelines to provide evidence-based care for common clinical presentations, especially when these illnesses present as a singular problem. However, for all of the reasons cited above, many clinicians struggle to apply results from singularly focused studies to their multifaceted practice.

Subsequently, some researchers have shifted outcome measures, moving away from efficacy (performance of a narrowly defined intervention in a tightly controlled setting with a very specific patient population) to effectiveness (performance of an intervention in the real world). Researchers increasingly include patient-reported outcomes (Lavallee et al., 2016) and practice-level outcomes as they relate to broad quality metrics (Peek et al., 2014).

These shifts necessitated development of new, clear definitions of practice models and clinically meaningful measurements. For example, the development of a shared Primary Care Medical Home (PCMH) model definition facilitated the creation of quality benchmark measures for primary care practices seeking this recognition (Stange et al., 2010). In turn, the need to define the PCMH spurred development of clear definitions of integrated care (Peek, 2010). These definitions of best practices and other sources informed efforts to create measures of practice quality, with patient-reported and valued characteristics increasingly emphasized (Etz et al., 2019). Research on models of care such as the PCMH and its elements (including integrated behavioral health) exemplifies these shifts in research focus.

Researchers increasingly focus on understanding *complex adaptive systems* (Begun et al., 2003). This term describes the synergy of elements that work together to support excellent care. W. L. Miller, Crabtree, and colleagues (2010) applied the concept of complex adaptive systems to primary care and described it as a combination of the core elements of the practice (e.g., resources, structure, processes), adaptive reserve (e.g., practice resilience factors such as relationships), and sensitivity to and alignment with the local environment. To understand complex adaptive systems, researchers used natural "experiments" to compare care models, collecting myriad types of data as practices evolved. They collected data that informed a systemic understanding of care-level interactions (whether individual, family, or practice) in order to measure and understand the adaptive nature of primary care practice (Peek et al., 2014). The complex adaptive systems of healthcare recognize and focus on the interrelatedness of care elements and interactions that spur positive change.

Early research on integrated behavioral healthcare models sought to evaluate their effectiveness using RCT methods, comparing integrated behavioral health to standard care. Particularly, the Collaborative Care Model (CoCM) evolved out of research efforts to determine the efficacy of the model. Even with their limitations, RCTs—with their comparison to baseline or no-intervention groups—serve a crucial role in expanding our knowledge of what constitutes the best care, at the right time, to the right person or family, delivered by the right clinician.

As the benefits of integrated care are now established (Possemato et al., 2018), research has shifted to examining the effects of care elements, such as the population served, and particular clinical presentations, interventions, and team composition to inform best practices (e.g., Coventry et al., 2014; Sanchez, 2017). Research continues to discern the critical elements of integrated models and implementation processes as well as to investigate optimal dissemination and implementation processes (Overbeck et al., 2016; Simmons et al., 2017).

Success in these endeavors likely will require moving beyond model-based silos. There is substantial RCT evidence that CoCM improves patient experience and clinical outcomes and reduces costs for a focused group of populations and presenting concerns. Although the data to support the Primary Care Behavioral Health (PCBH) model is evolving, it already offers compelling evidence that this model of care provides significant benefits over standard care for a broad population of patients. Evaluating a blended CoCM–PCBH model in a practice reflects a level of complexity unlikely to be understood via RCT methodology alone. Research is sorely needed to guide those who seek to implement these models alone or together. Other questions include the following: What type or level of integration is best suited to specific populations and practice contexts? How do we motivate individual clinicians to alter practice patterns? What are the key elements to initiate and maintain team-based integrated care that optimizes patient, clinician, and practice outcomes?

Research on healthcare teams similarly is shifting from questions regarding its efficacy (e.g., Kiran et al., 2015) toward seeking best practices in implementation and strategies to maintain team-based care (e.g., Kyle et al., 2021). Multiple disciplines contribute to research on optimizing team functioning and the practice transformation process. Research on the effect of different structures and collaborative styles on team functioning and patient outcomes is particularly relevant to integrated care efforts (e.g., Wranik et al., 2019). Yet, many questions remain. We do not know what type of leadership is best suited to facilitate integrated care for particular populations or problems, but a recent summation of the literature concluded: "The importance of leadership to integrated primary care does not yet transcend the level of opinions" (Nieuwboer et al., 2019, p. 16). Clearly more research is needed; like so many other stories in systemic integrated care, this one is still being written.

Most traditional healthcare research and policy efforts do not address challenges that integration proponents face in shifting to a healthcare system in which integrated care is normative. Most current healthcare reimbursement structures and healthcare policy preclude progress, even as payers (particularly the government) work to support this movement in other ways. In parallel, our healthcare research infrastructure generally is not designed to support research that examines complex adaptive systems and models of care. In this context it has been difficult to shift from a focus on integrated model efficacy toward exploring the important elements of care provision and care model implementation to create much-needed, second-order change in the system. That being said, new models of research are being developed that do focus entirely on the populations and clinically significant outcomes that are important in 21st-century healthcare. These models offer promise for moving the needle forward with effective integrated care implementation.

In Part II of this book, we describe the benefits, explore the challenges, and offer strategies to overcome the challenges associated with the implementation of team-based integrated care.

TAKEAWAY POINTS

- Healthcare reform efforts to achieve the Quadruple Aim supported the emergence, evolution, and definition of integrated, team-based care models.
  - Integrated care, in particular, can improve physician and team well-being, in addition to patient outcomes.
- Systemic integrated care reflects a model of care that transcends professional disciplines and requires competencies that may not be included in traditional, discipline-based training.
- Evidence-based healthcare reformers and direct care clinicians struggle to apply results of research that used linear, reductionistic methodologies.
- The research community is evolving toward new research methodologies that better capture complexity in healthcare and healthcare system designs. These changes include
  - enhanced focus on patient-reported outcomes,
  - evaluating effectiveness in addition to or instead of efficacy,
  - evaluating models of care (such as systemic integrated care) and their elements rather than specific interventions, and
  - diversifying study samples and targets to enhance generalizability.

PART II

OVERVIEW: SYSTEMIC INTEGRATED CARE IMPLEMENTATION

Despite strong evidence of the benefits of integrated models of care, behavioral health integration is far from normative in primary or specialty care (Richman et al., 2020). As we noted in the introduction to the book, many elements of the system must come together for successful implementation. In Part II, we focus on this process of implementing integrated care. Implementation processes require a keen analysis of the changes necessary for success and the system's readiness and bandwidth for these changes. Therefore, we review processes and tools to support this assessment process as well as strategies to enhance systemic readiness to change.

The implementation process must assess and address inevitable barriers to change. Toward this end we review healthcare system elements that contribute to integrated care implementation challenges at various levels of the system. We also outline mitigation strategies to overcome these challenges, emphasizing the importance of engagement at each level of the system and customization of the process to align with local needs.

Finally, implementation requires a strategic plan based in systemic change management evidence and principles. A systemic approach fosters second-order change that shifts the essential nature of the system by realigning the interactions of the system's elements. Practice transformation ideally focuses on how the system elements interact and potentiate each other to form the whole. Appreciating the complexity of practice transformation in this way reduces the likelihood of unintended consequences and facilitates response to unexpected issues, facilitating necessary complex adaptations to contextual factors (Stroh, 2015).

We are guided in part by Lau and colleagues' (2016) systematic review that examined facilitators and barriers to the adoption of evidence-based models of care that involve complex interventions. They developed an evidence-based framework that describes four levels of healthcare sub-systems and identifies factors that influence implementation and practice transformation (see Figure 1). These factors are as follows:

• external contextual factors such as policies, incentivization, and dominant paradigms;

FIGURE 1. A Conceptual Framework of Key System Elements That Influence Implementation Healthcare

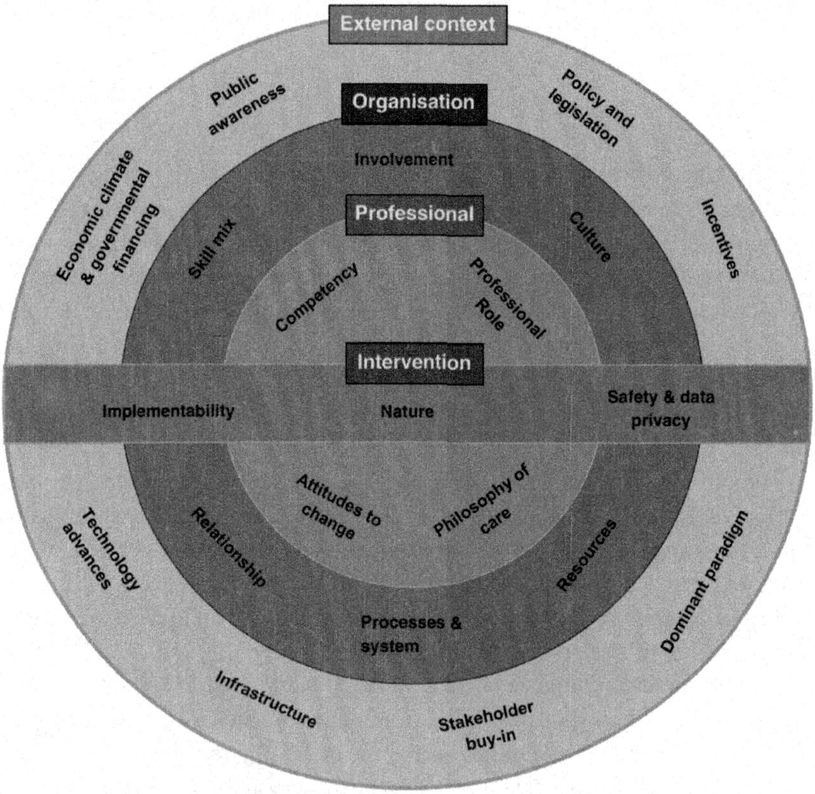

From "Achieving Change in Primary Care–Causes of the Evidence to Practice Gap: Systematic Reviews of Reviews," by R. Lau, F. Stevenson, B. N. Ong, K. Dziedzic, S. Treweek, S. Eldridge, H. Everitt, A. Kennedy, N. Qureshi, A. Rogers, R. Peacock, & E. Murray, 2016, *Implementation Science, 11,* Article 40, p. 31. Copyright 2015 by Springer Nature. Reprinted with permission.

- organizational-related factors such as culture, resources, relationships, staff mix, and engagement;
- individual professional factors such as the underlying philosophy of care and competencies;
- intervention characteristics including benefits; and
- the ease and adaptation to local circumstances (Lau et al., 2016).

Lau and colleagues (2016) were clear that many of these subsystem elements must change in a fundamental way for transformation efforts to have the intended effects in a lasting way. We this framework to the specifics of integrated behavioral health implementation, identifying key factors and how they relate to one another to foment or complicate change efforts.

The structure of this part parallels this breakdown of subsystems, with each chapter reviewing the barriers and facilitators at a specific level. Our proposed practice transformation strategies emphasize moving toward a shared mental model of care that produces the synergies between behavioral and physical health. Just as a systemically oriented therapist may work with a family to change how members interact with one another, we apply systemic and organizational change strategies to help a healthcare system, practice, or individuals within these systems begin to interact with each other differently toward improving care for those we serve.

Chapter 4, the first chapter in Part II, reviews contextual elements that inhibit integrated team-based care, primarily the medical/mental health bifurcation of our healthcare education system, reimbursement strategies, and policy structures. We note how these issues play a role in health disparities. Chapter 5 focuses on healthcare organizational factors, recognizing how practice culture, resources, relationships, staff mix, and engagement in the change process affect integration efforts. The chapter offers both practice assessment and intervention strategies, recognizing that organizational change is a process that takes significant time and effort. Finally, Chapter 6 aligns with Lau and colleagues' focus on individual clinician and staff factors. Integrated care implementation requires clinical and staff behavioral change across the board. "Unsticking" established workflows and habits can be challenging. As such, we discuss specific strategies to help build competencies and shared mental models (e.g., training). We recognize that these efforts are necessary but not sufficient. Implementation processes must also address inherent individual resistance to change and utilize relationship-based and systemic strategies to enhance motivation.

Reaping the benefits of integrated care requires systems to embrace a new culture of collaboration, a mental model based in the biopsychosocial approach, and realigned resources, relationships, and staff. The system must make structural changes in the way they meet their mission. For integrated care to become normative, the very DNA of our healthcare system must move away from a bifurcated view of mental health and physical health. Integration allows clinicians, practices, and healthcare systems to walk the walk of the biopsychosocial model and collaborative, patient-centered, team-based care.

Given the complexity of the integration process, no one resource can describe every possible strategy. Integrated behavioral health implementation has been the subject of numerous books and journal articles as proponents seek to disseminate best practices. Although our review of best practices expands on these resources by taking a systemic lens to the process of integration implementation, the following resources form an important complement by focusing on additional pragmatic elements in the implementation process:

- *Behavioral Consultation and Primary Care: A Guide to Integrating Services* (2nd ed.) by P. J. Robinson and Reiter (2016). This book provides a deep dive into how clinical services, roles, responsibilities, and mindsets change and how to measure the integration progress during the implementation process. In addition to reviewing the rationale for integration, Robinson and Reiter addressed common ethical and clinical "challenging moments." The book is rich with case material and clinical tools.

- *Integrating Behavioral Health Into the Medical Home: A Rapid Implementation Guide* by Corso, Hunter, Dahl, Kallenberg, and Manson (2016) focuses on the Primary Care Behavioral Health (PCBH) model. It guides the reader through the process of developing a business plan and care for integration, hiring and training behavioral health clinicians, working through billing issues, designing documentation and workflow processes, and monitoring implementation efforts over time. The guide is pragmatic and offers numerous resources that can be used to guide integration efforts (e.g., stakeholder lists, job descriptions, financial tools).

- *Integrated Behavioral Health in Primary Care: Your Patients Are Waiting* (S. B. Gold & Green, 2018) guides physicians and other clinicians through the process of integrating behavioral health into their practice. They focus on pragmatic issues and emphasize that behavioral health integration requires a reconstruction of primary care practice and delivery. In addition to providing the rationale for integrated care, the authors outline a step-by-step approach to integration and team-based care, with applications to specific situations and populations.

- *Integrated Care: A Guide for Effective Implementation* by Raney, Lasky, and Scott (2017) focuses on the Collaborative Care Model (CoCM) of integration. The book reviews some leadership and organizational change elements, clinician roles in CoCM including the psychiatric consultant, and policy and financial considerations in implementation. It also provides rubrics for measuring the impact of implementation efforts, with a focus on two "essential questions: 'Are we doing what we said we were going to do?' And, 'Are patients benefitting from our approach to care?'" (p. 244).

- *Patient-Centered Primary Care: Getting From Good to Great* by Blount (2019b) outlines the importance of patient-centered care. The book focuses on helping practices utilize an integrated team-based care model that includes the patient and family as part of the team, seeking a true partnership with patients. We share this vision of integrated primary care, one that emphasizes the role of the patient and family.

We also encourage the reader to access resources available through the Substance Abuse and Mental Health Services Administration's Center of Excellence for Integrated Health Solutions at https://www.thenationalcouncil. org/integrated-health-coe. This website is a compendium of best practices and integration resources focused on organizational readiness, building the business case for integration and workforce development. The center offers training, technical assistance, and connection to other sites to support integration implementation.

Another excellent resource is the Advancing Integrated Mental Health Solutions (AIMS) Center affiliated with the University of Washington. Their *Collaborative Care Implementation Guide* offers step-by-step considerations for integrated care implementation and is available at https://aims.uw.edu/ collaborative-care/implementation-guide. The AIMS Center website also includes information about billing and financing for CoCM, available at https://aims.uw.edu/resources/billing-financing.

4 HEALTHCARE EDUCATION, FINANCING, AND EQUITY

In this chapter, we describe the origins of long-standing schisms between mental and physical health. This systemic dualism is rooted in early philosophical attempts to understand the essence of or hypothesized distinction between our minds and bodies and the interaction of these concepts (Rozemond, 1998). Current research acknowledges that our thoughts and emotions mediate our experience of physical symptoms (Pennebaker, 2012), soundly rejecting the idea that the mind and body are separate. In this context we embrace a whole-person approach to care (Wade & Halligan, 2017). Yet our healthcare system too often continues to operate in a problematic dualistic manner (Mehta, 2011). Moving away from reactive, disease-driven care toward more proactive, prevention-oriented care requires structural changes that prioritize health behavior and mental health. "No health without mental health" has become a rallying cry (Prince et al., 2007).

So, why are medical and mental healthcare still delivered in largely separate systems? We begin to explore this question by examining various external contextual factors that continue to support this bifurcation. We examine how our healthcare educational system's foundational structures, practices,

https://doi.org/10.1037/0000381-005
A Systemic Approach to Behavioral Healthcare Integration: Context Matters, by
N. B. Ruddy and S. H. McDaniel

and mental models inculcate future professionals to think and practice in a bifurcated way. We then review how the profit-driven U.S. healthcare system, with its reimbursement structures and chronic underfunding of primary care and behavioral health, thwarts integration efforts. Finally, we recognize how integration efforts affect and are affected by systemic structural racism within our healthcare system and the only recently broadly acknowledged impact of social determinants of health.

For each of these areas, we discuss advocacy and change strategies. To be clear, no silver bullet strategies will eradicate the underlying issues in the external contexts that form our systems. Rather, strategies that support incremental progress toward integration are critical to healthcare improvement (Christian et al., 2018; Sikka et al., 2015). Ideally, these incremental strategies motivate and empower individuals to become engaged in improvement efforts. We have a long way to go, but the relatively recent acknowledgment of the need for change reflects progress.

EXTERNAL CONTEXTUAL FACTORS THAT CHALLENGES INTEGRATED CARE

In this section, we review various challenges to integrated care that are embedded in the larger healthcare system and its contexts. These include separate educational systems for medical and behavioral health professionals, healthcare policy and reimbursement structures that impede integration efforts, and the effects of systemic biases on healthcare provision.

Challenge #1: The Healthcare Education System and Workforce Readiness

Currently, many aspects of healthcare professional training are largely siloed by discipline, most commonly during early training that focuses on development of basic professional competencies. Although some trainees do experience interprofessional training early in their education, in general, early coursework and, in some cases, clinical training occur solely within a given discipline. Siloed education has been found to inhibit the development of team-based competencies (Reuben et al., 2004).

As trainees move through the educational process, the experiential clinical training that occurs later in the trajectory is more likely to expose them to other disciplines (Chakraborti et al., 2008). During practica, internships, residency, and fellowship, learning often occurs in multidisciplinary environments. Multidisciplinary training programs initially prospered in academic health centers (Rozensky, 2012) and, more recently, occur in other settings, such as university healthcare settings (Crumb et al., 2018) and the VA (Kearney et al., 2014). However, supervisory relationships tend to be dictated by discipline. In this context, physicians largely supervise physicians, nurses supervise nurses, social workers largely supervise social workers, and so on. These patterns may limit the development of knowledge and respect for other disciplines' cultures and competencies, which is a key competency for interprofessional practice (MacDonald et al., 2010). Overlapping clinical competencies across disciplines can contribute to a lack of role clarity and sometimes competition between disciplines (Hepp et al., 2015). These issues may negatively affect integration efforts because team-based care requires shared workflows and collaborative clinician and staff behavior that are difficult to establish if there is animosity or poor role clarity (J. Hall et al., 2015).

Tension can exist between instilling team-based competencies and ensuring that trainees adopt a personal sense of accountability for patient care. A sense of individual accountability may inhibit team collaboration as trainees seek to prove themselves in the clinical environment. For example, research reveals that, traditionally, many family physicians tend to see themselves as the leader of the team. Researchers Szafran and colleagues (2018) stated: "The findings suggest that moving family physicians toward more integrative and interdependent functioning within the primary care team will require overcoming the culture of traditional professional roles, addressing facilitators and barriers, and providing training in teamwork" (p. 169).

Our education systems also struggle to balance a strong sense of discipline identity with team-based care. As academic institutions work to teach teamwork skills (Klein & Falk-Krzesinski, 2017), the disciplinary tribalism and value placed on professional identity development can act as a counterpoint (Weller et al., 2014). Professional tribal norms are codified in discipline-based accreditation standards that tend to lean into a primarily biomedical or psychosocial focus.

The biopsychosocial approach is not always realized in today's medical education, in part because acquiring a massive volume of biomedical information is sometimes prioritized over psychosocial competencies (Lane, 2014). However, some medical training programs do instill an integrated biopsychosocial approach. These institutions prioritize interprofessional teamwork as exemplified by inclusion of faculty from many disciplines and biopsychosocial content in the curriculum. Instilling team-based competencies is particularly helpful. Whereas biopsychosocial practice is possible without interprofessional collaboration, our medical system's structure and the necessary breadth of competencies make it extremely challenging without an interdisciplinary team. Bloch's "dual optic" persists (Bloch, 1988, 2002).

Similarly, most behavioral health professional training programs are one-sided in their focus on psychosocial and mental health issues. For example, although accreditation requirements for psychology doctoral programs call for biopsychosocial coursework focused on biological bases of behavior, the requirements do not specify that psychologists have coursework focused on the interplay of chronic health issues and mental health or basic health behavior interventions (American Psychological Association, 2015). Too many behavioral health training programs do not have faculty with experience in healthcare and do not prepare students to work in interprofessional medical settings (W. Ward et al., 2018). Unlike medical and nursing schools that usually have psychologists on faculty, psychology programs rarely have physicians, nurses, or other health professionals teach their students. Similar patterns can be seen in other behavioral health disciplines including social work and family therapy (Fox et al., 2012; Gehlert et al., 2010). As Hoge and colleagues (2005) stated, "Competency development in behavioral health can be described as a patchwork quilt of initiatives that have been conducted independently" (p. 595).

Healthcare professional training requires extensive experiential components, yet opportunities for shared experiential training for behavioral health and medical professionals continue to be limited (Blount & Miller, 2009; Cubic et al., 2012). Most future behavioral health clinicians are unlikely to interface with nonpsychiatrist medical colleagues during the typical educational trajectory, unless their training program has a specific focus on health such as health psychology, medical family therapy, hospital social work, psychiatric nursing, or addiction specialties.

Some psychiatrists bridge the chasm between medicine and behavioral health, particularly those who provide traditional consult–liaison services or Collaborative Care Model (CoCM) services. In general, however, psychiatrists work primarily in specialty mental healthcare. Survey data reveal that many psychiatrists do not have direct experience in primary care yet are critical of primary care clinicians' ability to provide and adhere to standards of care of mental health issues (Ng et al., 2021).

Some movement has occurred toward a more biopsychosocial approach in academic circles; research focused on the biopsychosocial model has been on the rise over the past decade (Wade & Halligan, 2017). Research faculty increasingly collaborate across disciplines, in part because grant funding has shifted to require a team-based approach. Prior to this shift, faculty were less likely to collaborate across disciplines, and research on the interplay of behavioral health/physical health was more rare outside of health psychology and psychosomatic medicine (Young et al., 2008). Interdisciplinary research supported the development of new journals that focused on a biopsychosocial approach, expanding scholarly venues (e.g., *Family, Systems, & Health, Brain and Behavior, Medical Humanities*). This evolution illustrated how changing systemic financial and publication structures can result in a more holistic, integrated approach.

Ultimately, it is most useful to develop strong interprofessional experiences early in training, during the formation of mental models of care and normative concepts. When biopsychosocial, interprofessional team-based models are normative early in training, the task of helping clinicians and researchers prioritize these values and skills in practice becomes less of a challenge in integration efforts.

Challenge #1 Mitigation Strategies: Educational Strategies and Training Environments That Support Biopsychosocial, Team-Based Integrated Care

Over the past decade, educators have started to outline and implement strategies to improve interprofessional education. In 2010, the Interprofessional Education Collaborative (IEC) convened an interdisciplinary expert panel of medical professional educators. Their report, *Core Competencies for Interprofessional Collaborative Practice* (IEC Expert Panel, 2011), highlighted the importance of recognizing and instilling team competencies, stating that interprofessional practice is "key to the safe, high quality accessible, patient-centered care desired by all" (p. i). They outlined four competency domains: values and ethics for interprofessional practice, roles and responsibilities, interprofessional communication, and teams and teamwork. The report also recommended learning activities to instill these competencies. Although behavioral health disciplines were not represented on the panel, the report still serves as a helpful blueprint for the way forward and as a catalyst for change in healthcare education. Since this report, interprofessional education, including education across the physical/behavioral health divide, has become more common (Wade & Halligan, 2017).

Educators whose training programs continue to be siloed can work toward greater integration in their own institution. The first step is to audit curricula across relevant training programs, seeking opportunities for cross-pollination and collaboration. The review may reveal existing interprofessional education activities that can be expanded to include additional programs or departments. It is also helpful to learn specifics about existing cross-training, such as whether the cross-training encompasses required or elective training experiences, the context of the training (e.g., shared coursework vs. shared experiential training), and the degree of interplay among trainees of different disciplines. Faculty can collaborate across departments to build shared trainings or offer their expertise to expand training offerings in a different department. When the educational institution does not have programs that cross the behavioral/physical health divide, educators may need to look outward into the community for potential training partners. Healthcare clinicians in the community may also serve as educational consultants, adjunct faculty, or guest lecturers to bring the relevant expertise into an educational or training program.

As noted earlier, accreditation requirements can be a barrier to cross-training and instilling interprofessional cultural competence (Pecukonis et al., 2008). It may not be possible to implement new courses with a collaborative, interprofessional focus or to add degree requirements. Rather, educators can focus on embedding integrated care concepts and skills into existing coursework (K. F. Johnson & Freeman, 2014; Rozensky et al., 2018; Serrano et al., 2018). Case examples, clinical simulations, and coursework that heighten awareness of the connection between mind and body serve to prepare future healthcare professionals to consider the "bio," "psycho," and "social" aspects of care and to begin to integrate these various perspectives (Ward-Zimmerman et al., 2021). Exhibit 4.1 highlights curricular resources that can be integrated into existing curricula to expose students to integrated care and facilitate a biopsychosocial systems approach to teaching.

Dr. Timmons, a professor in a community mental health counseling master's training program, felt strongly that her students would benefit from more training in health topics and integrated care. While reviewing alumni surveys, she noticed that many graduates of the program were now working at the nearby regional children's hospital. Furthermore, these graduates stated that, although they loved the work, they wished they had more education prior to graduation. Dr. Timmons realized that creating a separate class on health-related topics and integrated care might be challenging, especially because students had so few elective courses. So, she met with all of the adjunct faculty who taught case conferences and provided supervision. She found about a third of these adjunct faculty had ties to healthcare and were excited to share their expertise. They worked together to identify opportunities to embed health issues and clinical strategies into existing case conferences. In addition, the health-based supervisors agreed to create a continuing education series for the other supervisors, which was offered to them as part of their compensation for

EXHIBIT 4.1. Selected Integrated Primary Care Curriculum Development Resources

Source	Website
AHRQ National Integration Academy Council	https://integrationacademy.ahrq.gov/about/academy-team
Alexander Blount, EdD	https://www.integratedprimarycare.com
AIMS Center, University of Washington Medical School	http://aims.uw.edu/resources-0
APA Curriculum for an Interprofessional Seminar on Integrated Primary Care	https://www.apa.org/education-career/grad/curriculum-seminar
APA Society for Health Psychology Integrated Primary Care Psychology Curriculum	https://societyforhealthpsychology.org/training/integrated-primary-care-psychology-curriculum Also available on Collaborative Family Healthcare Association learning hub: https://integratedcarelearning.talentlms.com/catalog/info/id:360
Beachy Bauman Consulting: PCBH Corner video library	https://www.beachybauman.com/pcbhcorner
Collaborative Family Healthcare Association	https://integratedcarelearning.talentlms.com
Collaborative Family Healthcare Association Behavioral Health Consultant Skills video library	https://www.cfha.net
Centers for Medicare and Medicaid Services	https://www.resourcesforintegratedcare.com
Mountainview Consulting	https://www.mtnviewconsulting.com/primary-care-lectures
National Council Center of Excellence for Integrated Care Solutions	https://www.thenationalcouncil.org/integrated-health-coe
University of Massachusetts Medical School Center for Integrated Primary Care	https://www.umassmed.edu/cipc

AHRQ = Agency for Healthcare Research and Quality; AIMS = Advancing Integrated Mental Health Solutions; APA = American Psychological Association; PCBH = primary care behavioral health.

serving as a supervisor. Dr. Timmons also worked with the faculty who oversaw experiential placements, linking her with those alumni who worked in healthcare settings. Within 3 years, the program established six new training sites in healthcare settings.

Exposing students to role models who work in integrated healthcare settings early in training may spark trainee interest and further exploration of this pathway. Training placements in integrated care settings heighten awareness of the benefits of integrated services and the power of sharing expertise in team-based care. Ideally, training programs will hire faculty with integrated care experience to serve as role models, develop curriculum, and provide clinical supervision to facilitate integrated care competency development. Inviting a guest speaker with expertise in integrated health-care can spark interest.

Increasing capacity for experiential training in integrated practices is another opportunity to instill these competencies early in training (Cubic et al., 2012; World Health Organization, 2010). Community-based clinicians in integrated settings can reach out to local training programs in their discipline to offer experiential learning. Training programs often struggle to recruit interprofessional experiential training sites so may welcome the offer. Programs that train medical and behavioral health trainees, such as experiential placements for behavioral health clinicians in medical residency programs, are particularly effective in preparing students for future inter-professional practice (Hoover & Andazola, 2012). Depending on the discipline in question, integrated practices can host students at different levels of training. Offering clinical supervision from multiple disciplines and/or group supervision that includes multiple disciplines also strengthens interprofessional training (Martin et al., 2014). Although trainees typically work with a supervisor from their own discipline, secondary or ancillary supervision can facilitate cross-disciplinary pollination in the supervisory relationship. This interprofessional supervision helps students understand diverse perspectives based in different disciplines and may help them develop additional competencies (e.g., a psychology trainee can learn relational competencies from a family therapist supervisor). Similarly, interprofessional group supervision creates ongoing clinical dialogue. Having trainees share clinical cases and problem-solve together may help them recognize other perspectives as well as consistencies in approach across different disciplines. These experiences help trainees integrate various perspectives into their work, help them to define their own competencies, and can flatten traditional hierarchies and role-bound behaviors that can interfere with collaboration.

Substantial grant funding exists to support interprofessional, experiential training. For example, the Behavioral Health Workforce Education and Training (BHWET) and Graduate Psychology Education (GPE) programs create opportunities for behavioral health trainees to work in primary care settings. The BHWET grants emphasize integrated primary care settings, with a focus on the underserved (Kepley & Streeter, 2018). Some grants, such as GPE and BHWET, provide training stipends for students, which can help to recruit students. Numerous U.S. foundations (e.g., Hogg Foundation, Robert Wood Johnson Foundation) have identified interprofessional education and practice as grant funding targets (Massachusetts College of Pharmacy and Health Sciences, 2021). Educators who seek these grants often must work with faculty from other programs to be successful, further sponsoring interprofessional collaboration. Creating these incentives for collaboration incubates relationships between faculty in academic medicine departments and arts-and-sciences-based training programs. Silos among different parts of a higher learning institution can be overcome with effort (Dhand et al., 2016).

> Dr. Kinders, a program director of a family medicine residency, hoped to begin hosting behavioral health trainees in the residency training practice. She hoped this would help the residency program align with accreditation requirements for integrated care and behavioral health training. She approached Mr. Kahn, a medical family therapist, who served as their behavioral health faculty. Mr. Kahn welcomed the opportunity to host students but knew there wasn't a family therapy training program in the area. Dr. Kinders and Mr. Kahn obtained a list of training programs in the state that had received GPE and BHWET funding and approached the program directors at each school. Although the psychology program that had GPE funding was too far away, they found a clinical mental health counseling (CMHC) program in an adjacent town that had been struggling to find interdisciplinary placements for their students. The CMHC program accepted supervisors based on licensure in the state, rather than discipline, which enabled Mr. Kahn to serve as a supervisor. The residency hosted two students each year and over the course of the grant was able to hire three students to help expand its integrated behavioral health services in the residency practice.

Shifting toward an interprofessional focus may help academicians connect to new professional communities whose mission is to support integrated care. Interprofessional organizations such as the Collaborative Family Healthcare Association (https://www.cfha.net) and the Society of Behavioral Medicine (https://www.sbm.org) grew to fill a void for people who wanted to explore the interstitial space between medicine and behavioral health disciplines.

Kirchner and colleagues (2019) noted that some organizations highly committed to integrated primary care have homegrown training programs to address these shortcomings in the formal healthcare education system. Fortunately, a number of these organizations now offer training to outside organizations. These training opportunities are discussed in more detail when we describe strategies to help individual clinicians adapt to an integrated primary care approach in Chapter 6.

Even clinicians who are not part of a formal training program can play a role in de-siloing our educational systems. Some strategies are simple, such as attending or presenting at a professional conference different than one's own discipline, potentially educating others, and networking. Clinicians can offer to present on integrated care in healthcare professional training programs. For example, medical professionals might present to behavioral health trainees regarding successful collaboration, psychotropic medications, or the impact of chronic disease on mental health. Behavioral health professionals can educate medical trainees on communication skills, management of behavioral health issues, health behavior change, behavioral management strategies for chronic issues such as pain, or health professional wellness.

To summarize, although there has been progress in interprofessional education and training, considerable change remains necessary to achieve training that supports a truly biopsychosocial approach to healthcare. There is no quick fix. However, small shifts that provide trainees with colleagues and role models from multiple disciplines can facilitate future interprofessional team care. Furthermore, academic faculty, researchers, and non–academically focused clinicians who reach across the aisle to collaborate with or provide educational assistance to other disciplines can model interdisciplinary collaboration. These collaborations ultimately may have the additional benefit of enhancing one's scholarly and clinical work as well.

Challenge #2: Reimbursement and Policy Barriers in Our Profit-Driven, Bifurcated Healthcare System

Many foundational issues that perpetuate mind–body dualism stem from our fee-for-service (FFS), disease-focused, profit-driven healthcare system. Broad agreement exists that our current trajectory of year-over-year healthcare cost increases is not sustainable. However, it has proved challenging to adequately address the systemic complexity that underlies these problems (Lipsitz, 2012).

Current reimbursement structures do not align with the priorities and values of integrated behavioral health (B. F. Miller, Ross, et al., 2017). Integrated care focuses on prevention, improved access, chronic disease management, patient-centered goals, and clinician wellness. These priorities run counter to larger system fixation on technological and pharmaceutical fixes for treating serious illness. In addition, FFS reimbursement does not align with the integrated service model and does not reimburse clinicians for key activities such as consultation with the care team, health behavior change programs, or population health assessment (B. F. Miller, Ross, et al., 2017; Pomerantz et al., 2009). FFS incentivizes behavioral health clinicians to focus on traditional individual psychotherapy, thereby reducing their availability to other clinicians and patients. In addition, codes and procedures for behavioral and mental health differ from those for medical services, complicating billing to support financial sustainability. The mantra "no margin, no mission" reflects the reality that healthcare services that do not at least break even are vulnerable. Services that cost the practice financially are especially difficult to maintain in underfunded primary care.

Although our review of financial issues focuses on the United States, other countries face similar integrated and collaborative care financing woes. From Norway, Rugkåsa and colleagues (2020) stated: "However, the funding system in effect penalizes collaborative work. It is difficult to see how policy aiming for successful, sustainable collaboration can be achieved without governments changing funding strategies" (p. 1).

Financial constraints spur many practices to use grant funds to cover implementation costs such as early salary support for the behavioral health clinicians, electronic health record (EHR) alterations, and training. Practices increasingly recognize the need for outside consultants or practice coaches to facilitate necessary workflow changes and staff training (Dickinson, 2015). As with all grant-funded projects, practices must then contend with long-term sustainability issues or risk losing progress toward integrated services when the grant ends.

There is some good news. The Centers for Medicare and Medicaid Services (CMS), which sets policy and reimbursement structures for the United States, increasingly recognizes that our current FFS reimbursement must change. CMS approved the use of health and behavior codes that allow behavioral health clinicians to bill for encounters that focus on health behavior problems without requiring a diagnosable mental health condition (Butler et al., 2008). This expands billable encounters to include those that focus solely on chronic disease management and health behavior change (e.g., smoking cessation). However, many payers reimburse at a lower rate for health and behavior codes and may be more likely to reject these claims, which incentivizes behavioral health clinicians in FFS practices to use primarily psychotherapy codes (Duke et al., 2012). In addition, some clinicians have experienced difficulty obtaining reimbursement for these codes secondary to payer rules or requirements that are challenging to navigate.

CMS also created payment codes for activities associated with care management for patients with significant impairment and/or serious mental health diagnoses. These codes reimburse practices on a per-member per-month rate. CoCM is an example of an approach using these codes (Wolk et al., 2021). To obtain reimbursement, the practice must create a registry of these patients, track their progress, and provide, at minimum, 20 minutes per month of "care management" services. This payment structure has been criticized because practices can struggle to cover costs of program requirements necessary to obtain reimbursement and typically need a large cadre of patients enrolled in the program for it to be cost-effective (B. F. Miller, Ross, et al., 2017). In addition, smaller practices often struggle to secure necessary capital to pay for program costs that may not be budget-neutral or profitable for some time (Overbeck et al., 2016).

To add to these challenges, the U.S. reimbursement system has very strict guidelines tying reimbursement codes to specific documentation. Healthcare EHR templates are not designed for documentation of integrated care (Cifuentes et al., 2015). These issues can be mitigated when a system has the capacity to create its own behavioral health templates or pay for their practice's EHR vendor to create them (Kessler & Hitt, 2016), but these documentation concerns can be a significant barrier for systems with less capacity or support.

Reimbursement issues reflect the reality that our primary care and behavioral health systems are chronically underfunded (Goroll, 2019; Saxon et al., 2018). These resource issues are severe in services for underserved populations, despite the greater needs secondary to the impact of social determinants of health such as food deserts, systemic racism, and housing insecurity (Daniel et al., 2018). Access to specialty mental healthcare is problematic, particularly in areas where there are few clinicians (Andrilla et al., 2018). The lack of resources in both primary and specialty care reduces practice bandwidth to make necessary changes and absorb any short-term implementation costs.

On the policy side, multiple national, state, and local healthcare policy issues can complicate integration implementation (Freeman, Hudgins, & Hornberger, 2018). The specifics vary across states and localities. In many states, the government agencies that oversee mental health, substance abuse, and medical services continue to operate in silos, resulting in conflicting regulations. Common challenges include regulations regarding space, resources, professional communication, and documentation. Regulations about clinical space can be vexing, expensive, and seemingly discriminatory, such as requiring separate check-in and waiting rooms for behavioral health or that specific resources be available (e.g., running water in every room).

Challenge #2 Mitigation Strategies: Systemic Reimbursement and Policy Reform Advocacy

Individuals within large systems often feel that they cannot influence reimbursement and policy issues. But, as C. J. Peek (2019) wrote:

> Policy development is often local—where clinicians live and work. Your own work can inform policy if you think of it as having policy significance—and bring it forward. You can influence policy as a clinician who is looking forward to fewer workarounds that result from delayed policy change. (p. 177)

The same can be said about reimbursement and advocating for change with insurance companies. Here we outline some strategies individuals might use to address these challenging issues.

The first strategy for sustainability is embracing non-FFS reimbursement strategies. This approach to healthcare funding is predominant in the rest of the world, and it is critical to supporting preventive, primary care, and integrated care programs. Many healthcare practices, particularly those in primary care, embrace a future with non-FFS reimbursement. Behavioral and medical clinicians must work together to advocate for federal and local policy and reimbursement changes. Using alternative reimbursement codes, particularly programmatic codes, is imperative to ensure these codes are not terminated secondary to poor adoption. Integration proponents recommend that billing and financial offices collaborate with payers to resolve credentialing issues and denied claims and advocate for alternative payment systems (Freeman, Manson, et al., 2018). This process is easier to maintain in large healthcare systems, a fact that may underlie the relative paucity of integration in small practices (Richman et al., 2020). Each practice and community is different, so the appropriate solutions and workarounds vary. Kirchner and colleagues (2019) provided checklists and factors to consider, including the payer mix and potential alternative funding sources.

Measuring the functioning of integrated services can help to guide opportunities for improvement, perhaps moving toward establishing the value of these models beyond the income they create based on direct care services. However, this appears to be a growing edge for practices. Muse and colleagues (2022) surveyed practices with integrated behavioral health services about their evaluation of clinical, operational, and financial elements of the service. They noted that fewer than half of the practices surveyed actively measured these elements, let alone how the services impacted the practice as a whole.

Those practices who find it necessary to use grant funding as they start integration implementation must ensure that they obtain sufficient financial support to cover startup costs. Until recently, grants often offered short-term assistance, assuming the practice would achieve financial sustainability within a year or two, an outcome that often takes several years. Integrated care advocates work to educate grant organizations about the length and cost of the implementation process, emphasizing that longer-term support is more likely to result in a sustainable shift. Second-order change does not come quickly or easily. Granting organizations and those who seek grants must ensure that the seed money is sufficient to create a stable, self-sustaining program.

> Ms. Jackson served as the practice administrator for a large federally qualified health center that served a diverse, vulnerable inner-city population. The practice had previously contracted with a community mental health center to provide services, but the linkage frayed over time. She worked with her grant acquisition team to secure funding to help the practice begin an integrated behavioral health service. When writing the grant proposal, the team included a 5-year timeline toward financial sustainability. In addition to requesting financial support for initial salaries, training, and so on, they included a budget line for a billing consultant who could help them track denied claims and work with payers to ensure payment for as many direct services as possible. They designed behavioral health services to meet the needs of specific clinical populations that tended to have high healthcare costs. They tracked the impact of integrated services on chronic disease outcomes and care costs, with a focus on emergency department visits and repeat hospitalizations. Over time, they were able to show that the salaries and other costs associated with the integrated behavioral health program were minimal, compared to the cost savings the system secured by reducing these associated costs.

Healthcare and behavioral health clinicians can make significant contributions with their professional advocacy associations by lobbying for reimbursement reform at the state and federal level. To be optimally effective, professional advocacy organizations should collaborate across disciplines, rather than focusing only on payment issues for their own discipline (Freeman, Manson, et al., 2018). There is progress in this area. Interprofessional organizations such as the Primary Care Collaborative (https://www.pcpcc.org) advocate at the federal level for an interprofessional, team-based primary care model, rather than for a specific discipline.

Similarly, advocacy organizations can help to address prohibitive policy and regulatory issues. Prior to starting an integration effort, it is critical to understand issues with relevant state and local health regulations and policies (Freeman, Hudgins, & Hornberger, 2018). The regulatory issues are complex, so collaborating with the legislative arm of a professional association, an interprofessional advocacy group, or experts in healthcare law is helpful. Legal experts also can determine if perceived barriers actually are codified in the law. Because of the complexity of many regulations, even people who work within the system may believe policy myths or interpret existing policies idiosyncratically. Healthcare advocates can highlight inconsistent or contradictory rulings across or within agencies (Jacobi et al., 2016). These inconsistencies represent opportunities to clarify and drive policies that enhance comprehensive patient care.

Seeking a legislative champion for needed policy and funding changes also helps. Many legislators are interested in behavioral health, particularly access to care and impact on public safety. They may welcome guidance from clinicians and advocacy organizations on how government can address these issues. Additionally, health professionals can become involved in the electoral and political process to support candidates likely to prioritize meaningful healthcare reform.

A legislative champion can help integrated care advocates be aware of opportunities for change—the regulatory space is dynamic and ever-changing. For example, the Coronavirus Aid, Relief, and Economic Security (CARES) Act (2021) may have a significant impact on medical records. The "open notes" provision gives all patients direct access to their medical records, with only a few exceptions (Salmi et al., 2021). The intent is to improve patient engagement and to give patients information and the opportunity to correct any errors in their medical records (OpenNotes, 2021). These new regulations may motivate behavioral health and medical clinicians to prepare notes in collaboration with a patient and family or, at a minimum, with a new sensitivity for how the record may be perceived by the patient and family. The VA has piloted open-notes programs, but the impact on patient care, particularly integrated care, has yet to be studied (Blok et al., 2021).

> Dr. Zimmerman felt strongly that integrated care was the future. Although she had not been involved with her state's social work professional organization in the past, she decided to begin to attend conferences and network to share her convictions about integrated care. Within 2 years she was elected to the board of the organization and became president a few years later. As a member of the board, she was able to convince the organization to partner with the state psychology association and the state primary care association to work together to craft and support legislation and payment reform that facilitated integrated care implementation. The collaboration across discipline-based professional organizations proved

critical. Legislators recognized that no one discipline was lobbying for special treatment and were swayed by both empirical data and compelling stories about the benefits of integrated care. The primary care association had a professional lobbyist on staff, a resource neither behavioral health professional organization could afford. Dr. Zimmerman invited representatives of the psychology and primary care associations to serve on a panel for her presidential address, during which they shared their experiences and how joining forces had enabled them to achieve legislative victories that might have taken years longer, or never occurred at all, without collaboration.

Challenge #3: Systemic Bias and Healthcare

The U.S. healthcare system reflects and perpetuates the historical systemic racism that continues to permeate the United States in the early 21st century. Health disparities across different races and cultural backgrounds are well-established (Baciu et al., 2017). Historical mistreatment of racial minorities, such as in the Tuskegee studies and the origins of the HeLa cell line, underlies deep mistrust by many people in our healthcare system. Care disparities have been found throughout the healthcare system (Derose et al., 2011), including in the treatment of pain (Ly, 2019) and pediatrics (Flores & Committee on Pediatric Research, 2010). The behavioral health system has not fared better, with minoritized populations accessing services at low rates because of mistrust, cultural beliefs that often do not support seeking psychotherapy, and barriers encountered when they do seek services (Cook et al., 2017). These issues, coupled with the interplay of structural racism and poverty, severely affect the physical health and mental health of millions of Americans.

In addition, until recently most research was conducted with White male participants, rarely including women and people of color despite clear biological differences in health and disease (Schiebinger & Stefanick, 2016). The mental health fields are no stranger to sexism as well, reflected in the history of mental health research and clinical practice (Ussher, 2013). As we seek to level the healthcare playing field, we must attend to the ways racism and sexism pervade healthcare professional education, healthcare provision, and the very assumptions that underlie many epistemologies of health, mental health, and the role of women and families (Candib, 1995). As recently as 2020, the Commonwealth Fund acknowledged needed changes in healthcare education, primary care access and provision, and representation of women and people of color in healthcare leadership and policymaking

(Commonwealth Fund Task Force on Payment and Delivery System Reform, 2020). Women's health is particularly politicized, and issues in women's health likely were exacerbated by the COVID-19 pandemic in part because many women left the workforce (Lindberg et al., 2020).

The evidence is also clear that sexual and gender minorities experience bias in our healthcare system as well as health disparities (Medina-Martínez et al., 2021). Again, these issues are evidenced in the mental health system (Rees et al., 2021). Research examining individuals who are both sexual gender and racial minorities noted that bias and health disparities are particularly problematic for those with intersecting minority identities, citing "double discrimination" (Robertson et al., 2021).

Challenge #3 Mitigation Strategies: Addressing Inequities in Healthcare

No quick fixes are available for the effect of systemic racism, sexism, and other biases on healthcare, but training health professionals from diverse populations and integrating services can significantly lessen these disparities. Some healthcare and academic health systems have created programs to support a training pipeline for underrepresented minorities, recognizing that systemic barriers must be mitigated and trainees must be supported throughout the training trajectory (Wilbur et al., 2020).

Integrated services are in and of themselves a strategy to improve the system's ability to address social determinants of health, thereby improving population health for vulnerable communities (O'Loughlin et al., 2019). Placing behavioral health services in primary care may significantly improve access to care for African American and Hispanic patient populations (Flynn et al., 2020; Wielen et al., 2015). In order to potentiate these benefits, integrated care advocates can partner with community leaders and racial justice advocacy groups to ensure that patients are aware of integrated services and their advantages. In addition, these partnerships can facilitate community needs assessments to reveal and address issues that affect the health of marginalized populations. Clinicians often have established relationships with community groups, such as churches, to facilitate population health efforts, and integrated care advocates may build on these existing relationships.

The impact of integrating services on health and mental health outcomes for sexual and gender minorities has not been evaluated. However, there is emerging literature on the adaptation of lesbian, gay, bisexual, transgender, and queer (LGBTQ+) affirming care to integrated behavioral health services (Heredia et al., 2021). The healthcare community is working to improve healthcare for sexual and gender minorities via enhanced education (Sekoni et al., 2017) and development of best practice guidelines (Fredriksen-Goldsen et al., 2014). Advocates can utilize these guidelines and training elements in integrated care implementation. In addition, they can work with LGBTQ+ advocacy organizations to ensure awareness of local concerns and needs and to convey a commitment to reducing bias and stigma.

Toward these same ends, behavioral health clinicians can work with their systems' leadership to ensure that patient advocacy and advisory boards have a true voice in systems decisions that affect the community. In addition, leaders and professionals can advocate for hiring practices that ensure clinicians and staff mirror the community they serve. Finally, they can ensure that system and practice leadership are aware of culturally and linguistically appropriate services (CLAS) standards and seek to implement them and monitor their appropriate use. CLAS standards provide a road map to implement care elements that improve care for all patients, regardless of cultural background or disability. They focus on creating a healthcare environment that strives to meet community-specific needs and reduce health disparities rooted in race, class, gender, and socioeconomic status (Booth & Lazar, 2015). The U.S. Department of Health and Human Services website (https://thinkculturalhealth.hhs.gov) provides a detailed review of these guidelines.

Another strategy to improve care for marginalized populations is to ensure that primary and specialty healthcare provide appropriate trauma-informed care. Exposure to some types of trauma is significantly higher in minoritized groups, as are rates of diagnosable posttraumatic stress disorder (PTSD). Despite higher rates of PTSD, Black and Hispanic people are less likely to seek treatment (Roberts et al., 2011). Research also indicates that the experience of racism itself is a source of trauma for many African American, Latinx, and Asian people (Kirkinis et al., 2021). To provide trauma-informed care, a practice must ensure care meets the following criteria:

- illustrates trauma awareness and acknowledgment;
- emphasizes safety and trustworthiness;
- provides choice, control, and collaboration;
- focuses on strengths and skill building; and
- exhibits sensitivity to cultural, historical, and gender factors in care (Purkey et al., 2018).

As with the CLAS standards, members of the healthcare team with strong expertise in this area can ensure the practice is aware of these issues and implements training and practice standards that align with the needs of all minoritized groups and vulnerable populations.

Dr. Timmons' expertise and teaching focus in the CMHC program was trauma-informed care and culturally appropriate care. Her focus had always been on the application of these concepts to behavioral healthcare settings. However, as she collaborated with the adjunct faculty who worked in healthcare settings, she realized that her expertise could be applied there as well. She educated herself about how these issues play out in healthcare settings and developed continuing education for faculty on these topics. The adjunct professors were keen to bring these strategies back to their work settings. Dr. Timmons was invited to four community-based practices to conduct staff training. The reviews were very positive, and the chief diversity, equity, and inclusion (DEI) officer from the local health system became aware of the well-received trainings. Ultimately, Dr. Timmons worked with the DEI officer to develop and implement trainings for staff and offered consultation regarding opportunities to address shortcomings in practices throughout the health system.

SUMMARY

External contextual factors often underlie large system issues that support mind–body bifurcation and can seem immutable. Yet, the integration of behavioral health into healthcare is, in and of itself, a powerful way to create change. People who are committed to integration can band together around this shared mission. To support integrated healthcare, we must advocate for continued evolution of our healthcare education system. We must implement training opportunities for professionals to work together during their education and experiential training programs. We must address and change healthcare policies and reimbursement structures that reflect healthcare's bifurcation. We must name and work to change the systemic racism that plagues our society and its healthcare system, using integrated care as a tool to improve care for people from all cultural and socioeconomic backgrounds.

Over the past 50 years, we have made a great deal of progress via advocacy and system change in these areas. The next chapter reviews how proponents can support integrated care at the local healthcare system and practice level. Each new healthcare system and practice that integrates behavioral health is a step closer to making this model of care normative and moves us closer to a tipping point toward a more effective, integrated model of healthcare overall.

TAKEAWAY POINTS

- External contextual factors foundational to our healthcare financing and education systems complicate efforts to implement systemic integrated care models.

- Health disparities based in systemic racism and sexism, as well as bias against LGBTQ+ individuals, persist; systemic integrated care models may play a role in reducing these care and outcome inequities.

- Systemic integrated care advocacy requires a strategic approach to address challenges to implementation based in these external contextual factors.

- Though these factors may seem immutable, advocates can engage in efforts to shift our payment and education systems and to reduce healthcare disparities. Strategies include
  - communicating with billing and payer experts to seek reimbursement for systemic integrated care activities,
  - encouraging use of non-FFS reimbursement options that focus on quality,
  - tracking the impact of integrated services on the Quadruple Aim, and
  - seeking opportunities for discipline cross-pollination in clinical, educational, and research efforts.

5 ORGANIZATION AND PRACTICE LEVEL INTEGRATION

Tackling large systems' dualism between medical and behavioral healthcare can seem overwhelming. Progress in changing these contextual factors can be slow, except when there are large-scale changes in policy and/or financing of healthcare. In recognition of these realities, we take a "think globally, act locally" view on manifesting change in one's own health system or practice. In this chapter, we review barriers that occur at the practice level and strategies that can facilitate movement toward integration. Of course, the degree to which the organization as a whole is ready to change must be considered and strategies selected and adapted based on this readiness (Corso et al., 2016).

Literature from industrial and organizational (I/O) psychology provides best practices in organizational change management. I/O psychology research examines how to shift organizational structures, processes, and strategies to optimize organizational functioning using a systemic view. The field of change management recognizes that systemic homeostatic mechanisms resist change efforts. Around 1970, corporate America turned to I/O psychologists for assistance with change processes as companies worked to adapt to an

https://doi.org/10.1037/0000381-006
A Systemic Approach to Behavioral Healthcare Integration: Context Matters, by
N. B. Ruddy and S. H. McDaniel

ever-changing business climate. About 40 years later, healthcare considered these principles in seeking to improve systems of care (e.g., Parmelli et al., 2011). These practice transformation efforts parallel strategies in family therapists' work with families.

Behavioral health integration is a substantial change for a healthcare organization. This chapter provides a road map for this change, recognizing that organizational change, like individual and family change, tends to follow recognizable patterns. We review organizational factors that affect the system's ability to move toward integration as well as strategies to facilitate that change. We also describe Peek's (2008) three-world model of integrated care, which emphasizes the importance of creating alignment between the clinical, operational, and financial aspects of the care system.

CHANGE MANAGEMENT 101

Systems have powerful homeostatic mechanisms such that change is not easy to initiate, propel, or maintain (Butts & Carley, 2007). Yet adaptability is often imperative to respond to ever-changing market landscapes. Taking these principles into account, Kotter (1996) outlined eight foundational elements necessary to foment change:

- Establish a sense of urgency about the need to achieve change—people will not change if they cannot see the need to do so.

- Create a guiding coalition—assemble a group that has power, energy, and influence in the organization to lead the change.

- Develop a vision and strategy—create a vision of what the change is about and tell people why the change is needed and how it will be achieved.

- Communicate the vision for change—tell people about the why, what, and how of the changes, in every possible way and at every opportunity.

- Empower broad-based action—involve people in the change effort and get people to think about the changes and how to achieve them, rather than thinking about why they do not like the changes and how to stop them.

- Generate short-term wins—to see the changes happen and work is pivotal, recognize the work being done by people who are achieving the change.

- Consolidate gains and produce more change—create momentum for change by building on successes, invigorating people, and developing them as change agents.

- Anchor new approaches in the culture to support long-term success and institutionalize changes. Failure to do so may allow hard-won changes to slip away because people tend to revert to the old homeostasis with its comfortable habits.

These concepts have been applied in myriad settings, including healthcare (Donnelly & Kirk, 2015). These tenets for change are "baked into" the processes and strategies we present in this chapter to facilitate the adoption of integrated care. The following example illustrates how they might be applied to a change management efforts toward integration:

Dr. Fernandes is a clinical psychologist who was trained in integrated care settings throughout her graduate work, internship, and postdoctoral fellowship. She moved to a community where integrated care was not yet established. She initially joined a group private practice and emphasized her expertise in helping people manage chronic illnesses. She networked with health professionals in the community, building relationships through clinical collaboration. She eventually connected with three medical clinicians (a cardiologist, an endocrinologist, and an internal medicine nurse practitioner), all of whom expressed an interest in building integrated care relationships. The three clinicians worked for the same hospital, and one was married to the medical director at the hospital. Dr. Fernandes recognized that these individuals could serve as internal champions for integrated care and began to coach them on how to advocate for integrated services.

Dr. Fernandes asked the cardiologist who was married to the medical director to arrange a meeting with his wife. During her meeting with the medical director, she learned that the hospital was struggling with attracting and retaining physicians. She also learned that the hospital had lost significant revenue related to poor outcomes in patients with diabetes and rehospitalization for patients with congestive heart failure. The rehospitalization issue was particularly troubling to the medical director and chief financial officer because hospitals currently do not get paid for subsequent hospitalizations if the patient is readmitted less than 30 days after initial discharge.

Dr. Fernandes then helped the medical clinicians develop compelling arguments for integration based on these issues. Their message emphasized how integrating behavioral health improves clinician satisfaction and patient outcomes. They crafted a proposal focused on the administration's pain points. First, they suggested embedding care managers in the cardiology outpatient practice, advocating for implementation of the Collaborative Care Model (CoCM) for individuals with concomitant depression and congestive heart failure. They presented data on how this program could be financially sustainable based on per-member per-month fees and emphasized how avoiding even a few readmissions could save significant money. Second, they suggested that Dr. Fernandes begin to offer services at the diabetes center, with a focus on patients with poorly controlled disease. Again, they emphasized how she might help the practice improve patient outcomes. The proposal clearly defined Dr. Fernandes's role and did not link her salary to fee-for-service (FFS) reimbursement. Instead, they asked the hospital to fund the position for 2 years, during which they would track the impact of her work with a specified group of patients and Dr. Fernandes would seek grant funding. Dr. Fernandes's role also included practice transformation efforts in both practices to ensure that the CoCM and Primary Care Behavioral Health (PCBH) models were implemented to full effect.

Two years later, Dr. Fernandes was able to show that the patients with whom she worked at the diabetes center evidenced significantly improved HbA1c outcomes and were more adherent to prescribed medical regimens. A small grant from a local foundation supplemented her salary. In addition, the implementation of CoCM in the cardiology practice reduced hospital readmissions for people with congestive heart failure by 20%. The medical director noted that this outcome, alone, paid for CoCM and that the program was financially net positive for the system.

Dr. Fernandes then suggested that the system begin placing behavioral health clinicians in primary care practices, starting with the practice in which the internal medicine nurse practitioner worked. During the prior 2 years, Dr. Fernandes worked with the practice to set the stage for integration, providing education to staff and clinicians. In addition, the practice started to screen all patients with the Patient Health Questionnaire-9 (PHQ-9), raising awareness of the high percentage of patients who were struggling emotionally. Dr. Fernandes also networked with behavioral health clinicians employed by the hospital in traditional specialty mental health. She became acquainted with a social worker who previously worked in an integrated primary care practice and wanted to return to this setting. The hospital agreed to reassign the social worker to the internal medicine practice, funding her position with a mix of traditional psychotherapy and other FFS revenue from groups, such that she had 3 half-days a week for unscheduled consultation services. This social worker used her existing relationship with the specialty mental health administration to create a pathway to services for patients who needed more intensive or longer term services beyond what she could provide in primary care.

The previous example illustrates how building coalitions, addressing system pain points, and measuring the impact of innovations can create a slow wave toward integrated care. These shifts do not happen overnight and often result from a mix of relationship-building, data tracking, funding innovation, hard work, significant patience, and leadership vision.

THE ROLE OF THE LEADERSHIP TEAM IN INTEGRATION EFFORTS

Systemic second-order change—change in the very DNA of the system or practice—is necessary to initiate, propel, and (particularly) maintain substantial changes such as integrated healthcare. Success generally requires significant culture shifts, sometimes even a change in the core philosophy of the practice or health system (Corso et al., 2016; Parmelli et al., 2011). In business circles, a common refrain is that "culture eats strategy for lunch." As illustrated in the example above, strategies to create second-order change must be aligned with the specific context of an existing system (Graetz & Smith, 2010). In some cases, these shifts reflect larger system priorities, with organizational leadership leading the charge (Raney, Lasky, & Scott, 2017; P. J. Robinson & Reiter, 2016). In other cases, the move toward integration occurs more organically, with practice members themselves pursuing an integrated model to address practice issues. Implementation processes, including practice selection and leadership and practice engagement strategies, benefit from attention to the genesis of the implementation effort, and they can inform the appropriate implementation strategies and targets for these strategies.

Engaging the leadership team in implementation efforts is key, as is application of leadership best practices in the implementation effort itself. Kotter (2017) differentiated leadership as qualitatively different than management, arguing that true leaders establish and change culture. He defined leadership in the following ways:

- Leadership anticipates and responds proactively to change.

- Leadership supports a vision that aligns with the needs of stakeholders in healthcare (e.g., patients, clinicians, payers) and specifies a functional strategy to achieve that vision.

- Leadership aligns people, communicating a shared vision (as part of a shared mental model) to all. Communication is key to ensure everyone is swimming in the same direction.

- Leadership motivates people, in part by aligning the organization's vision with stakeholder values. Stakeholders help decide how the system will reach this vision. Leaders also provide clear feedback on performance and celebrate success.

As Kotter's model outlines and our story illustrates, integrated care implementation needs leadership with a clear vision they can communicate clearly to others (Lardieri et al., 2014). A clear vision enables leaders to overcome external contextual barriers such as reimbursement and policy issues with unique and innovative strategies aligned with the system's needs. Leadership can work collaboratively with staff to define and align roles, logistics, and workflows to address organizational barriers. To address professional-level barriers, leaders must understand that ongoing training is very important to maintain integrated care, along with onboarding training for new clinicians and staff. Often, leaders also need to align financial incentives to leverage improvements in quality indicators that are likely with integrated care. Leaders must help clinicians demonstrate these benefits and then communicate them throughout the system, emphasizing benefits for complex patients with multiple comorbidities, including serious mental illness (Minkoff & Parks, 2015).

As noted earlier, the role leadership plays in the process can vary depending on the genesis of the implementation effort. When individuals inside the practice are driving the effort, engaging system leadership to support integration is imperative. When system leadership drives the decision to integrate services in a more top-down manner, the implementation process must engage practice members and recognize and address resistance in a collaborative fashion.

The systemic concept of "the body follows the head" also holds true for the culture or environmental tone of the organization. A true leader exemplifies a value-based, relationship-focused style that enables shared decision making, when possible, throughout the organization. Collaborative leadership helps to create an environment that supports a collaborative stance with patients, emphasizing patient- and family-centered care and the value of service to the community as the organizational north star (Blount, 2019b; McDaniel et al., 2005). In turn, a culture that empowers clinicians and patients to cocreate care based in the patient's values can enhance patient engagement and quality of life. McColl-Kennedy and colleagues (2012) found that patients had the best outcomes in settings with a high level of team management and a culture of partnering based on collaboration, interprofessional learning, and connection between staff, clinicians, and patients. These patients evidenced improved quality of life, satisfaction with care, and enhanced behavioral intention for positive health behaviors (Sweeney et al., 2015).

To successfully achieve these changes, leaders—as the executive subsystem—work to create the necessary administrative structure and motivation to engender systemic change (Rawson & Moretz, 2016; Whitebird et al., 2014). deGruy and Khatri (2019) emphasized that achieving "complex adaptive leadership" requires leaders to take on the role of disruptor. Furthermore, they argued that practice-level data, the "measurement of internal state" (p. 107), is crucial in identifying change targets and measuring the impact of change efforts. In our example, Dr. Fernandes's leadership used subtle disruption techniques that aligned with the values of the system. She initially focused on building relationships with medical clinicians, establishing the value of her expertise and involvement in care via clinical collaboration. She listened to system leaders and illustrated her understanding of their worries by designing interventions that addressed key concerns, with attention to the financial bottom line. She customized her approach to each practice, based on her understanding of the different needs of the cardiology, endocrinology, and primary care settings. She leveraged her relationships with internal champions by offering consultation services. She tracked data to show the impact of organizational integration efforts, attending to clinical outcomes, clinician and patient satisfaction, and financial consequences. Her strategies often presented integrated services as a potential solution to vexing problems and addressed potential barriers via relationship development, training, and other means of disrupting the status quo.

Some organizations are more able and likely to embrace change than others. In "Changing the Way Organizations Change: A Revolution of Common Sense," Dannemiller and Jacobs (1992) outlined a simple but compelling formula for the likelihood of change. They noted that change typically occurs only when there is

- sufficient dissatisfaction with the current state;
- a clear, desired change end state; and
- a set of clear, actionable "next steps" to begin the change process.

Based on Beckard's (1975) principles of organizational change, the following points outline key strategies that can be used to implement behavioral health in healthcare settings. Again, we use Dr. Fernandes's successful integration efforts to illustrate each point.

- Find the pain points (dissatisfaction with status quo) in these settings related to mental health and health behaviors.
  - Dr. Fernandes helped medical clinicians with challenging patients. She also addressed the administrator's difficulties with unpaid hospital readmissions and poor outcomes for patients with diabetes.

- Create a clear vision of the desired state by conveying how systemic bio-psychosocial, team-based care addresses these issues. Define integrated care and illustrate the link between integration and the desired state.

  - Dr. Fernandes advocated for different implementation solutions that directly addressed differential practice needs. She ensured that her role was not dependent on clinical income, which freed her up to engage in practice transformation efforts rather than direct clinical service.

- Provide a roadmap that leads to integration, with a specific focus on early steps, and set clear expectations regarding both the benefits and the complexity of the integrated care implementation process.

  - Dr. Fernandes implemented screening in the primary care practice to heighten awareness of unmet patient needs. She obtained seed money for the first 2 years of work, then obtained additional grant funding to continue practice transformation work, which highlights that these changes do not occur overnight.

- Recognize the inevitable reluctance because of competing agendas. Some resistance is positive in that it helps propel change by creating a counterpoint. However, overwhelming resistance or too much reluctance from powerful individuals or aspects of the system can derail practice transformation/implementation efforts.

  - Dr. Fernandes established relationships with hospital leadership, early innovators in different practices, and eventually with staff and other clinicians in those practices by using her expertise to make their lives and those of their patients easier.

CHANGE MANAGEMENT AND IMPLEMENTATION SCIENCE IN HEALTHCARE

In healthcare, clinical and system design is best rooted in any available evidence-based treatments (EBTs). Implementation and dissemination research has identified nine key elements to ensure that healthcare processes are rooted, as much as possible, in evidence:

- select the appropriate implementation team;
- identify an appropriate EBT;
- recruit staff to be trained in the EBT;
- conduct preservice training on the specific EBTs;

- bring in expert consultation and coaching to perform the new skill;
- evaluate staff to assess the level of new skill use;
- evaluate the organization's performance of the new skill via program evaluation;
- use the program evaluation to give administrators feedback to inform decision making; and
- identify systemic financial, organizational, and staffing resources needed to support new skills and practice patterns (Fixsen et al., 2005).

As noted earlier in Chapter 3, the complexity of primary care clinical work in particular can muddle the link between EBT and real-world implementation of integrated care (Sederer, 2009). As A. Miles (2015) noted about evidence-based medicine (EBM):

> EBM has never quite fully understood that people who have become ill present not as a collection of organ systems, one or more of which may be dysfunctional requiring scientifically indicated technical and pharmacological interventions, but rather as integral human beings with narratives, values, preferences, psychology and emotionality, cultural situation, spiritual and existential concerns, possible difficulties with sexual, relational, social and work functioning, possible alcohol and substance abuses and addictions, worries, anxieties, fears, hopes and ambitions, personal life goals and aspirations—and much more. Scientific medicine can, by its nature, address only a fraction of such concerns, illustrating the limits of science in medicine, limits which directly and unequivocally preclude the very notion of a science-*based* clinical practice. It was for this reason that in 1995, *The Lancet* called loudly for EBM to be put "in its place," so that the "E" of EBM might inform complex clinical decision making and not dictate to it. (p. 985)

In short, science that informs system change, clinical system redesign, and implementation can guide our work. However, one must always consider the applicability of the evidence to a given situation. Is this the best practice for this presentation, for this person, at this time, in this context? For example, Dr. Fernandes knew that decades of research had established links between heart attack, congestive heart failure, and depression (Barefoot & Schroll, 1996; Liblik et al., 2021). She also knew that patients with concomitant depression and cardiac disease have significantly worse clinical outcomes, including higher rates of hospitalization (Sundquist et al., 2005), poor quality of life in both patients and family members (Mårtensson et al., 2003), and increased mortality and morbidity (Celano & Huffman, 2011). She used this evidence to develop the care model implementation plan and to compel leadership to support the new care model.

Science can inform implementation and practice, but it does not create a set, clear path. Uncertainty is ubiquitous in healthcare, particularly in primary care. This uncertainty is a practice and clinical pain point that can be mitigated to some degree by interprofessional team practices. For example, the COVID pandemic generated massive uncertainty, and clinicians noted this lack of clinical clarity as a specific stressor (Larry A. Green Center, 2021). "Long haul COVID" is a perfect example of the types of clinical uncertainties and complexities that healthcare clinicians face every day, highlighting the need for an interprofessional team (Pavli et al., 2021). Yet science does point the way. To reduce uncertainty, health system and practice change agents can use local data, generated by a repeated measurement of a target indicator, to determine if the intervention is having the intended effects. Dr. Fernandes tracked data to show that her efforts were improving care. Data collection facilitates change by removing (or at least reducing) the clouds of uncertainty and ensures that necessary adjustments are made throughout the practice transformation and implementation process.

CHANGE MANAGEMENT IN THE "THREE WORLDS" OF HEALTHCARE DELIVERY

Illustrating that context matters, C. J. Peek (2008) described three separate worlds within healthcare delivery systems that must be coordinated for successful change management: clinical, operational, and financial. The clinical world focuses on the type of care needed and how to improve the quality of care. The operational world focuses on processes such as workflow, staffing, and space usage, aspects of the work that ensure that healthcare is well-executed. The financial world focuses on the value of care delivered and the literal bottom line.[1]

It is easy to imagine how these worlds can collide. Clinicians want to focus on the best clinical outcomes and may feel burdened by the financially focused administrators who are simply trying to keep the doors open. Operationally focused administrators may be stymied when clinicians balk at changing practice patterns to become more efficient. Financially focused administrators may be frustrated when an operational person focuses on staffing while billing problems negatively affect the bottom line. In other words, each group has its own priorities, all of which are crucial to the

---

[1]Peek (2008) also highlighted a "hidden" fourth world in his model, noting that our healthcare education system plays an important role (see Chapter 3).

success of the healthcare system and practice such that failure in one area will cause failure in all three. Seeking a balance among competing demands helps the system deliver on its mission. Poor clinical functioning will result in poor care, poor financial functioning will result in closing the practice, and poor operational functioning will result in poor service, inefficiency, and waste (Peek, 2008).

> Dr. Fernandes initially attended to clinical concerns by collaborating with the health system's medical clinicians, developing relationships that eventually served to get her foot in the door of the organization's leadership. She addressed operational issues with her subsequent work, establishing new care models and crafting a leadership role to oversee integrated care implementation. She attended to financial consider-ations by focusing on populations that cost the organization money and offering a care model that has the potential to directly address the source of financial losses (hospital readmissions for depressed patients with cardiac disease). Dr. Fernandes ensured that her data tracking established the impact of organizational change on these worlds, rec-ognizing the importance of evidence-based practice and practice-based evidence.

Integration efforts ideally begin with a practice needs assessment that determines the system's facilitators and barriers in the financial, operational, and clinical realms. Representatives of each perspective should be involved in planning and identification of metrics to evaluate the implementation process. This representation of all areas ensures that issues are identified early and gives the implementation team an opportunity to highlight how integration benefits align with priorities, helping to engage key leaders who are pivotal to success (B. F. Miller et al., 2009).

The remainder of this chapter is organized around Peek's (2008) three-world model. We discuss common operational, financial, and clinical facilita-tors and barriers to behavioral health integration and mitigation strategies for each barrier. Implementation efforts must consider how these worlds intersect at both the larger healthcare system and the individual practice levels. Prac-tices within the same healthcare system may face very different challenges to implementation, depending on practice culture, population served, available workforce, payer mix, and other factors (Chapman et al., 2020).

> Dr. Fernandes's story didn't end with the initial implementation efforts described above. In the following sections, we jump forward in time to 5 years later. Dr. Fernandes is now the chief integration officer for the healthcare system. The hospital where she started her work was

acquired by a larger hospital chain that is now seeking ways to adopt integrated models in both primary care and outpatient specialty care practices. Impressed with Dr. Fernandes's inroads, the larger organization hired her as part of the leadership team and gave her a budget to increase integrated care. Dr. Fernandes worked with the system's grants team to expand this budget and set about developing a system-wide integration implementation strategy.

Operational Systems Barriers and Facilitators for Change

Many aspects of daily practice functioning must be adapted for successful integration. Here we review key elements of these shifts, including strategies that support success. We discuss processes to assist with

- site selection,
- adaptive reserve and bandwidth for change,
- physical space,
- documentation,
- workflow,
- team huddles,
- scheduling, and
- marketing integrated care to patients.

Site Selection

For each state, locale, health system, and individual practice, it is vital to understand and address issues related to site licensing and service accreditation. The organization's classification or type (e.g., ambulatory care center vs. Federally Qualified Health Center) has implications for the services offered and payment structures available. Federally Qualified Health Centers have a complex reimbursement structure different than that of an ambulatory practice associated with a hospital system or a private practice setting (Kautz et al., 2008). Currently, these payment structures are evolving; they are sometimes value-based but often fee-for-service (FFS). Local, regional, and state regulations must be considered as well (Freeman, Hudgins, & Hornberger, 2018). To integrate behavioral health into primary or specialty care, the site may need to obtain a different type of licensure, particularly if they plan to seek reimbursement from a public payer such as the Centers for Medicare and Medicaid Services (Corso et al., 2016).

Site selection should depend on organizational characteristics that can facilitate or complicate successful implementation. Each clinical system is a microcosm, with different values, priorities, and cultures. As we discussed earlier, it is not unusual for the push toward integration to come from within the practice. Practice members may have experience with integrated care previously or become aware of integration efforts in other practices. In these cases of practice self-selection, the readiness assessment focus can be on leadership engagement and increasing the engagement and motivation across various clinicians and staff within the practice. In contrast, sometimes integration efforts are more top-down, with leadership driving the change. When organizational leadership seeks practices to serve as early adopters of integration, they must attend to practice culture and readiness to change. Practice measures that assess practice readiness and enhance the likelihood of success are listed in Exhibit 5.1.

Prioritizing sites that are certified Patient Centered Medical Homes (PCMHs) may enhance success. By definition, these practices have an existing information and communication infrastructure. Many PCMH practices have established mental health screening, patient registries, and case management capabilities for chronic diseases. Patient registries and case management programs help identify patients in need of chronic disease management assistance. Existing screening protocols identify patients struggling with mental health issues, including those who might otherwise avoid detection. These existing processes

EXHIBIT 5.1. Measures of Practice Readiness for Integrated Care

Source	Measure	Website
AIMS Center, University of Washington	Integration Readiness Checklist	https://aims.uw.edu/sites/default/files/Integration%20Readiness%20Checklist_120419.pdf
Agency for Healthcare Research and Quality	Atlas of Integrated Behavioral Health Care Quality Measures	https://integrationacademy.ahrq.gov/products/lexicon
Integrated Care Leadership Program, Center of Excellence for Integrated Care	Readiness for Integrated Care Questionnaire (Scott et al., 2017)	https://psycnet.apa.org/doiLanding?doi=10.1037%2Fort0000270
Resources for Integrated Care (CMS and IHI)	Behavioral Health Integration Capacity Assessment Tool	https://www.resourcesforintegratedcare.com/tool/bhica
University of Massachusetts Medical School	Practice Integration Profile	https://www.practiceintegrationprofile.com

AIMS = Advancing Integrated Mental Health Solutions; CMS = Centers for Medicare and Medicaid Services; IHI = Institute for Healthcare Improvement.

can facilitate case-finding for the behavioral health clinician and reflect a proactive care culture already attuned to prevention and early intervention, clinical workflow, team-based care, and chronic disease management (Corso et al., 2016).

Practices that have achieved a level of PCMH certification also may have an established team-based model of care. PCMH practices are more likely to employ other clinicians in addition to physicians such as nurse practitioners, nutritionists, and behavioral health clinicians (Hing et al., 2017).

PCMH practices also are less likely to have high levels of clinician burn out than are non-PCMH practices (K. M. Nelson et al., 2014). This is especially important to implementation efforts because clinician burnout and the adaptive reserve available in a practice are negatively correlated. High levels of burnout may undermine change efforts (Goldberg et al., 2021). In the context of the COVID-19 pandemic, levels of healthcare professional burnout skyrocketed (Larry A. Green Center, 2021; Restauri & Sheridan, 2020). Behavioral health professionals played key roles in developing and implementing policies and programs to prevent and manage burnout in support of their colleagues during this difficult time, reflecting another benefit of interprofessional integrated care (Karekla et al., 2021; Tosone, 2020).

Change fatigue and limited adaptive reserve are endemic in healthcare (Nutting et al., 2010). Some practices with COVID burnout welcome the help that comes with behavioral health integration; others may need to stabilize the financial health of their clinic before enlarging their team.

Integrated services are more likely to thrive in practices with a general culture of whole-person, biopsychosocial care. A systemic biopsychosocial, team-based care approach reflects a "shared mental model" of care (McDaniel et al., 2005; Raney, Lasky, & Scott, 2017) that is critical to the success of implementation efforts. Ideally, medical clinicians view psychosocial issues as foundational to good healthcare. They also view behavioral health clinicians as colleagues with expertise that helps them and their patients. Behavioral health clinicians in these practices need to be mindful of the impact of social stressors and trauma on the health and mental health of both patients and other health professionals.

Biopsychosocially oriented clinicians and staff are more likely to welcome and champion integration efforts. Strong champion administrators, clinicians, and support staff can promote the integrated model and manage internal resistance or pushback within their own peer group. Often champions share stories of successful patient care that include collaboration with the behavioral health clinicians. These stories help motivate less enthusiastic practice members to consider team-based care and collaboration (Corso et al., 2016).

Practice selection, then, involves considering the system's needs and its bandwidth for change. If practice members feel overwhelmed by current expectations and workload, they may struggle to muster the energy and effort that adaptation and change require, even if they agree with the plan. When the majority feel they are unable to do one more thing, any change initiative is going to meet resistance (W. L. Miller et al., 2010).

Addressing Adaptive Reserve Issues

Jaén and colleagues (2010) described a variety of methods to address adaptive reserve and change bandwidth issues by using qualitative and quantitative measures to monitor progress from baseline throughout implementation. They used quantitative chart reviews to track care outcome and patient experience indicators. They used qualitative measures to elicit implementation issues and practice members' experiences of the implementation effort. Their research was part of a highly resourced national demonstration project that likely outstrips the evaluation capabilities of a typical practice. However, practices can select and track specific measures of interest and ensure that practice members have an opportunity to share their experiences to inform ongoing implementation processes.

Adaptive reserve issues also can be addressed by engaging in successive approximation of integrated services. Some integration efforts start with a colocated model that funds a mix of brief psychotherapy and behavioral health consultation primarily through FFS. In these practices, grant funding can be useful for clinician training and practice consultant fees. Demonstrating the value of integrated services can whet the appetite of those in the practice to increase a range of behavioral health interventions, including those that are not billable.

Many systems that seek to implement a fully integrated model need initial grant funding (Hornberger & Freeman, 2015), and outside consultation (Bareil et al., 2015; Roderick et al., 2017; Siantz et al., 2021) is often necessary. However, the practice's history with grant funding must be considered. Some organizations have "grant fatigue." In other words, jaded practice members have seen many grant-funded projects come and go. They may automatically assume that the program will last only as long as the grant money does and resist making significant, second-order change. A transparent sustainability plan and emphasis on how behavioral health integration can help long-standing problems may motivate people to see the effort that practice transformation entails as worthwhile.

Addressing Space Issues That Impact Operations and Workflow

Ideally, the spatial layout of the practice stations the behavioral health clinician in the clinical space. Truly integrated services are difficult to establish when the behavioral health clinicians work in another wing or floor of the building. In the busy world of healthcare, a behavioral health clinician who is not visible and easily accessed is "out of sight and out of mind." Anything less than working shoulder to shoulder with the rest of the healthcare team may sideline psychosocial issues. In addition, embedding the behavioral health clinician in the medical workspace reduces the patient's sense of stigma in seeking services and ensures that the behavioral health clinician is readily accessible for warm handoffs, joint appointments, and crisis management (Corso et al., 2016; Crowley & Kirschner, 2015). Grant funding or practice investment may be needed to support adaptations to physical practice space that align with integrated services (Gunn et al., 2015).

Addressing Documentation Issues to Facilitate Communication

Some electronic health record (EHR) systems are designed solely for medical care and lack necessary templates and other resources for behavioral health clinicians. Unless the health system utilizes an EHR that has mental health documentation easily adapted for integrated care, funding also may be needed to develop appropriate documentation processes for integrated care (Cifuentes et al., 2015; Dickinson, 2015). In addition, as with other health professionals, behavioral health clinicians need training in appropriate use of EHRs and documentation adapted for integrated care.

> Dr. Fernandes realized she couldn't possibly integrate services at every outpatient site. She worked with system leadership to identify practices with the right combination of clinician interest, patient population need, change bandwidth, and strong leadership to stack the deck in favor of success. Administrators from their suggested list completed practice-readiness measures that further clarified which practices were most likely to succeed. Interestingly, word about Dr. Fernandes's work got around such that primary care practices started to compete for her attention to win the opportunity to develop integrated behavioral health services.
>
> Each year, Dr. Fernandes chose four new practices with whom she would collaborate to begin the integration program. She was clear that she could not manage more new practices in the context of her ongoing work to maintain integration efforts at more established

practices. She learned the importance of maintenance the hard way, when integration established at a few sites fell apart after personnel changes.

In each new site, she identified administrative and clinical champions and helped them identify specific patient needs that aligned with available grants. Each grant proposal centered on integrated care implementation, often to address a specific issue of concern to that population. One primary care practice served a rural population devastated by the opiate epidemic so they sought funding to integrate medication-assisted therapy and wraparound substance use disorder services. A pulmonary outpatient treatment center obtained funding to support embedding a family therapist in the pulmonary rehabilitation service to engage families in care, address social determinants of health, and address health behavior issues such as smoking cessation. In addition, Dr. Fernandes advocated with system leadership for additional financial and operational support to help these practices achieve financially sustained integrated services before the grant expired. As she worked with administration to develop an organizational infrastructure, it became clear that each practice needed "boots on the ground" assistance. So, each practice had an integrated care coordinator who had some administrative time allotted to carry out the integrated care development process within each practice. These individuals were charged with developing a customized integrated plan adapted to the specific culture and baseline clinical processes at each practice.

In existing sites, Dr. Fernandes worked closely with behavioral health clinicians to monitor their stress levels and provide support. She created a career path for behavioral health clinicians such that those with interest could begin to supervise other behavioral health clinicians with less training and experience and be promoted and compensated for these activities. Dr. Fernandes also tracked behavioral health clinician activities to ensure fidelity to their integration model and counseled clinicians who preferred more traditional approaches to return to specialty behavioral healthcare. She also closely monitored reimbursement, ensuring that the coding and billing expert continued to track claims to ensure that payer shifts did not threaten the financial sustainability of the integrated services. Finally, Dr. Fernandes made sure that all new medical clinicians and practice administrators understood integrated care and their role in helping it thrive in their practice.

Shifting Clinical Workflows to Align With Team-Based Integrated Care

As the review of various implementation models in Chapter 1 illustrated, practices with more integrated services function differently than do those with colocated or separate behavioral health services. Adjusting how patients "flow" through the practice affects the success of implementation efforts. There is no one "right" workflow, but a recent study of successful integration efforts (M. M. Davis et al., 2019) found four essential elements:

- Identify patients who would benefit from integrated care. This process is accomplished via screening, chart review, case management, and staff and clinician flagging of the patient during a team huddle.

- Provide close to real-time engagement with these patients and transition them to the integrated care team. Real-time services help patients in their moment of need, rather than at a later date based on a traditionally scheduled clinician's availability.

- Provide integrated care treatment. Integrated care treatment is delivered in a qualitatively different way than in specialty mental health to align with the pace of the healthcare setting's workflow.

- Monitor immediate treatment outcomes and adjust treatment when needed. Measurement-based care processes track patient progress over time to ensure patients receive care that "moves the needle." Measurement also determines when services are no longer needed, freeing up the behavioral health clinician to be available for other patients in greater need.

Workflows and staffing plans determine the who, what, when, and where of integrated practice (M. M. Davis et al., 2015). These plans need to be communicated overtly, coupled with accountability for clinicians and staff. Ultimately, the goal is to ensure that every patient who enters the practice needing behavioral health intervention gets assistance in real time or, at a minimum, leaves with a clear, time-sensitive follow-up plan. Real-time care is one of the major differentiators of integration and likely drives many of its benefits.

Implementing Consistent Team Huddles

Team huddles prior to clinical sessions and debriefs after sessions support integrated care and provide continuous quality improvement (Shaw et al., 2012). During the initial huddle in a primary care setting, the team may select the lead team member for each patient based on relevant expertise and relationship with the patient (Fiscella & McDaniel, 2018). This leader then facilitates the team's planning about the patient and family. Postsession huddles review what went well and any challenges that occurred in that day's clinical session. They also can serve to assign responsibility for follow-up and discuss any challenging encounters and care issues.

Regular huddles have been associated with improved teamwork and more supportive practice climate (H. P. Rodriguez et al., 2015), particularly postsession huddles that debrief care (Tannenbaum & Cerasoli, 2013). Although this type of brief planning may seem intuitive, it can be difficult to establish as part of the daily routine because immediate clinical tasks can take priority in the workflow over planning that may be more useful in the long term. The use of technology, such as handheld mobile devices, allows for staff and clinicians to take a simple survey about the day at the various times that their days end, providing the benefits of debriefing (Fiscella & McDaniel, 2018). Debriefs are more common in specialty care, such as the intensive care unit and operating rooms, where clinicians and staff may have workflows and work schedules that build in time for reflection at the end of a procedure, an operation, or a session—again focusing on what went well and what improvements they would like to make next time. Planning and debriefing huddles facilitate more effective and efficient practice and can ensure team-based care planning customized to each patient's needs.

Fine-Tuning Scheduling Processes
Appointment scheduling is another seemingly simple practice characteristic that is, in reality, quite complex and important to integration efforts. Across healthcare, tension exists between sufficient patient volume that provides adequate financing and access to the population served with sufficient time with each patient and family. Similar tension occurs between offering appointments quickly and maintaining continuity for patients with a given clinician. Continuity supports chronic disease management (Cabana & Jee, 2004) and relationship-based care (Blount, 2019b; McDaniel et al., 2005). Team-based care, in turn, facilitates relationship-based care in that continuity occurs with the team of clinicians, rather than with just one clinician.

> Dr. Fernandes targeted the primary care network to instill integrated care workflows. She convinced the administration to pay for mandatory training for all practice administrators that educated them on the value of integrated care, along with specific strategies they might implement such as behavioral health screening. Training helped

motivate the administrators to support implementing universal mental health screening, with clear workflows and roles for positive-screen follow-up in real time.

Dr. Fernandes was surprised how difficult it was to establish huddles. First, clinicians failed to attend, and many of them who did devolved into a recitation of the names of patients coming in and what medical equipment should be in each room. To support huddles, the health-care system agreed to adjust all primary care clinicians' schedules so they and their staff could have 20 minutes prior to each patient care session (i.e., at the beginning of a morning or an afternoon) to engage in a care team huddle. The system paid for refreshments to be served at some huddles, creating a variable reinforcement schedule to maintain attendance. Where needed, clinicians who rarely came to huddles were reminded of their responsibility to attend. Key huddle members were trained to moderate huddles to ensure they focused on identifying patients who struggled emotionally or with chronic disease management, crafting a shared plan for each patient. Each practice administrator tracked how often these huddles revealed a patient who would benefit from behavioral health intervention in real time. Tracking this practice metric helped convince administration to hire multiple behavioral health clinicians to address these otherwise unmet needs.

Schedules for behavioral health encounters must be adapted, particularly if the practice previously offered colocated services that aligned with specialty mental health models. Specifically, the length of patient encounters with a behavioral health clinician also must be adapted for integrated care (Reiter et al., 2018). In general, integrated behavioral health encounters are shorter than those in specialty mental health settings. The goal is to give the patient and family the time they need (typically anywhere from 5 to 45 minutes) but be as brief as possible to provide access and meet the behavior health needs of the population served by the practice. Some systems seek a middle ground by scheduling one or two behavioral health patients an hour for brief (20-minute or so) encounters. This leaves time for other consultations, follow-up documentation, and other patient-related issues during the rest of the hour. Other systems with multiple behavioral health clinicians ensure at least one clinician is always available in real time for arising needs and consultations. Practices must find a balance between scheduled appointments and unscheduled time to be available for real-time services. Even during scheduled appointments, interruptions are normative to ensure real-time availability. Follow-up may be with the medical clinician or both the behavioral and medical clinicians, depending on the problem.

Ensuring Patients Are Aware of and Understand Integrated Services
Some practices actively market integrated care services to patients and families. For example, they may include information about the embedded services in materials distributed when patients enroll in the practice. With an eye to health literacy (Willis & O'Donohue, 2018), the description can help patients understand how the services are different than specialty mental health and how the behavioral health clinician can be of assistance to any patient. The behavioral health clinician is profiled in the same manner as medical clinicians, including training, special competencies or interests, and availability. Similar information can be included in practice newsletters, electronic portals, and informational materials in the waiting and exam rooms. The presence of integrated behavioral health services helps to market the broader practice, highlighting the benefits for patients and communicating the practice's commitment to whole-person, family-oriented care.

Dr. Fernandes worked with the organization's marketing director, Mr. Brown, to find synergies between the integration work and community marketing outreach as well as marketing integrated care to established patients. Mr. Brown reported that their market research revealed community members who sought help with unmet behavioral health needs, having been frustrated with access to the behavioral health services at a competing health system. Mr. Brown also spearheaded a marketing campaign that emphasized the role of relationships in care, vying to position their healthcare system as the counterpoint to a highly regarded but very technically focused health center about an hour's drive away.

Mr. Brown helped Dr. Fernandes create integrated care marketing tools for existing patients that emphasized the benefits of integrated care and explained how patients could access services. These tools were embedded in patient communications, including links on the patient portal, articles in the patient-focused newsletter, and flyers and posters throughout practices that had behavioral health consultants. In addition, Mr. Brown helped Dr. Fernandes create integrated care marketing materials for staff and clinicians. He even convinced the administration to hold an integrated care engagement contest with a pizza party prize to incentivize staff and clinicians to identify patients for the behavioral health clinicians and to engage in follow-up consultation.

Financial Systems Barriers and Facilitators to Change

The change management literature is clear that, for change to occur, the desired state must create relief from identified operational and clinical pain points and not create strong resistance (Dannemiller & Jacobs, 1992). In our profit-driven healthcare system, most change efforts begin (and some end) with a financial cost–benefit analysis. Establishing the financial support for integration is a key step to avoid resistance from administration. Here we review the following strategies:

• track all impacts of integrated care models on the bottom line;
• set clear, realistic financial benchmarks that evolve over time;
• seek value-based contracts; and
• track behavioral healthcare claim payment and denials.

Ideally, the business improvement plan for integrated care considers the financial impact of these services on patient care outcomes and clinician stress and turnover (B. F. Miller et al., 2013). Integrated services generally improve the quality of care and are perceived positively by medical clinicians (Torrence et al., 2014), variables that are extremely important to practices with value-based or cost-sharing contracts. These contracts are becoming increasingly common, as reimbursement systems are slowly shifting away from FFS payment (McConnell, 2019). One key measure can be the percentage of patients who are referred to integrated services, which can highlight prior unmet needs. Tracking follow-through with in-house behavioral healthcare can show how these services improve access to care. Pomerantz and colleagues (2008) found that integrating behavioral health services in primary care sharply reduced the no-show rate for behavioral health referrals. Vogel and colleagues (2012) noted the same impact, with referral no-show rates falling from 28% to 10% when the practice moved from colocated to integrated services, increasing access by offering services the same day.

In an FFS environment, abject profitability of services matters. Financial benchmarks should be set with realistic but slowly increasing revenue expectations over time, toward at least eventual budget neutrality (Corso et al., 2016). Primary care practices, especially, rarely have deep pockets to fund services that are not budget neutral, no matter how much they value the services. Sometimes specialty practices can afford to cover the delta between reimbursement and cost of services. Often behavioral health clinicians need to be both creative and flexible to meet population health needs and budgetary goals, working closely with the financial administrators to track progress.

Kolko and colleagues (2019) conducted a survey of primary care clinicians in which reimbursement for integrated services was ranked the number one barrier to integration. As noted earlier, successful billing and coding strategies vary across markets, so it can be helpful to consult a billing and coding expert in integrated services (ideally one with an established relationship with payers). A consultant can work closely with payers to break the code of what services that payer will and will not reimburse and how to complete billing forms (e.g., which Current Procedural Terminology® [CPT] and location codes to use, if any billing modifiers are required on the claim).

Kathol and colleagues (2014) emphasized the importance of seeking value-based payment, as opposed to FFS, to ensure sustainability of integrated behavioral health. They noted seven components of value-based contracts necessary for financial sustainability:

- a shared payment pool for behavioral health and medical benefits;
- targeted clinical interventions and programs for complex patients;
- proactive, embedded on-site behavioral teams;
- use of stepped-care models in recognition of patient behavioral health needs beyond the scope of primary-care-based services;
- measurement-based outcomes;
- EBTs for behavioral health interventions; and
- care management for most complex patients.

They argued that these elements both align with patient care best practices and facilitate financial sustainability.

Tracking claims and seeking explanation for denied claims also help develop maximally successful billing and coding processes that align with payer expectations (Freeman, Manson, et al., 2018). This process may also inform treatment modality choices, such as whether group interventions or care management services are preferentially reimbursed and can help cover costs. Clearly the effort to submit claims in the necessary format for reimbursement takes time and effort, especially in the beginning of implementation. Therefore, prioritizing this process is important for achieving financial sustainability.

Dr. Fernandes had an existing relationship with the Chief Financial Officer, Ms. Knowles, who was promoted into the systemwide role after her hospital was acquired. Ms. Knowles respected Dr. Fernandes and valued how she had been able to implement integrated services in generally budget-neutral ways. She also believed that integrated care was a better service delivery model that ultimately saved the system money. Ms. Knowles created a new role and hired a billing and coding expert to focus specifically on chasing reimbursement for integrated care services. She also sought to strike deals with various payers that would support integrated care, negotiating higher rates for behavioral health services that were delivered in the primary care setting. In addition, Ms. Knowles and Dr. Fernandes consistently educated other administrators about the importance of value-based payments to the ultimate financial health of the institution. They argued that the system would benefit from being an early adopter of these payment schemes because they could adapt care to patient needs (reducing costs) and begin to evaluate which types of value-based payment contracts were financially beneficial and which were not.

Clinical Systems Barriers and Facilitators of Change

Shifting to integrated care models requires many changes to clinical mindsets as well as to assessment and intervention strategies. We review the actual clinical changes clinicians must make in the next chapter. Here we review the following shifts in the practice's clinical approach:

- population health focus,
- stepped-care protocols and processes, and
- alternative service delivery processes.

Shifting to a Population Health Focus

Integrated behavioral health services focus on meeting the mental and behavioral health needs of a population—either all the patients of a health system or focusing on those in a particular practice. This shift in focus can be challenging for traditionally trained behavioral health clinicians who may be accustomed to focusing only on those patients who actively seek behavioral health services and identify their presenting concern as emotional or relational.

Building a clinical practice to meet the needs of a population begins with a needs assessment in the practice and community to reveal unmet needs (Druss & Mauer, 2010). The needs assessment should expand beyond mental health concerns to encompass health behavior interventions; chronic disease management; psychotropic medication; substance use, misuse, and disorder assessment and intervention; and relationship problems. Ideally, the process reveals opportunities for prevention efforts and means of reducing health disparities (Kringos et al., 2010). It also helps the practice measure those issues that cannot be managed in the healthcare setting, such as serious mental illness, substance use disorder (if the practice does not have embedded addiction services), eating disorders, and intransigent relation-ship problems. This information helps the practice recognize where they need to strengthen community partnerships and referral relationships to achieve stepped care, which is crucial to integration success (McGrath & O'Donohue, 2015). This is yet another role for the embedded behavioral health clinicians, who may initiate and foster communication and relationship-building with specialty mental health (Greene et al., 2016).

Implementing Stepped-Care Protocols
Stepped-care protocols are clinical pathways that work to ensure patients receive care at the right level at the right time. SBIRT (screening, brief inter-vention, refer to treatment) is one type of stepped-care protocol. Screening and other assessment processes identify patients in need and stratify risk. Low-risk patients stay in usual care. Moderate-risk patients initiate in-house brief interventions. If these interventions are successful, they return to normal care; if not, they are referred for specialty care. High-risk patients are referred to specialty care after an assessment and often receive in-house brief interventions while awaiting access to specialty care. Importantly, the model also emphasizes the need to use the lowest level of care necessary to be effective to ensure that higher levels of care are available as needed (Babor et al., 2007; Hargraves et al., 2017; Moyer, 2013). We discuss the clinical strategies inherent in a stepped-care protocol in Chapter 6.

> Dr. Fernandes worked closely with the behavioral health clinicians who transferred into primary care. Her goal was to ensure as many patients as possible received real-time services when they had a need. She helped the clinicians develop new clinical strategies that aligned with primary-care-based services, including an emphasis on family support, chronic disease management, and health behavior change.
>
> Dr. Fernandes also worked with both the primary and specialty care behavioral health clinicians to implement a stepped-care protocol. Initially, there was pushback from the Director of Specialty Mental Health Services, Ms. Ivanenko. She feared that her budget would be cut if all the services moved to primary care and was upset because Dr. Fernandes hired away some of her best clinicians. Dr. Fernandes emphasized that the clinicians could not manage all the patients who presented in primary care, so they needed Ms. Ivanenko's help to collaborate with specialty care and to create pathways for patients who needed more. Dr. Fernandes also collaborated with Ms. Ivanenko on hiring decisions and apologized for not starting this way. As their relationship improved, Dr. Fernandes discussed the importance of

stepped care. She worked with Ms. Ivanenko to enhance bidirectional communication between specialty behavioral health and primary care. In addition, she emphasized the need for these patients to return to primary care as soon as possible to create capacity for new patients in specialty behavioral healthcare services because they always have a significant waiting list. Over time, this waiting list for specialty behavioral health services was cut in half as patients moved more seamlessly between primary care and specialty care behavioral health services. This process also helped to clarify unmet community needs that could be managed only in specialty care. Dr. Fernandes and Ms. Ivanenko collaborated on lobbying the administration and eventually the state for additional adolescent inpatient beds to address a rise in adolescent suicidality in the years since the COVID-19 pandemic began.

Ultimately, the collaboration between the two services enhanced commitment to whole-person, comprehensive care. The behavioral health specialty services began to routinely take full health histories on new patients and refer them for medical consultation as appropriate. Two primary care nurse practitioners agreed to offer primary care services in the day treatment programs for individuals with serious mental illness, establishing "reverse integration" services.

Implementing Alternative Practice Modalities

Increasingly, practices are embracing digital behavioral health interventions as a way of extending services. Telehealth, computer-delivered psychotherapeutic interventions, psychotherapy apps (Hoffman et al., 2019; Sinsky et al., 2021), and ECHO (Extension for Community Healthcare Outcomes) programs that offer tele-education and consultation to practitioners all can expand access to care (Jacobs et al., 2019). Research is ongoing to understand the best applications of these methods (Raney, Bergman, et al., 2017).

The COVID pandemic ushered in a new era of telehealth acceptance, with the use of telehealth expanding exponentially (Sockalingam et al., 2020). Some believe telehealth is here to stay (Volk et al., 2021), whereas others question the long-term impact (Haque, 2021). Proponents tout its ability to improve access to care to rural populations (Hills & Hills, 2019) and potentially reduce health disparities for minorities (Egede et al., 2020). Telehealth also facilitates access to care for patients who have special needs (e.g., homebound patients, older adults, children with developmental disorder and their families; Jacobs et al., 2019).

In addition to psychotherapy, telehealth consultation is a foundational element of CoCM, expanding access to evidence-based, optimized psychotropic medication management through psychiatric consultation with primary care physicians (Fortney et al., 2007; Raney, Bergman, et al., 2017). Waugh and colleagues (2019) noted that telehealth can enable a remotely located psychiatrist to complete direct evaluations of patients and provide consultation with the primary care medical and behavioral health clinicians who implement the plan. Similarly, psychologists and other behavioral health clinicians provide telemental health services for patients and consultation with physicians. Research supports the use of telehealth with a wide variety of mental health concerns (Turgoose et al., 2018; Varker et al., 2019).

Maintaining team-based, whole-person care via telehealth is not easy. As practices shifted to telehealth abruptly during the COVID-19 pandemic, interprofessional communication and collaboration typically declined when clinicians were not in the same space. Sinsky and colleagues (2021) described these challenges and offered practice-level strategies to maintain team-based care even when clinicians were not together. Although not focused specifically on behavioral health integration, they noted the need to clarify workflow issues, track collaboration, and conduct mock shared virtual visits to facilitate team cohesiveness.

Dr. Fernandes used the COVID-19 pandemic as an opportunity to expand telehealth services in the integrated services. She offered clinicians and staff training to help them implement telehealth successfully, emphasizing the importance of ongoing collaboration and communication even when clinicians were remote. She worked with the EHR and telehealth vendors to seek technological solutions to collaboration challenges. For example, the EHR added an instant alert and messaging function that allowed clinicians to engage each other in real time. The telehealth vendor provided all clinicians with clear instructions on how to add another clinician to an ongoing encounter, which allowed them to engage in virtual warm handoffs and shared appointments.

Telehealth is not the only technological innovation to consider. Digital screening processes help identify patients in need of behavioral health services. They augment information garnered from huddles, including chart review for specific patient characteristics and histories and verbal screening (Balasubramanian et al., 2015). Digital screening can streamline the use of multiple tools to drill down into the patient's concerns at the time of initial presentation and stratify risk, facilitating SBIRT processes (Byrd et al., 2018). Digital screening provides a way to track to target from baseline to enable measurement-based care (Mulvaney-Day et al., 2018). The process of using validated instruments to measure patient symptoms, functioning, goal attainment, and satisfaction informs service planning. Measurement-based care also can reveal success stories to motivate staff and clinicians to further support integration.

Data on patient and clinician service utilization, ideally in dashboard format, helps guide implementation (Corso et al., 2016). Tracking the number of warm handoffs, referrals, specific clinical presentations, and treatment outcomes can reveal variability in medical clinician use of integrated services, guiding leaders to access additional training for all clinicians or targeted consultation with specific clinicians.

THE PROCESS OF PRACTICE INTEGRATION

Across the board, implementation research indicates that the process of large system change occurs in stages. Building awareness of this reality and proactively setting appropriate expectations are critical. The EPIS model identifies four stages in practice transformation: exploratory, preparation, implementation, and sustainability (Aarons et al., 2011). These stages parallel Prochaska's readiness-to-change model, which is usually applied to individual behavior change (precontemplation, contemplation, preparation, implementation and maintenance; Prochaska & Velicer, 1997).

Attending to the practice's current stage of practice transformation guides selection of change management strategies and tracks progress (J. D. Smith & Polaha, 2017). Of course, change is rarely linear. Just as individuals recursively cycle through stages of change on their way to sustained change, healthcare practices and health systems evolve toward implementation in fits and starts. This type of recursive process requires ongoing monitoring to capture the complex outcomes involved in practice transformation (Hinde et al., 2020). In this vein, research on CoCM implementation found large variation across practices (Solberg et al., 2013). Researchers tied these outcomes to variation in real-world limitations such as a practice's ability to reduce financial barriers and effectively train staff.

In 2015, D. J. Cohen, Davis, Balasubramanian, and colleagues conducted a comparative case study in which they observed primary care practice operations, interviewed and surveyed practice members, and reviewed clinicians' implementation diaries in 11 practices undergoing integration implementation. Five factors, along with practice context, influenced the outcome of the integration efforts:

- primary location of the integration staff,
- a shared mental model by the medical and the behavioral health clinicians,
- integration reach (the likelihood a patient who screened positive received interventions),
- warm handoffs for on-site behavioral health services, and
- stepped care, when needed.

Four of the five elements relate to real-time access to care, reflecting the importance of prioritizing patient care that gives the services patients need, when and where they need them.

SUMMARY

Implementation of behavioral health is not an overnight process. It often evolves over many years, alongside shifts in professional relationships and the health system itself. A three-worlds approach to address operational, clinical, and financial barriers to integration facilitates success. Systemic financial barriers can be particularly problematic but often can be overcome with creativity, flexibility, and persistence. Like any second-order change, integration efforts require buy-in from various groups within an organization and significant time, energy, and resources to manifest second-order change that is self-sustaining.

Organizational change cannot be maintained if the individuals who implement the work of the organization do not adapt. Therefore, in the next chapter, we shift to a discussion of the changes clinicians and staff must make in the way they offer clinical care.

TAKEAWAY POINTS

- Shifting to an integrated care model requires healthcare systems and practices to make second-order changes in their financial, operational, and clinical functioning.

- Many integration barriers can be mitigated or even overcome. However, this process takes time and resources, so stakeholders must have appropriate expectations, change bandwidth, and motivation to support this process.

- Leadership plays a particularly key role in change processes, ideally working collaboratively to engage stakeholders and attending to systemic change management and readiness principles.

- Practice staff and clinicians ideally share a biopsychosocial mental model of care and view integration efforts as aligning with practice and patient needs.

- Systemic assessment to understand practice needs and pain points can inform integration planning to ensure that the proposed care model and programming address areas important to stakeholders.

- Measurement of patient symptoms, goals, and outcomes helps to guide and validate integrated care efforts.

6

SHIFTING PRACTICE BEHAVIORS OF CLINICIANS, STAFF, AND ADMINISTRATORS

At the practice level, significant changes in routines and behaviors by every member of the practice are required for the second-order change necessary to achieve integrated care (deGruy, 2015). Toward this end, this chapter focuses on understanding and influencing individual behaviors and mental models of care. We review key competencies for clinicians in integrated care. We also discuss ways to evaluate a clinician's suitability for integrated care and training opportunities to support the transition. These individual skills and characteristics are based on the science of teams and teamwork, with a focus on strategies to establish highly functional teams. We also describe the inevitable challenges and strategies to overcome these challenges as clinicians work together to provide integrated, biopsychosocial, team-based care.

The implementation process initially is designed to align enough with current clinical practices to be acceptable, then to build new competencies and leverage peer influence to shift practice culture in ways that support systemic change. Ultimately, the goal is to help administrators, clinicians, and staff adapt their daily routines and behaviors to provide patient-centered, biopsychosocial health through behavioral health integration and team-based care. We begin

https://doi.org/10.1037/0000381-007
A Systemic Approach to Behavioral Healthcare Integration: Context Matters, by
N. B. Ruddy and S. H. McDaniel

this discussion by focusing on clinicians because they often must make early and significant change.

CHALLENGES TO INTEGRATION EFFORTS: CLINICIAN FACTORS

Clinicians' practice styles vary, with some more aligned with integrated, team-based care than are others. Clinician beliefs and practice patterns can be difficult to alter, so early efforts may need to focus on increasing motivation for change, including openness to clinical beliefs and patterns that can support integrated care (Dickinson, 2015; L. A. Green et al., 2007). These baseline beliefs should be considered when assessing practice readiness and staffing selection decisions. The goal is to influence key practice members and develop a strategy that considers the impact of individuals' inclination (or disinclination) toward an integrated model. Where clinicians fall on the following continua often influence this process:

- reflective practice,
- biopsychosocial approach,
- systemic thinking,
- comfort with team-based care, and
- behavioral health clinician "fit" with primary care culture.

Level of Reflective Practice to Inform Needed Change in Practice Patterns

Davies (2012) defined reflective practice as continually and systematically engaging in a process of self-review regarding one's practice and making necessary adjustments as needed, based on this reflection. Brandt (2014) described it as "learning to learn" (p. 293). Reflective clinicians recognize the impact of their own personal and professional history on patient care and relationships with clinical colleagues. The ability to turn a mirror on oneself, recognize opportunities for improvement, and engage in these opportunities facilitates practice transformation of many types, including integration.

Building a reflective practice is normative in behavioral health clinician training and practice, where self-reflection is often a focus of supervisory processes (Bennett-Levy & Thwaites, 2007). Fortunately, it is becoming more common in medical clinician training (Epstein et al., 2022), but it is not as ubiquitous as for mental health professionals (Mann et al., 2009; McDaniel et al., 2005). We discuss how a behavioral health clinician's level of reflective practice affects their ability to adjust to, or "fit," primary care culture later in this chapter. Here, we focus on this continuum as it relates to medical clinicians.

In general, research shows that physicians believe they provide excellent care and tend to have relatively set clinical practices. Yet, these established patterns of care may not be informed by evidence-based clinical guidelines. For example, Gabbay and le May (2004) used the term "mind line" to describe

> collectively reinforced, internalized tacit guidelines that are informed by brief reading, but mainly by their interactions with each other and with opinion leaders, patients, and pharmaceutical representatives, and by other sources of largely tacit knowledge that build on their early training and their own and their colleagues' experience. (p. 1016)

Clinicians, whether medical or behavioral health, with a rigid "mind line" show a low awareness of and motivation for the need for change (Stevens, 2013). They generally do not engage in reflective practice. In addition, many efforts aimed at changing the practice patterns are experienced as imposed from the outside and not collaborative (P. V. Miles et al., 2013). Many physicians and some behavioral health clinicians perceive the use of quality metrics and associated incentives to change practice patterns as potentially harmful, rather than helpful, to excellent care provision (J. Ryan et al., 2015). Given these factors, implementation efforts must assess and directly address clinicians' interest in change.

Level of Commitment to a Biopsychosocial Approach

Clinicians who embrace a biopsychosocial approach, rather than a bifurcated health model, are generally more amenable to integrated care models (Baird et al., 2014). Bifurcation can result in viewing medical issues as the sole purview of the medical clinician and behavioral health issues as the sole purview of the behavioral health clinician. This practice pattern is antithetical to comprehensive, team-based care that requires flexible clinician roles to be determined by the patient's need at a given encounter (Blount, 2019b).

For medical clinicians, an exclusively biomedical approach may negatively affect one's ability and willingness to implement relevant behavioral health screening, recognize opportunities for collaboration, and prioritize behavioral health and social issues that have a direct effect on adherence and outcomes. Even biopsychosocially oriented medical clinicians may be more comfortable and therefore more focused on biomedical conceptualization and management.

Similarly, behavioral health clinicians may be more comfortable in the psychosocial realm and even push back against the role of biological processes in patient presentations out of a concern for "overmedicalizing" or pathologizing the patient. The behavioral health clinicians' practice stance may affect their ability and willingness to engage in health behavior conversations as well as their comfort with facilitating adherence to medical regimens to support chronic disease management. It may also affect their comfort in supporting medication adherence for psychotropic medication, a key role in integrated care settings.

Level of Systemic Thinking and Understanding of Systemic Conceptualization

Clinicians vary in their familiarity, understanding, and abilities regarding systemic thought and practice. Individually oriented clinicians may struggle to engage family supports and contextualize a clinical presentation (Rosland & Piette, 2010). Systemically informed clinicians are attuned to how changes in one aspect of care affect the whole system, in both patient care and practice functioning (Marlowe et al., 2012; McDaniel & Fogerty, 2009). In this way, a systemic lens can support teamwork, highlighting parallel processes and complementarity in the patient–family–healthcare dynamic and how team members interact with one another.

Level of Comfort With Team-Based Care

Some clinicians may struggle to share care, even when a different discipline might best serve the patient. In a 2015 survey of primary care clinicians, 90% of nurse practitioners and physician's assistants viewed team-based care as a positive change, whereas only 30% of physicians shared this view. In fact, 40% of physicians felt that team-based care had a negative impact on care quality (J. Ryan et al., 2015). This opinion may reflect a sense of personal accountability and physicians' sense of ultimate and ethical legal responsibility (P. V. Miles et al., 2013; E. Miller, 2020), stances that may be embedded during medical training. When medical clinicians or practice staff rigidly adhere to a traditional view of physician as the only leader, true team-based care is unlikely (Rosenberg et al., 2017).

Team-based care requires that clinicians and staff understand and appreciate each other's relevant expertise. Most practices currently include a traditional team of physicians, nurse practitioners, nurses, medical assistants, secretaries, and other medical support staff. These professionals function as a unit and inevitably see many patients with behavioral health issues in their everyday work (Kessler & Stafford, 2008). These existing roles and workflows must then shift to make space for the behavioral health clinician. The behavioral health clinician, in turn, must be mindful of entering an established team and commit to learning about and respecting the roles of every member of the practice, including administration and staff.

Furthermore, clinicians must trust other members of the team. Trust and reflective practice may predict the successful adoption of innovative practice changes (Lanham et al., 2016). W. L. Miller and colleagues (2019) noted that building trust, sharing learning, connecting team members via reflection, and creating shared mental models ("sensemaking") are processes that help to build the adaptive reserve necessary for positive change.

Level of Behavioral Health Clinician Preparation and "Fit"

Ideally, a practice that is newly implementing integrated care will hire behavioral health clinicians with interest and experience in integrated care or, at least, in medical care. In their implementation guide, Corso and colleagues (2016) emphasized the importance of getting "the right people on the bus" (p. 127).

The shifts a behavioral health clinician must make to be successful in integrated care settings are easier for some than others. Nash and colleagues (2012) noted that certain behavioral health clinician personality and professional attitudes portend success in primary care. Some of the foundational elements important for a clinician's in this role include

- interest in and willingness to adapt to primary care culture and practice;
- flexibility, tolerance, and resilience;
- ability to communicate clearly and concisely;
- ability to project a professional, self-assured, assertive practice style;
- ability to conceptualize broadly and contextually;
- ability to engage in self-reflection toward self-improvement;
- understanding and appreciation of the relevant expertise of various health disciplines;
- support of multicultural and diverse identities;
- ability to understand and integrate the complex legal, ethical, professional, and practice issues inherent in primary or specialty care;
- respect for patient privacy in the context of team-based care;
- interest in interprofessional collaborative care and team-based care;
- valuing of patient safety, quality improvement, cost-effective care; and
- understanding of the importance of evidence-based, patient-centered population healthcare.

Unfortunately, a shortage exists of behavioral health clinicians with integrated care training or expertise (Serrano et al., 2018). In addition to seeking the foundational characteristics outlined by Nash and colleagues, practices often need to provide or support training to instill the behavioral health competencies reviewed in Chapter 2 (Glueck, 2015).

Larger healthcare practices may have an interprofessional behavioral health team. A behavioral health team can benefit all behavioral health clinicians by reducing a sense of isolation, creating opportunities for peer supervision and case consultation, and sharing responsibilities to reduce stress. As with any interprofessional team, it is important that clinicians work collaboratively and respectfully, recognizing and respecting the differential competencies of other behavioral health disciplines (Dickinson, 2015). Toward this end, the implementation team and the members of the care team themselves should define clear roles and workflows that align with the specific skills and preferences of each team member. They must address differences in ethical codes and norms around confidentiality in their communications about shared patients (Hodgson et al., 2013; Runyan et al., 2018) As part of this process, the group also needs to develop processes that address conflicts or confusion related to role ambiguity overlapping competencies and variation in ethical code and norms.

The shift from a mental health to a primary or specialty care culture can feel like moving to a foreign country, both exciting and uncomfortable at times. Initially, behavioral health clinicians will feel challenged as they adjust to new language and a much faster pace (Rizq et al., 2010). Despite these necessary shifts, many behavioral health clinicians thrive in the fast-paced healthcare environment, feeling a sense of accomplishment and fulfillment from "meeting people where they are." They find that the shared responsibility and mission inherent in team-based care reduces stress and increases the joy of practice. For the people for whom it is a fit, integrated care is an opportunity to take one's skills and apply them in a whole new way. But fit alone is not enough. Ensuring clinicians successfully adapt their practice style and skill set is foundational to the integration process (Willard-Grace et al., 2014).

TRAINING STRATEGIES TO SUPPORT INTEGRATED CARE

Shifting attitudes, knowledge, and skills to support integrated care takes time and effort. These shifts affect every function in the office, including administrators, medical clinicians, behavioral health clinicians, and staff. In this section we review key elements of training for each of these groups.

Training Strategies to Engage Leadership and Administration

Practice leaders need to have a clear understanding of the integrated care model. This understanding includes benefits to patients, families, and clinicians; financial and operational issues; and realistic timelines for implementation. Healthcare leaders often become advocates once they understand and experience the model. They may develop an elevator speech to describe the benefits of integrated models in order to sell the model to others in leadership. They also may benefit from collaborating with systemic integrated care leaders to strategize change management and consider the operational, clinical, and financial changes necessary for success (Peek, 2008). Strong leadership and a clear strategic plan are key factors in the success of an implementation process (Swavely et al., 2020). Leaders may find additional support by creating a peer group or learning collaborative where they can share challenges and strategies with other leaders (Okafor et al., 2018).

Training Strategies to Engage Staff

Engaging and educating staff (particularly front-desk staff, case managers, and billing and scheduling staff) can make or break integrated care efforts (Anastas et al., 2019). Staff must understand they are essential members of the team and play a key role in integration.

Initially, staff may perceive change as additional work. A survey of medical assistants in newly integrated practices did report a perceived increase in workload but also improved job satisfaction (Sheridan et al., 2018). Emphasizing how integration will benefit patients and the practice is imperative. Staff generally realize that a small proportion of challenging patients have an outsized impact on their overall stress level. Ideally, the behavioral health clinician acts as a staff ally by helping successfully manage these patients as well as other staff pain points.

Collaboration and structured training sessions can help the behavioral health clinician develop positive relationships with staff. Staff typically need training regarding how to introduce screening instruments, describe new services, and introduce behavioral health clinicians. Research indicates that the introduction and description of a screening instrument affect patients' perceptions of the value of screening (Hsieh et al., 2021). Consequently, it helps staff to have flexible scripts to employ in these interactions, methods to respond to patient resistance, and triggers for when and how to seek consultation from the behavioral health or other primary care clinician. O'Malley and colleagues (2015) found that eliciting staff input regarding workflow redesign and sharing quality improvement data improves their buy-in.

Training for Medical Clinicians

Medical clinicians are the economic engine of the practice, so extensive training that takes them away from patient care may not be economically viable. Yet, medical clinician training is critical to success (McDaniel et al., 2005; Roderick et al., 2017). Given time constraints, training can occur in existing grand rounds, other teaching rounds, seminars, or lunch-and-learns, along with brief training tips shared during team huddles or other meetings. Brief educational activities, or "academic detailing," can be an important way to disseminate best practices (Van Hoof et al., 2015). Many residencies now have behavioral health professionals on their faculty, which promotes the development of a shared mental model with behavioral health clinicians providing integrated services. Continuing medical education (CME) credits for training in integrated models, biopsychosocial care, and team-based care are helpful incentives. For example, the AIMS (Advancing Integrated Mental Health Solutions) Center that supports Collaborative Care Model (CoCM) implementation offers 2 hours of CME for medical clinicians who complete an online, self-paced training to learn about CoCM, their role, and benefits to patients (AIMS Center, 2023e). The University of Rochester offers a 5-day intensive in integrated care for health and mental health professionals. Many of the groups listed in Exhibit 2.4 offer trainings in addition to the teaching and learning resources cited there.

Key focus areas for medical clinicians include population-based behavioral health, clinician roles, functional assessment, and behavioral health assessment tools (P. J. Robinson & Reiter, 2016). Medical clinicians can learn to recognize collaboration opportunities that cover the full scope of practice for integrated care, including health behavior change and chronic disease management as well as common mental health disorders. In addition to structured training sessions, these shifts can be supported with dialogue about this expanded referral focus embedded in daily practice, clinical consultations, and live coaching.

Medical clinicians may benefit from coaching on how to introduce the behavioral health clinician to the patient as part of their care team. A medical clinician's perspective on behavioral health and the behavioral health clinician's role on the team can make or break the success of integrated care. A warm handoff can be very useful, in which the medical and behavioral health clinicians briefly see the patient together (Blount, 2019a; McDaniel, Doherty, & Hepworth, 2014). Medical clinicians often have an established relationship with the patient, so their support for integrated care can facilitate patient engagement.

Blount (2019a) suggested training medical clinicians use the mnemonic of SSRI (situation, skill set, relationship, indicators) in a warm handoff or shared appointment with a behavioral health clinician. These elements highlight important behavioral components of the patient's expanded care team or "passing of the relationship" (p. 147). He stated the medical clinician should include the following points:

- Situation: Overtly share the patient's situation that resulted in the behavioral health clinician being part of the care team.

- Skill set: Describe the skill set of the behavioral health clinician to highlight how adding them will be of assistance to the patient and family.

- Relationship: Outline how the behavioral health, medical clinician, patient, and staff will work together in the overall treatment plan.

- Indicators: Explain how the team will work together with the patient and family to monitor the patient's progress and ultimately determine when behavioral health services are no longer warranted.

Finally, training should support reflective practice by ensuring regular team meetings, clinical huddles, and, when possible, debriefing sessions. For both Primary Care Behavioral Health (PCBH) and CoCM team meetings and regular case conferences are critical for reviewing a patient's progress and exploring opportunities for improvement (Fiscella & McDaniel, 2018; Raney, 2017). These dialogues can highlight missed opportunities for collaboration and enable dialogue about shared patients and team functioning. Helping clinicians reflect on their internal reactions to patients (or each other) may identify struggles where consultation or conversation with the team may be helpful.

Training to Engage and Prepare Behavioral Health Clinicians

Fortunately, many skills transfer from traditional or specialty care to integrated care. Behavioral health clinicians transitioning to integrated care are not starting over. Rather, they are adding new concepts and skills and adapting how they apply their foundational knowledge and skills. Competencies in systems theory, mental health diagnosis, human development, relationship development, cultural humility, and assessment of psychological and social factors in functioning as well as cognitive behavior therapy, mindfulness, and relational interventions all play key roles in helping patients.

Even so, training for behavioral health clinicians is often initially a heavy lift. For example, the AIMS Center offers a 9-hour remote training to orient behavioral health managers, significantly longer than the 2 hours of initial training for primary care clinicians (AIMS Center, 2023d). Broadly speaking, the training categories:

- the basics of interprofessional care: typical team roles, the training and competencies of different disciplines, ethical considerations in team based car, the culture of healthcare, services offered, patient-centered medical home concepts, and the role of primary and specialty care in the larger healthcare system;

- the basics of integrated behavioral healthcare: understanding various models of integration, benefits of integration as it relates to the Quadruple Aim, and best practices to support integration efforts at the individual and practice levels;

- integrated care clinical assessment and intervention: functional assessment, the patient's readiness to change, and brief, pragmatic evidence-based clinical strategies that focus on patient and family goals and address the medical clinician's questions or concerns;

- measurement-based care: developing and implementing a measurement-based treatment-to-target program, using measures as a routine part of clinical care and care planning;

- collaboration and consultation: time-sensitive consultation, the benefits of collaboration, confidentiality in team-based care environments, sharing accountability for clinical successes and failures, and helping staff with challenging situations via training and real-time assistance;

- chronic disease management: basic information regarding common chronic conditions, functional assessment, the chronic care model, and motivational interviewing regarding behavior change;

- population-health-focused behavioral healthcare: transitioning to brief encounters, outreach, screening workflow, case-finding, and participating in quality improvement initiatives;

- cultural humility training: understanding health disparities and underlying factors, culturally based health beliefs, and the impact of the medical culture and environment on the patient's experience; and

- a systemic orientation to clinical work and implementation efforts: engaging family members and other social supports and understanding the system of healthcare, as well as the local system of the clinical team, and teamwork (Horevitz et al., 2013; Lekas et al., 2020).

In their orientation and training, Cherokee Health Systems in Tennessee emphasizes the importance of the behavioral health clinician's role in sometimes serving as the first-contact clinician (*accessible*), working with a broad array of presenting concerns (*comprehensive*), and aligning with other care professionals (*coordinated*) as part of a long-term partnership (*continuous*; Khatri et al., 2017).

Dobmeyer and colleagues (2016) described the training program developed by the Department of Defense, highlighting the many new competencies behavioral health clinicians often must develop to be successful in integrated care settings. They emphasized the importance of clinical skills to serve patients and offer useful consultation to medical colleagues. However, they also outlined methods to instill competencies in practice management, documentation, administration, and team-based care. In describing the various trainings that were implemented in different branches of the military across time, they illustrated how training can be customized to setting, clinician and patient population, and other factors to create a phased training approach. The article also highlighted how training evolved over time to prepare a workforce that could implement various models of integrated care. As the Department of Defense worked to make integrated care normative, they created and implemented a training structure that formally measured progress and recognized individual development and achievement of competencies.

Early adopters of integrated care models have developed extensive in-person and remote training programs. In-person trainings may optimally spur initial learning for clinicians new to healthcare settings. Remote training may be best suited to introducing and shoring up content areas such as chronic disease management and specific assessment and intervention strategies (e.g., motivational interviewing). Remote training also may extend in-person resources. For example, Project ECHO (Extension for Community Healthcare Outcomes—"moving knowledge, not people") provides "virtual integration" via remote psychiatric and psychological consultation and liaison services embedded in remote training for clinicians (Sockalingam et al., 2018).

Large health systems, such as the Veterans Administration (VA), have found success using a hub-and-spoke method of dissemination. In this model, the VA first trains regional leaders, who in turn train behavioral health leaders from each VA site, who in turn train all primary-care-based behavioral health clinicians. In this way, they are able to provide ongoing training that supports integration and tracks the impact of their efforts. This systematic approach recognizes that integration is a process that must be nurtured over time (Kearney et al., 2020).

Ongoing supervision, as well as peer supervision and consultation groups, can help disseminate best practices in behavioral healthcare, in team-based care, and in behavioral health consultation. In addition, regular meetings with other behavioral health clinicians can counteract any sense of isolation some may feel in healthcare settings and serve as a venue for processing ethical issues that may arise as part of integrated care provisions (Williams et al., 2015; Runyan et al., 2018). Ensuring behavioral health clinicians feel supported and connected can improve retention over time (B. F. Miller et al., 2014). These processes also help behavioral health clinicians identify and address challenges, track progress, and share successes, enabling them to build and adapt their skills over time.

Many behavioral health clinicians find the shift to brief encounters particularly challenging, as it requires them to adapt many aspects of the patient encounter. Most of these shifts can be measured by the Primary Care Behavioral Health Provider Adherence Questionnaire (PPAQ; Beehler et al., 2015), which was developed in the VA. The PPAQ helps clinicians reflect on routine integration behaviors. Some are essential to success (e.g., brief encounters) whereas others interfere with model adoption (e.g., staying in one's office rather than the clinical space). As clinicians adapt their practice to integrated care, the PPAQ can identify opportunities for improvement and spur dialogue regarding best practices.

Training leadership, staff, and clinicians to work together differently is only part of the practice transformation process. Integration directly influences and is influenced by the interplay and relationships among individuals in the practice. In the next section, we review change management strategies that can leverage these relationships.

BEYOND TRAINING: SYSTEMIC STRATEGIES FOR PRACTICE TRANSFORMATION

Training is necessary but not sufficient for successful practice transformation (L. A. Green et al., 2007). A systematic review found that interventions that restructure practice operations, modify peer-group norms and expectations, and restructure professional relationships are most effective in changing individual clinician behavior toward evidence-based practices (M. J. Johnson & May, 2015). Ultimately, integration efforts must address the intersection of the practice styles of individual practice members and attributes of the practice itself while emphasizing evidence-based care and models that ensure treatment team accountability to provide quality care.

Behavioral health clinicians can and should serve as members of the practice transformation team. Organizational change management strategies parallel systemic interventions that behavioral health clinicians employ with groups and families. Drawing on this expertise is yet another way that behavioral health clinicians support integration. It also helps behavioral health clinicians develop important relationships in the practice and ensure they clearly understand their own and others' roles in achieving and maintaining an integrated care practice.

Change management and implementation elements that facilitate success include

- optimizing practice selection,
- defining the desired end state,
- defining an "effective team,"
- building a reflective team culture,
- targeting early adopters among staff and clinicians, and
- garnering engagement in the change effort.

Select a Practice Interested in Engaging in Integration

We alluded to the importance of practice selection in Chapter 5, but it bears repeating. Sometimes, practices self-select to be part of integration efforts in an organic process. However, when a large system seeks to integrate practices, the first step in a systemically informed integrated process is careful practice selection. We recommend consulting Exhibit 5.1 in Chapter 5 to select the available measures to discern practice readiness, based on prior change efforts, adaptive reserve, and the practice's interest in integrated care. Attention to the attitudes of practice leadership toward change can be important, given the degree to which their buy-in can portend the change's success or failure (Garland et al., 2010).

Define the Desired End State

There is no one-size-fits-all model of integrated care, so a dialogue that establishes a north star for desired improvements is an important first step. Key practice members are important in a discussion of the desired end state (Blount, 2019a). Ideally, this end state is based on a thorough practice and community needs assessment. Integration typically does not occur in one fell swoop; it is an evolution. Full integration typically results from multiple change initiatives that implement integration elements over time. For example, the initial goal may be increasing mental health screening rates. Once that goal is achieved, the goal of the next change initiative may be increasing team-based care for patients with poorly controlled diabetes. Ongoing dialogue creates a roadmap for change that represents goals of financial, operational, and clinical stakeholders. This roadmap ensures that individuals on the team share the same mental model for the end goal.

Clarity of purpose and mission highlights a potential benefit of CoCM: The model provides a very clear end goal with clear roles, processes, and expectations (Raney, 2017). On the other hand, some practices might find more success adopting aspects of PCBH integrated care, working toward a fully integrated practice over time. As we noted in Chapter 1, the evidence indicates that real-world applications rarely align perfectly with any one model (Buchanan et al., 2022). Customization to address practice pain points can serve as a strategy to engage individual practice members in the effort by addressing the "What's in it for me?" question overtly. As Peek (2019) noted, a balance between anything goes and standardization is likely key.

Define What It Means to Be an Effective Team

Achieving a high level of team functioning is a common denominator for all models of integrated care. Simply put, teams are more effective than are individual efforts, particularly when good outcomes require multiple types of expertise, as in healthcare (Salas et al., 2018). Industrial/organizational psychology researchers have studied the essential elements of excellent teams extensively. Most mention five core elements (Goodwin et al., 2018; Salas et al., 2005):

- Team leadership: The team has flexible but clear leadership that supports innovation and prioritizes team morale and functioning.

- Mutual performance monitoring: A systemic feedback loop with all members of the team creates the opportunity to both give and receive performance feedback to other members of the team, also referred to as "360-degree feedback."

- Backup behavior: Team members monitor the need to help each other as needed and pitch in and provide backup when they have the relevant expertise.

- Team adaptability: Team roles and processes adapt to shifts in practice need and situations as they arise, returning to normal state when appropriate.

- Team orientation: Members view themselves as a team and prioritize activities that enhance team functioning. The administration supports this sense of team.

In general, teams function best when they have a shared mental model of care, a sense of identity, relationship continuity with clear roles and workflows, common goals, and open communication (Salas et al., 2018; Tannenbaum & Salas, 2020). Psychological safety, defined as the team's shared belief that it is safe to take interpersonal risks without fear of backlash (Ilgen et al., 2005), is particularly central to optimal team functioning as it enables the team to resolve conflicts, learn from each other, address problematic patterns and errors, and improve performance (Frazier et al., 2017; Salas et al., 2018).

High-functioning teams require nurturance and maintenance. Best practices for team-building include regular meetings to enhance trust and psychological safety, adequate staff, physical work proximity, and shared training (Allen et al., 2018; Ghorob & Bodenheimer, 2015; Salas et al., 2015). Research on primary-care-based integrated care teams found that, in general, the same success factors apply (Fiscella & McDaniel, 2018). Implementation research on CoCM found evidence that clear roles, training, and communication between clinicians were particularly important (Wood et al., 2017).

Blount (2019b) used the metaphor of a squad versus a team to describe how clinical leadership roles need to shift to address the complex, varied problems addressed in healthcare. A squad is a group of people with a defined leader and roles who share a purpose. A team, alternatively, can have flexible leadership and malleable roles to address the issue at hand. Traditionally, medical teams have had a squad structure in which the physician is always the leader of the team. This is reflected in early (and some current) medical home descriptions that call for a "physician-directed team" (American Academy of Family Physicians, American Academy of Pediatrics, American College of Physicians, & American Osteopathic Association, 2007). Yet, transitioning to a more flexible team structure is important to provide truly patient-centered care, which often also reaps important staff and clinician benefits from the integrated care model (Crabtree et al., 2010).

Building Reflective Team Practice Culture

To create a practice environment that engenders supportive relationships, all team members must feel they have a voice in the practice, with autonomy and opportunities for ongoing learning. Trust underlies a sense of team cohesion (Fiscella & McDaniel, 2018). Building relationships takes time, but time is in short supply in healthcare settings. Ideally, leaders prioritize time for team-building and reflection, given its protective factor in lowering burnout (Willard-Grace et al., 2014) and guiding practice improvement (Balasubramanian et al., 2010). Team-building and reflection may be especially important for practices that work with underserved complex populations, in terms of team functioning, patient outcomes (Mulvale et al., 2016), and preventing clinician burnout.

Strategically Target Early Adopters Among Staff and Clinicians

The adoption of innovation has been the subject of a great deal of research. Across the board, people tend to respond to change in ways that settle out along a normal distribution, as illustrated in Figure 6.1 (Rogers, 1995).

The perspectives of the people that make up a healthcare team impact the change process. It can be tempting to focus on the practice members who embrace change. However, one of the key takeaways from the research is that innovators, while typically on board for change from early in the process, are not the key to success. Innovators may be perceived as prone to "impulsive adoption" and therefore often lack credibility with their peers (Balas & Chapman, 2018). Therefore, change management experts suggest targeting influential early adopters who are open to change but do not jump on the bandwagon quite so easily (Varkey et al., 2008). Early adopters can then share their positive experiences with late adopters and others who wait to adopt change until later in the process (e.g., the "late majority") to engender openness to innovation. Positive peer testimonials that embed patient and clinician benefits of integration into a clinical story are sometimes more compelling than any data point or in-service (Varkey et al., 2008). In effect, winning over innovators, early adopters, and people who adopt change shortly thereafter (e.g., the "early majority") helps the practice reach a tipping point. The tipping point reflects the phase of practice

FIGURE 6.1. Distribution of Innovation Roles

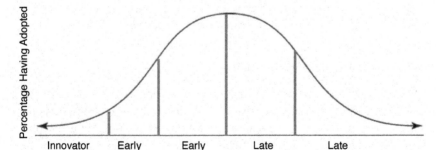

From *Diffusion of Innovations* (4th ed.), by E. M. Rogers, 1995, p. 285. Copyright 1995 by Free Press. Reprinted with permission.

transformation when the system begins to regard the change as normative, resulting in second-order change.

Regarding late adopters, change management experts recognize some people will very slowly, if ever, embrace this type of second-order change. Fortunately, these late adopters are not necessary for successful systems change, as long as they do not preclude others from practicing differently (Gotham, 2004). Behavioral health clinicians can approach a late adopter in a manner akin to how they approach a patient in precontemplation. In other words, do not try to convince them, work to develop a collegial relationship, and wait patiently for a critical incident in which one's clinical expertise can ease the late adopter's reticence. Sometimes a strong clinical relationship or even one critical patient care encounter can create a practice shift.

Garnering Engagement in the Change Effort

As we have noted, engagement in the change process across all job functions is important (Colquhoun et al., 2017). Because change requires both motivation and knowledge, practice members need to know they will have the resources and training they need to be successful (Higgs & Rowland, 2005). A kickoff meeting can set the stage to achieve these goals. The meeting serves to introduce the implementation and training plan, provide a rationale for change, and answer staff and clinician questions. The meeting may set a somewhat festive tone (food never hurts) and build excitement for integrated care based on the benefits for patients, staff, and clinicians.

Clear goals, performance measures, and incentives for change also support integration engagement. For example, staff can be incentivized via financial bonuses or recognition events to engage in huddles and screening and explain the behavioral health clinician's role in a way that results in successful referrals. Medical clinicians can be incentivized for warm handoffs, referrals, and shared appointments. Behavioral health clinicians can be incentivized for population-focused care and collaboration with other team members. These individually targeted strategies facilitate behavioral shifts that can coalesce into an integrated practice.

SUMMARY

For a practice to transform from separate services to colocated services and ultimately a more fully integrated practice, the people in the practice must change how they go about their work. Fortunately, not every person needs to support integration efforts, but there must be support across various roles in the practice. Training people how to do their job differently is necessary but not sufficient to achieve practice transformation. They must also be motivated to change and understand their role in the change process. Understanding the change management process facilitates practice transformation and provides a road map to success.

TAKEAWAY POINTS

- Integration implementation requires individuals within a practice to adapt their work roles and patterns.

- Approaching implementation strategically with awareness of individuals' readiness to change, motivation, and ability to shift patterns can facilitate second-order change.

- Training is necessary to develop new competencies and a shared mental model of care, but it is not sufficient as a lone implementation strategy.

- Leadership engagement can make or break implementation efforts.

- A systemic, evidence-based approach is important to optimize team functioning.

PART III
OVERVIEW: A SYSTEMIC LENS FOR INTEGRATED CLINICAL SERVICES

In Part III, we focus on a systemic lens for clinical assessment and intervention in integrated, team-based care. Many healthcare clinicians associate a systemic lens with family therapy, in part because much of the literature on systemic clinical strategies has focused on family relationships, broadly defined. As such, our discussion in this part largely focuses on the impact of family on health and well-being.

We use the term *family* in the broadest sense possible. By family, we mean not only relatives but also friends, members of one's spiritual community, and so on. We also differentiate patients' personal and professional support systems. *Personal supports* are those people who are socially connected to the patient and care about their well-being. *Professional supports* are those people who offer professional services to the patient, including social service representatives; professionals in the mental health, substance use, and healthcare systems; and other professional helpers such as clergy. True team-based care requires clinicians to rally all relevant sources of support for the patient and to respect that the clinical care team in a healthcare setting is but one part of the patient's overall support network. Utilizing a systemic lens to leverage the "team" in the broadest possible sense strengthens care and empowers patients and families to chart a course forward, even in the face of difficult health and mental health challenges.

Although the assessment and intervention strategies discussed in this part can be used by healthcare professionals of all types, we concentrate on interactions between behavioral health clinicians, patients, and family members.

Our goal is to highlight how the integrated behavioral health clinician role shifts with a systemic approach to care, in part by illustrating the role with descriptions of clinical strategies and examples.

We also focus on family-centered care because healthcare policy experts increasingly recognize the need to ensure the family's perspectives and priorities are considered in care planning. The Institute for Patient- and Family-Centered Care (IPFCC) defines family-centered care as having four core concepts:

- honoring patient and family perspectives and choices in the context of their values, beliefs, and cultural background,

- sharing information with patients and families in a way they can use to facilitate engagement in care and decision making,

- encouraging patients and families to engage in care at the level they choose, and

- engaging patients and families in policy decisions and practice and healthcare decisions that affect their care (e.g., program development, implementation and evaluation, facility design; IPFCC, 2021).

The goal is to move toward a collaborative relationship with families to improve care quality and safety, enabling family members and other support people to serve as allies in healthcare.

Although we focus on families in Part III, we emphasize that all levels of the system affect interactions between healthcare clinicians and patients. Macrolevel factors such as our healthcare reimbursement, education, and delivery systems directly affect healthcare at the micro level of the clinician–patient encounter. Clinicians are human, and as such they bring their implicit biases and health beliefs (usually based in a Western disease-focused model) to each and every patient encounter. Naming these influences and attempting to address how these factors can negatively affect care reflects a systemic lens for healthcare.

There is little debate that families and social support networks play a large role in health maintenance and caregiving for people with health issues. Yet, in our linear, individually oriented system, the healthcare encounter typically focuses on the individual. Much of the guidance for behavioral health clinicians in integrated care settings reflects this individual focus. As integrated care evolved, the clinical how-to guides generally focused on assessment and intervention with individuals, most commonly utilizing cognitive behavior strategies. C. L. Hunter and colleagues' (2017) book *Integrated Behavioral Health in Primary Care: Step-by-Step Guidance for Assessment and*

Intervention exemplified this approach and continues to serve as a seminal text that helps behavioral health clinicians transition to primary care. Here we hope to expand the lens of the clinical encounter, offering strategies to provide systemically informed integrated care.

Individually oriented strategies addressing specific motivational issues, health behaviors, and symptoms can be incredibly helpful in healthcare, particularly as we seek to improve a patient's daily functioning. Research conducted in community-based primary care practices shows robust effects sizes for brief cognitive behavior therapy for patients struggling with anxiety and depression (Bogucki et al., 2021). Furthermore, integrated brief cognitive behavior therapy services have shown a small but significant improvement over typical primary care for depression and anxiety (Twomey et al., 2015).

To be clear, we advocate a both/and approach. We argue that integrating relational factors strengthens and expands the clinical focus and options. Considering the impact of family relationships and larger systems on a patient's health and wellness serves to expand the purview of the behavioral health clinician. The family may be a source of untapped strength or significant stress. They can support a treatment plan or disagree in a way that puts the patient in a loyalty bind between the healthcare clinicians and family members. Flying blind regarding the family's perspective puts the clinician at a considerable disadvantage.

Toward these ends, we describe clinical assessment and intervention strategies that enable clinicians to recognize and leverage the role families play in health and illness. We review the use of a developmental, systemic lens to understand the impact of health conditions on networks of social support and of social support on health conditions. From this foundation, we describe systemically focused clinical assessment and intervention strategies that facilitate engaging social support networks toward positive change.

Chapter 7, the first chapter in Part III, describes general concepts and systemic strategies gleaned from the medical family therapy literature that transcend the population served. The chapter guides clinicians in expanding their focus to include family health beliefs, relational patterns, and illness scripts based in family lore. It also describes how families can affect the patient's response to ill health and how ill health can affect the family. We describe clinical techniques that help families successfully manage the impact of illness and address harmful patterns.

Chapter 8 presents an umbrella review of literature on the impact of families on health. We also summarize the literature on family-oriented clinical programs to address healthcare and caregiving issues. The chapter more specifically reviews systematic reviews of the literature on medical family therapy with couples and families facing illness. This "review of reviews" highlights emerging evidence regarding best practices in medical family therapy as well as the large gaps in our knowledge.

Chapters 9, 10, and 11 apply these general concepts to different healthcare settings and the populations they serve (primary care medicine, pediatrics, and women's health). In each chapter, we describe how the context of care and its common clinical presentations affect the role of the behavioral health clinician. We apply the systemic clinical concepts described in the general overview to the specific population served and present relevant literature regarding best clinical practices. We then hone in on a segment of these common clinical presentations to illustrate the application of these concepts.

We begin with an overview of healthcare for adults, with a specific focus on chronic disease management from a family lens. We shift to integrated care in pediatric settings, where the focus is more often on prevention and early intervention, and discuss strategies for families who have a child with neurodevelopmental issues. Finally, we focus on the role of the behavioral health clinician in women's health. After a discussion of common clinical presentations, we offer strategies behavioral health clinicians can use to help families who experience pregnancy loss.

7 CLINICAL THEORY, STRATEGIES, AND RESEARCH

This chapter serves as a broad overview of a biopsychosocial systemic approach to the design and provision of direct clinical services. We begin by outlining the various lenses and mental models that are foundational to this work. We then describe the metaframework of medical family therapy. We link foundational medical family therapy concepts to the challenges families face in living with illness, describing various areas of focus for clinical encounters. We then outline how these concepts are operationalized with families in integrated healthcare settings and within the healthcare team itself.

FOUNDATIONAL LENSES FOR MEDICAL FAMILY THERAPY AND SYSTEMIC INTEGRATED CARE

It is critical that a systemic lens is not interpreted as focusing on family only. Rather, a systemic biopsychosocial lens integrates factors at multiple levels of the system—from our cellular system to individuals, families, and our society and culture writ large. A broader systemic perspective contextualizes

https://doi.org/10.1037/0000381-008
A Systemic Approach to Behavioral Healthcare Integration: Context Matters, by
N. B. Ruddy and S. H. McDaniel

the patient in their social milieu, acknowledging and respecting the impact of social factors and interpersonal relationships on health. This approach requires healthcare professionals to recognize the impact of poverty and racism on rates of chronic illnesses (National Center for Health Statistics [U.S.], 2016) and healthcare outcomes (Tai et al., 2021). This approach also emphasizes that the patient's and family's values, goals, and priorities should guide care. Systemic biopsychosocial care is more patient-centered, rather than clinician-centered, care.

Over the past 2 decades, it has become more normative to include psychological factors in the assessment and management of healthcare issues as the link between mental health and physical health became more salient. We also now know there is a significant link between the patient's quality of interpersonal relationships and health outcomes (D. Carr et al., 2014). Hence, we argue that healthcare must again expand its purview to embrace a systemic approach to relational issues. Acknowledging the importance of social relationships can spur clinicians (both medical and behavioral health) to build relational assessment and intervention competencies in their approach to care. These approaches support patient care based in empathy for the physical as well as the psychological and relational challenges of various health issues.

The contextualization inherent in this lens also requires a developmental approach. The focus on the developmental arc of children and their families makes this normative in integrated pediatric settings. Yet these same developmental factors are critical to integrated care across the lifespan. The family life spiral model (see Figure 7.1; Combrinck-Graham, 1985) melds individual

FIGURE 7.1. The Family Life Spiral

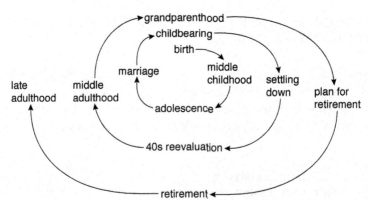

From "A Developmental Model for Family Systems," by L. Combrinck-Graham, 1985, *Family Process*, 24(2), p. 141.

and family developmental tasks, highlighting inherent points of tension. For example, the spiral reflects how an adolescent's need for individuation and identity development may overlap with the middle-aged parents' physical and emotional transitions and elderly grandparents' needs for support. In this scenario, the child and parent are navigating biological transitions fraught with parallel emotional manifestations at the same time. In addition, as the child seeks individuation, the parent may need support as they attempt to simultaneously parent an adolescent, care for an ailing parent (Boyczuk & Fletcher, 2016), and seek work–life balance (Hammer & Neal, 2008). Like any model that attempts to outline "normative" development, the spiral's alignment with racial and ethnic majority pathways must be considered a limitation of the model's generalizability to all populations (Goldenberg et al., 2017). Yet it can be a helpful framework to consider how the developmental tasks of the family and individuals within the family interact.

This developmental context intersects with the adaptations necessary when living with health issues. As Combrinck-Graham's (1985) spiral suggests, facing a serious illness at different stages in the individual and family developmental trajectory poses different family issues. Consider the very different challenges posed by a child with an illness, a parent of young children, a middle-aged empty nester, or an elderly grandparent. Many health issues shift the developmental arc of the individual, requiring the family to adapt their relationships and roles over time. Clinicians need to consider these developmental issues to fully understand the individual's and family's experience of health and illness.

Toward this end, ideally every member of the healthcare team recognizes the differential psychosocial demands of various health conditions. Rolland's (1994) "psychosocial illness typology" offers a conceptual frame, another lens, to facilitate this task. This typology recognizes that illness characteristics—such as the pace of illness onset, course over time, prognosis and outcome, and impact on functioning—demand different coping strategies from families. These illness demands intersect with individual and family relational functioning and developmental tasks. Some illnesses intersect with developmental tasks in a particularly challenging way, such as a debilitating illness in an adolescent that requires increased family support and closeness just as the adolescent seeks individuation. Recognizing this complexity helps guide assessment and intervention. For example, a family living with an illness with a sudden onset, unpredictable course, and high care needs requires different assistance than a family facing an illness with a slow onset, clear course, and low care needs.

Empirical evidence aligns with Rolland's typology. For example, Usuba, Li, and Nowrouzi-Kia (2019) compared disease burden and family challenges across many chronic conditions, noting that pain conditions and mood disorders are most impactful on health-related quality of life, with stroke being the most disruptive to daily life.

In the second edition of his book, Rolland (2018) expanded the typology into the Family Systems Illness Model. This expanded model recognizes the systemic interaction of three dimensions: typology of illness as described above, time phases of the illness, and family functioning as it relates to illness adaptation. Each time phase of the illness (crisis, chronic, and terminal) poses different challenges, requiring families to make serial adaptations over time. The illness developmental arc occurs in parallel with individual and family development, creating a complex intersection of tasks and adaptations. Naming these intersections and normalizing the challenges over time can help the family cope with this complexity. Rolland also emphasized that the family's baseline functioning, adaptability, strengths, and resilience form critical factors in the family's ability to manage the health condition successfully.

Rolland (2018) noted that the interplay of illness phases and types forms an "expanded system comprised of four interlocking triangles" (p. 51). The model is illustrated in Figure 7.2. The patient is in the middle of the system,

FIGURE 7.2. Rolland's Family Systems Illness Model: Therapeutic Triangles With Chronic Conditions

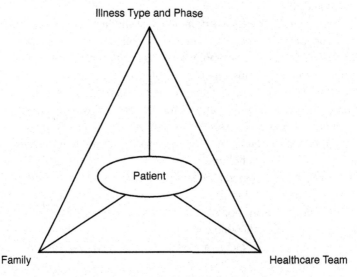

From *Helping Couples and Families Navigate Illness and Disability: An Integrated Approach*, by J. S. Rolland, 2018, p. 52. Copyright 2018 by Guilford Press.

surrounded by the personal social support network and the professional support network. The illness itself is a "fourth member of the system, having a personality (based on the patterns of onset, course, outcome, disability and predictability), and a developmental life course (the illness time phases)" (p. 51). These intersecting factors help the healthcare team work with the family to reveal the impact of the health issue on the patient, family, and their social network.

Research supports this expanded model. In a study of families who perceive themselves to be "living well" with chronic disease, C. A. Robinson (2017) found a five-phase recursive process for families:

- fighting the illness,
- accepting the illness,
- living with the illness,
- sharing the experience of living with the illness, and
- constructing a new life around the illness.

The first two phases focus on the family's relationship with the illness itself, as they slowly respond, adapt, and accept demands of the illness. The third phase reflects the family's internal process to reconfigure around the illness and integrate it into daily life. The fourth stage represents the need to establish new connections and develop a sense of meaning in the illness. The fifth stage describes the family establishing a new normal in which the illness is no longer front and center in daily life. Within the family, each individual's process can set the stage for a sense of synchrony or conflict as family members enter different phases of coping or acceptance of the health condition at different times. This reality is apparent when helping families make decisions at the end of life—often some family members welcome the end of a loved one's suffering, while others are not ready to let go (Caswell et al., 2015).

Understanding these frameworks is an important precursor to engaging in medical family therapy, especially when the work occurs in an integrated healthcare setting. Next, we review the concepts that form the undergirding of therapeutic encounters between patients, families, behavioral health clinicians, and the broader healthcare team.

MEDICAL FAMILY THERAPY KEY CONCEPTS

The field of medical family therapy is a relatively young discipline. The seminal book *Medical Family Therapy* by S. H. McDaniel, J. Hepworth, and W. J. Doherty was published in 1992, with a second edition in 2014 (McDaniel,

Doherty, & Hepworth, 2014). Professional competencies to guide training for medical family therapy were outlined in 2018 (American Association for Marriage and Family Therapy, 2018). Medical family therapists represent a broad array of disciplines, including family therapists, psychologists, counselors, primary care medical clinicians, nurses, and psychiatrists.

Medical family therapy is a biopsychosocial systemic metaframework that recognizes the utility of the range of family and individual interventions (e.g., cognitive behavior therapy, trauma-informed therapy, problem-solving or solution-focused therapy, emotion-focused couples therapy). Many of the key concepts parallel those of family therapy for myriad other issues. However, the metaframework highlights specific considerations for work with families living with illness within each of these concepts. This section reviews key considerations that guide medical family therapists as they help families live and function well in the context of physical illness, pulling from both the first edition of *Medical Family Therapy* (McDaniel et al., 1992); the second edition, *Medical Family Therapy and Integrated Care* (McDaniel, Doherty, & Hepworth, 2014); and the casebook, *The Shared Experience of Illness: Stories of Patients, Families and their Therapists* (McDaniel et al., 1997). Two subsequent titles, *Medical Family Therapy: Advanced Applications* by Hodgson and colleagues (2014) and *Clinical Methods in Medical Family Therapy*, edited by Mendenhall and colleagues (2018), also inform our discussion.

Now we review a set of concepts and mindsets that guide medical family therapy:

- balancing agency and communion,
- fostering resilience,
- improving communication,
- managing conflict,
- respecting defenses,
- finding meaning in the illness,
- addressing spiritual elements,
- exploring the illness narrative,
- establishing a new normal,
- supporting a non-illness-related identity, and
- addressing loss.

Supporting a Sense of Agency and Communion for the Patient and Family

Medical family therapy seeks to increase agency and communion for patients, families, and health professionals who face the physical, emotional, ethical, and financial challenges of living with illness (McDaniel et al., 1992; McDaniel,

Doherty, & Hepworth, 2014). A sense of *agency*, or effectiveness, reflects a sense of individual power in managing the illness's effects on daily life, family, and friends. *Communion* refers to strengthening emotional and spiritual bonds that can be frayed by illness and disability. It's the sense of being cared for, loved, and supported by a community of family members, friends, and professionals. It also refers to individual or communal beliefs about illness and loss that relate to spirituality or religion (W. D. Robinson et al., 2020).

Supporting Agency

Helping families achieve a sense of control and self-efficacy is key not only to helping families cope with illness but also to supporting their engagement as key members of the treatment team. Medical family therapists can help families learn to differentiate what is and what is not controllable about the illness experience. They can encourage the patient and family to focus on those aspects that can be controlled and accept those elements that are beyond their control. Solution-focused strategies can help families identify opportunities for agency and highlight how some aspects of the illness's impact on life can be mitigated.

Hassle factors and care fragmentation in our healthcare system can reduce family's sense of agency (White & Newman, 2016). Medical family therapists can help patients and families navigate the healthcare system, which can engender trust and reduce understandable frustration. This navigation is particularly important for patients from marginalized groups who may begin from a place of mistrust based in systemic racism within the medical system (Jaiswal & Halkitis, 2019). The medical family therapist may address system fragmentation by facilitating communication within the healthcare team and resolve disagreements or issues within the team that threaten to affect the patient and family. Medical family therapists may be particularly attuned to patterns of team interaction that mimic those of the patient's family or social system, reflecting strong pulls toward systemic parallel process.

Frustration with our healthcare system can be particularly challenging for caregivers, increasing life disruption and care load (Wolff & Jacobs, 2015). Integrated care teams can help by engaging caregivers, assessing the caregiving burden, and offering support. Improving social support and self-care are key elements to caregiver well-being (Adelman et al., 2014; Fu et al., 2017). In addition, asking all patients if they offer care to others or are affected by an illness in their family can reveal opportunities to be of assistance and decrease health issues for the caregiver (Swartz & Collins, 2019).

Supporting a Sense of "Communion"

Serious illness or disability is an existential crisis that can isolate people from those who care for them (Hoyt & Stanton, 2018). Families often become very focused on the illness and neglect social relationships, feeling that others in the "well world" cannot understand their experience. Some illnesses impair the individual's and family's ability to maintain social connections because of impacts on functioning or highly unpredictable symptoms that make planning and implementing social events difficult. This isolation can have significant health consequences. While normalizing these challenges, the medical family therapist helps the family overtly note the impact of the illness on social connection and strategize ways to create new or maintain old relationships.

Medical family therapists seek to mitigate or resolve conflict, building a web of support for the patient to facilitate self-management in the face of changes imposed by illness (De Maria et al., 2020). Collective conversations can help everyone grieve what they have lost as well as honor their shared experience, facilitating communion. Communication, connection, meaning, and spirituality are foundational parts of the concept of communion.

Taken together, agency and communion provide an integration of individual autonomy in a relational context (Bakan, 1966). Helgeson's (1994) research showed that a balance between agency and communion is related to positive health outcomes, whereas unmitigated agency or communion is related to negative health outcomes. Hence, it is important for integrated health clinicians to focus on connection and emotional support as well as opportunities to help the patient feel a sense of control in managing the condition (McDaniel, Doherty, & Hepworth, 2014).

Fostering Resilience

Walsh (2015) conducted seminal work on how family belief systems support resilience in the face of adverse events, such as illness. She noted that therapeutic strategies that facilitate family resilience include helping the family engage in meaning making regarding the adversity, supporting a positive outlook to the future, and supporting the family's sense of spiritual well-being. Prime and colleagues (2020) noted how these resilience strategies relate to family coping during the COVID-19 pandemic, highlighting that a systemic, multifactorial approach is necessary to lessen the potential long-term effects of the pandemic on children and families.

Improving Communication

Family communication is an important target for medical family therapy intervention. Reduced communication and support in response to an illness has been shown to adversely affect intimate relationships (Traa et al., 2015). Family members may avoid discussing important issues with the ill person out of fear of causing stress and exacerbating the illness or causing guilt. The person with the illness may take on a stoic role out of concern that the illness is stressing others or for fear they will be seen as complaining. The medical family therapist can normalize these patterns as well as seek to help the family find a communication style that balances the need for both privacy and connection.

Medical family therapy also facilitates communication regarding difficult emotions related to the illness. The intrusion of an illness is a unique stressor that can elicit fear, anger, shame, and other challenging emotions. Processing these feelings can be particularly fraught because of a desire to protect one another or because the feelings generate a sense of guilt. The goal is to find a pragmatic therapeutic balance that normalizes these intense experiences. It can be helpful to acknowledge and normalize feelings of anger and resentment related to role shifts and lifestyle changes imposed by the illness. These feelings can be particularly intense if family members feel that the patient bears responsibility for their illness or disability because of insufficient self-care, poor health habits, or ignoring medical advice.

Rolland (2018) stressed rebalancing relationship skews brought on by illness. This includes enhancing relational coping that views the illness as everyone's issue to manage, not just the patient's. Redefining the illness as "ours" acknowledges that the patient *and* the support network need to adapt.

Managing Conflict

Illness has been likened to a new, unwanted family member. The illness itself can be the third point in a triangle of conflicts or it can serve as a distraction or barrier to resolving painful, underlying problems. In these situations, the illness becomes a significant defense, such that clinicians must consider how the illness itself may become part of the homeostatic mechanism of a family. The therapist can help the family recognize how the illness has come to complicate the resolution of family issues and conflict and can help the family develop new strategies to improve conflict resolution and overall relational satisfaction and connection.

Respecting Defenses

Medical family therapists often focus on patient and family strengths and take care to respect the function of defenses. For example, denial that does not negatively affect adherence to the prescribed medical regimens can be adaptive, helping everyone involved deal with the practicalities of everyday life. Also, differing levels of acceptance and understanding of the illness may underlie what appears to be denial in the family. Living with a medical condition requires an acceptance process, with each member of the support system falling along a continuum of denial and acceptance. These differences can counterbalance each other or can become rigid and polarized, resulting in conflict. Medical family therapists can elicit and respect family members' differing beliefs. This helps the individuals within the family share covert feelings, fears, and perspectives. Once in the open, they can be processed, and the clinician can help all the family move toward acceptance.

Finding Meaning in the Experience of Illness

Individuals and families often struggle to understand "why us?" Exploring the meaning of the illness to the patient and the family helps to find areas of hope or resilience, sometimes rooted in spirituality. Potentially harmful "meanings" include a sense that the illness is a deserved punishment or that the patient and family are powerless to affect how they respond to an illness. These interpretations are particularly difficult when attempting to motivate self-management (Beverly et al., 2012; Halding et al., 2011). Alternatively, illness meanings that help define a purpose in the illness experience can reduce the sense of "why me?" ultimately enhancing a greater sense of acceptance (Palacio G. et al., 2020). Medical family therapists can elicit unspoken beliefs about the illness and work to address those beliefs that have the potential to exacerbate relational issues or complicate illness management.

Addressing the Spiritual Elements of the Illness Experience

Medical family therapy includes a focus on beliefs and meaning, which often includes spirituality.[1] Acknowledging the role of spirituality in illness coping reflects research that links spirituality and health (Zimmer et al., 2016), along with many families' desire to discuss their beliefs about these links (Best et al., 2015). Often, a family's faith community can be an important source of social support during a difficult time. Clearly, any discussion of spiritual beliefs must be guided by the patient's and family's interest and comfort level, with care and consideration regarding their cultural background (Sulmasy, 2009).

---

[1] Some medical family therapists prefer to use the term *biopsychosocial-spiritual* (Delbridge et al., 2014).

Using Narrative Strategies to Support Agency and Communion

Williams-Reade and colleagues (2014) outlined how four elements of narrative therapy can be applied specifically to empowering families facing illness. They suggested deconstructing the illness experience, taking care to reduce the degree to which family members' illness narrative is "problem-saturated" and shifting the focus to the family's sense of meaning regarding the experience. Helping the family externalize the problem supports the family's nonillness identity and helps them see the problem from different perspectives that can help them consider new possibilities and understandings. Williams-Reade and colleagues described a process of "mapping the effects" of the illness and illness-related problems on their lives. Finally, they recommended helping the family to reauthor their narrative, to consider new or unique outcomes, and to reinforce a narrative that the family might find more helpful as they seek to live with a health condition.

Helping the Family Adapt to Illness Demands and Establish a "New Normal"

As Rolland's model suggests, families must make adaptations to successfully manage a medical condition. In general, adaptation to health-related stressors requires families to shift roles and become more flexible, particularly when the health condition has a significant impact on the person's physical and emotional functioning. This is especially true when the family member who becomes ill is the person in the family who typically serves in the primary caretaker role.

Medical family therapists help families overtly discuss the ways the illness has intruded on their lives. Families often designate a specific point in the illness journey that differentiates before and after the illness became part of their family. Therapy often focuses on helping the family establish a new normal, supporting the family's adaptation to this new reality and acknowledging their adaptation challenges. The therapist can help the family identify the successful adaptations they have made to enhance the family's sense of agency. In addition, the family can be urged to discuss those adaptations that have been more difficult or concerns family members may harbor regarding future intrusions of the illness on daily life.

Therapy also may emphasize any silver linings when and if the family shows readiness to acknowledge positive shifts. For example, many families note a new closeness to one another or a new appreciation of both the fragility of life and the health that enriches it. Therapists can provide psychoeducation regarding posttraumatic growth, noting how a sense of meaning in the experience and a narrative that emphasizes adaptation and growth as a possibility can engender a more positive experience. The concept of supporting posttraumatic growth has been supported by research with individuals facing cancer (Casellas-Grau et al., 2017) and HIV (Ghabrial et al., 2019).

Recognizing the Family's Nonillness Identity

It is also important to remember that life goes on for many, even as the family's life is disrupted by illness. Especially with chronic illness, it is important to maintain family rituals and special events to support the development of children and family members who are not ill. Medical family therapists help families cope with other life stressors, recognizing that the family's own adaptive reserve may be depleted by the stress of living with a family member with a health condition. Medical family therapists can elicit these other stressors, normalizing how illness can exacerbate routine stressors such that they become problematic.

Addressing the Impact of Loss

Loss comes in many forms with medical conditions, depending on the ways the illness intrudes on daily life and functioning. Families may be facing the loss of a loved family member with a terminal illness. An illness that causes functional impairment requires grieving not only the functional losses but also beloved hobbies, hard-earned skills, and a sense of usefulness. Illnesses that cause little functional impairment still involve the loss of one's general sense of being a fully healthy person, and it may remind the family of their own mortality. Grief and loss associated with illness can affect mood and hamper social connection. Medical family therapists offer patients and those who care for them a place to begin a process of anticipatory grieving and acceptance.

Anticipatory grieving can be particularly important if the illness is likely to be terminal. Medical family therapists facilitate family discussions regarding end-of-life advanced care planning based on family values and preferences. These discussions reduce psychological distress and improve satisfaction with care (Houben et al., 2014). Studies show surviving family members are more satisfied with the care of the deceased when their loved ones are able to die at home, engage in hospice, and not have an intensive care unit admission in the last 30 days of life (Wright et al., 2016).

Medical family therapists play an important role in end-of-life discussions, because clear, overt discussion of end-of-life issues is not guaranteed in our healthcare system. Qualitative research with families facing a terminal cancer diagnosis revealed three patterns of perceived communications with the healthcare team about the transition from active cancer treatment to palliative care (Norton et al., 2019). Some families noted they had overt conversations that led to a shared understanding of this transition. However, many noted that they felt communications from the treatment team never shifted away from a treatment goal of "beating the odds," so that they did discuss end-of-life care but did not realize that death was imminent. Sadly, some families did not recall any overt discussion of end-of-life care planning, feeling their family member was "left to die."

MEDICAL FAMILY THERAPY IN INTEGRATED CARE SETTINGS: ASSESSMENT AND INTERVENTION STRATEGIES TO SUPPORT CARE TEAMS AND PROVIDE SYSTEMIC FAMILY-ORIENTED CARE

In healthcare settings, the pace and brevity of services may not be consistent with ongoing medical family therapy. However, many relational therapy and systemically targeted strategies can be embedded into brief services. Even one or two family consultations can lead to lasting and meaningful improvement in well-being, symptom reduction, and functional status (Bryan et al., 2009). For example, engaging family members in medical visits has been associated with improved outcomes in care for patients with heart failure (Cené et al., 2015).

Many medical family therapy strategies can be adapted to integrated, team-based care environments. In this section we review elements of practice structure and clinical strategies to facilitate engaging families as the unit of care. The goal is to make a systemic approach normative by removing barriers to family engagement in daily practice. In addition, we discuss how a medical family therapist or family-oriented behavioral health clinician can help the care team embrace a systemic model of care. Ideally, every member of the care team sees patients and families as partners of the team, ensuring that family members feel their perspective and experience is valued by the healthcare team.

Clinical Assessment Strategies to Support Systemic Integrated Care

Although integrated care encounters tend to be brief, this brevity does not preclude assessment of relational factors as part of routine healthcare. In fact, gathering relational and family information ultimately can save time, enabling clinicians to garner supports and raise awareness of family issues or health beliefs that might interfere with optimal care. In this section, we review strategies to include family factors in the assessment process.

Screen for Family Issues
Existing family assessment tools such as the McMaster Family Assessment Device can be used to screen for family issues (Van Fossen et al., 2022). Just as the Patient Health Questionnaire-9 (PHQ-9; C. L. Hunter et al., 2009; Kroenke et al., 2001) has been adopted as a mental health check, these measures may eventually be useful as a relational health check. As we noted earlier, we support expanding the purview of medical care to become more inclusive of relational and social elements. Routine screening can facilitate this goal, much as routine mental health screening increases the likelihood emotional concerns will be addressed. At a minimum, assessing family functioning conveys to patients that their relational life matters to the clinical team and is relevant to optimal healthcare. The screening process and results can set the stage for a dialogue about social support and relationships. In addition, the results of the screening tool can serve as a baseline for relational functioning. Repeated use of the screening tool over time can facilitate measurement-based care, a hallmark of integrated healthcare. Research on the feasibility and usefulness of these measures is ongoing. As with screening for individuals, even families who express distress on these measures may not be amenable or ready to seek relational therapy or assistance (Van Fossen et al., 2022).

Engage Family Members and Elicit the Family Perspective
Clinicians can invite family members and other supports to future appointments or engage in them in real time—patients have a family member in the waiting room at about one third of visits (Russell et al., 2008). Clearly, patient preference about who attends appointments and what is shared must be respected. Clinicians ensure that the patient remains at the center of the interview. Patients often appreciate the presence of a friend or family member to ask clarifying questions, provide information, and serve as a second set of ears about diagnosis and treatment planning. A shared encounter enables the clinician to monitor the tone of the support person's input to care, helping to shape it toward "autonomy enhancing" behaviors such as clarifying medical information and engaging the patient in the encounter (Wolff & Jacobs, 2015).

   When the patient's friends or family are not able to attend appointments, they can be included using telehealth or written communication. This enables family to ask questions, offer perspectives, and engage in shared decision making to the degree desired by the patient. The family member may offer important insights to the patient's functioning and may be able to support a treatment plan they helped create.

Occasionally patients do not want to include others. At a minimum, even without their presence clinicians can elicit the significant others' perspectives using circular questioning and other questions that bring them into the room at least figuratively. Questions for the patient such as "What would (family member) say if he/she were here?" elicit opinions of people important to the patient. This information can provide fodder for motivational interviewing by revealing change others want the patient to make. Alternatively, the information might reveal that others question the diagnosis or treatment plan and may need to be engaged more directly. Exhibit 7.1 offers questions that can elicit the family perspective and communicate to patients that their family and support system are important in their care.

Assess and Address Readiness to Change

Readiness to change for the individual *and* their supports is a key factor in helping patients change their health behaviors (Prochaska et al., 2005). Attending to both the individual's and family's willingness to make changes can elicit how family members are likely to support or resist change. For example, if a patient is advised to make dietary changes, it is important to ask who shops and prepares meals, ensuring they are on board for the changes. This type of support is important in myriad health behavior change efforts. For example, research clearly shows family and support systems affect smoking cessation, such that people who have a "quit buddy" and who do not live with someone who continues to smoke are far more likely to quit or reduce smoking (Holt-Lunstad & Uchino, 2015).

Understanding the family's level of readiness to change also can help the medical team set appropriate care expectations and reduce clinician frustration. If the assessment reveals a low level of engagement in the change efforts by the patient and family or significant others, the medical clinician may well be the only person motivated for change. Under these circumstances, the medical family therapist can shift toward a more consultative role to support the medical clinician by coaching them in methods to enhance the family's motivation for change and to manage any frustration the medical clinician experiences with the family's choices.

Develop a Timeline of the Health Issue

Creating a timeline of the illness as part of the assessment process can facilitate a biopsychosocial understanding of the patient's experience. Expanding

EXHIBIT 7.1. Questions to Elicit Patient's and Family Members' Illness Perceptions

For the patient

- What do you believe causes the problems?
- How do your symptoms impact daily life?
- How did you come to realize something was wrong?
- What was the process of obtaining a diagnosis like for you?
- What were the experiences of others you've known with this type of problem?
- If others in your family have had this problem, how did things go for them?
- What are your hopes for the treatment?
- What are your fears about the treatment? About the problem?
- What do you think you can do to make things better?
- What would likely make things worse?
- What parts of the problem do you believe will not change, no matter what you do?
- How do you feel about the care you've received so far?
- How difficult has it been for you to adjust your life to the problem?
- Do you see any ways that the problem has actually been helpful to you?

For family members

- How has the family managed with changing family "jobs" to adjust to the illness?
- How does the family decide who will help the patient as needed? Does that family talk about the need for help and formulate a plan overtly?
- To what degree does the family talk about the illness and its impact on family members?
- What questions do you have about the illness? About the treatment for the illness?
- What aspects of the care plan do you agree with? Disagree with? Think will be difficult to implement?
- How do family members feel about the care the patient has received so far?
- What do you expect to happen with the problem in the future?
- What lifestyle or management changes do you believe the patient needs to make? To what degree do other members of the family intend to make these changes as well?
- How has the illness affected the stress level in the family? Relationships?

Adapted from "Illness, Family Theory, and Family Therapy: I. Conceptual Issues," by L. C. Wynne, C. G. Shields, and M. I. Sirkin, 1992, *Family Process, 31*(1), pp. 3–18.

the focus of the timeline to include other major life events can reveal connections the patient has (or has not) made between the health issue and other life events. A timeline ideally includes information about the onset of the illness; illness symptoms; diagnostic process and diagnosis; treatments that have been suggested, tried, or desired; and the emotional and practical impact of the issue. Emotions and opinions regarding previous and ongoing interactions with the healthcare team and system are also helpful to understand.

Stretching the timeline into future expectations can elicit unspoken hopes, fears, and expectations.

The timeline conversation can be streamlined when the clinician gathers some information via chart review prior to the encounter. Clinicians can present their understanding of the timeline and ask for further patient and family input. Starting with a draft timeline orients the patient and family to how life events might have influenced their health. This process also gives families a chance to set the record straight when they disagree with the documentation. The dialogue elicits missing information as well as patient and family perceptions of events. This process not only thickens the narrative of their experience but may reveal points of difference between the care team and the family that underlie tensions or misunderstandings.

Construct a Collaborative Genogram

Gathering genogram information results in an expanded illness story and contextualization of current concerns (McGoldrick et al., 2020). Genograms are always useful as a pictorial representation of the patient's web of relationships. They are particularly important when the health condition has a genetic element and/or occurred in many family members. The patient and family may have an "illness script," a set of predetermined beliefs, expectations, or fears about the health condition based on prior experience or family lore. The genogram conversation can elicit information about the family's history and traditions in dealing with illness, health professionals, and the healthcare system. Given time constraints, clinicians can ask a few questions each visit, gathering genogram information over time and documenting it in the health record. A new clinician then can quickly scan a genogram for an overview of family information that can facilitate patient- and family-oriented treatment planning.

Ensure Assessment Focuses on Function and Relates to Patient Values and Goals

Functional assessment elicits how life has changed for the patient and family in the context of the illness, with a specific focus on its impact on work, relationships, and leisure/pleasure activities. Including the family in this conversation provides additional perspectives for both the patient and the clinician. Family members may have a different perspective regarding the most paramount issues or may not truly understand the impact of the patient's health issue. Eliciting both patient and family "pain points" related to the illness's impact on the patient's functioning can facilitate goal setting based on what matters most to both the patient and their family. Family support increases when they have input into the process of treatment planning (Mueller et al., 2020).

In a similar vein, eliciting both the patient's and family members' perceptions of preillness functioning, strengths, and challenges helps the clinician understand the patient's life before the illness. This process clarifies the impact of the illness, highlighting adaptations that have occurred or could occur. It also enhances the clinician's knowledge of the patient as a whole person, their strength, and their communities. Families often appreciate the opportunity to describe their individual and relational strengths and recognize how they have successfully adapted to the illness and other stressors.

Assess Beliefs About the Causes, Meaning, and Treatments for Health Conditions

Health beliefs are firmly rooted not only in one's individual family but also in their larger cultural fabric. Learning about the patient's and family's culture and its effect on their approach to the illness experience informs care. For example, the plan might shift if the discussion reveals health beliefs that engender blame or conflict. The discussion also might reveal that the patient is using culturally based alternative treatments—important information for the care team. Similarly, the family may believe that the prescribed treatment is not appropriate or could be harmful. These views can influence the patient's likelihood to follow the prescribed regimen. This information about beliefs and adherences is very helpful to the care team. In some circumstances, the medical family therapist can serve a crucial role in negotiating an effective treatment plan that aligns with cultural and family health beliefs.

Use Continuity of Care to Facilitate Ongoing, Comprehensive Evaluation

These assessment processes and tools are not a checklist for the initial encounter. Rather, clinicians gather bits of information over time and weave it into a coherent narrative. Behavioral health clinicians seek information from many sources, taking care to confirm information with the patient and significant others. Because of their long-standing relationships with patients, medical clinicians are often a repository of important information for their behavioral health colleagues. The process of a patient sharing their illness narrative and hearing how those who care for them have experienced the illness is powerful and therapeutic in and of itself. Ongoing measurement of important biopsychosocial outcomes reveals progress or the need for revision of treatment.

Clinical Team Interventions to Support Systemic Integrated Care

All assessment is an intervention, and all interventions are also assessments. The assessment process can set the stage for clinicians to engage the family in a way that emphasizes their role as key members of the healthcare team. Here we note how medical family therapy techniques described earlier might be adapted to an integrated healthcare setting.

Plan Team Care

Together the team can identify ways the family will need to adapt and adjust to a new normal. A shared team understanding of these challenges can facilitate consistent conversations with the family regarding needed chronic disease management and illness adaptations. For example, each team member can use similar motivational interventions to help the family make necessary lifestyle changes.

In parallel, the care team can collaborate to engage family members and professional supports to ensure a shared understanding of necessary adaptations and how they will support a positive outcome. A shared message from multiple clinicians may help to engage reluctant family members in the change efforts. When family members are unable or unwilling to engage in these health behavior shifts, the team can work to help the patient cope with and manage this resistance to change. Finally, the team can work with family members to elicit and address barriers to change, helping the family generate strategies that align with their values and healthcare goals.

Elicit and Discuss Emotional and Relational Elements of Living with an Illness

Integrated care teams can also acknowledge and address the family's experience of illness as an emotional rollercoaster. Watson and McDaniel (2005) outlined a seven-step approach to address emotional reactivity in a couple facing illness. They recommend working to

- discuss the pragmatic and emotional impact of the illness;
- determine how emotional reactivity affects each area of concern and which areas cause the most anxiety and distress;
- refocus on the internal response to the illness and its meaning, rather than on how it affects daily living;
- discuss emotional reactions and the internal processes associated with them;
- connect the emotions to each person's personal history and vulnerabilities;

- facilitate separation of the current reaction from reactions to historical triggers; and
- develop alternative, adaptive responses to current stressors and triggers.

This process can be completed across multiple encounters, with other team members engaging in these discussions as well. Ensuring all care team members engage in these types of discussions helps patients and families process their experiences. If it becomes clear that the family is not able to make needed shifts in a brief encounter modality, they may need to be referred for medical family therapy in a traditional setting with longer sessions that occur more regularly.

Facilitate Use of Narrative

Rajaei and Jensen (2020) highlighted the use of narrative therapy strategies in clinical encounters to facilitate joining, inform assessment processes, and support a sense of agency and communion. They noted that the clinical team also can benefit from narrative techniques, particularly reauthoring their own narratives about their families and their role in healthcare. Thickening the narrative to include contextual factors can enhance cultural humility and compassion for families, which can, in turn, facilitate optimal team function. For example, a team might seek to deepen their narrative regarding a "nonadherent" family. This process may facilitate a reevaluation of the family's reasons for not following the treatment plan. Enhanced understanding of the family's decisions and behaviors may help the team be more collaborative in treatment plan development and implementation.

Williams-Reade and colleagues (2014) also described how attention to narratives may help the team. For example, they recommended that behavioral health clinicians use externalizing language and emphasize strengths and contextual factors during consultations and in clinical documentation. They also describe a process of reflective witnessing in which the behavioral health clinician can facilitate team member dialogues focused on patient progress in front of the patient. The goal is to emphasize team successes and engender camaraderie and support. They also noted that behavioral health clinicians can prescribe writing exercises (e.g., encouraging the family to write a letter to the care team) to reinforce the patient's narrative and further contextualize the patient's perspective.

Set Goals for Behavioral Health Encounters

Clinical medical encounters typically focus on one or two target areas collaboratively determined by the clinician, the patient, and the family. In parallel, integrated behavioral health clinicians typically select with the patient the target concern for a given encounter in the first few minutes of conversation. Ideally, the target is actionable and reflects the values and priorities of the patient and family. Often, the target is best addressed via cognitive behavior, motivation-enhancing, mindfulness, and symptom management strategies. However, these same interventions can be delivered in a way that engages the patient's family and enhances relational functioning. For example, a patient's partner can be taught breathing and meditation strategies alongside the patient as well as how to negotiate a schedule for practicing these skills together at home. Motivational interviewing strategies can be implemented with multiple family members to enhance readiness to change and overly acknowledge adaptation (Hodgson et al., 2014).

At the relational level, targets for visits often focus on helping people adapt to the changes that illness has thrust upon them. Together, the patient and family can set realistic, small goals that enhance their overall adaptation and functioning. The family may work to resolve preexisting issues that interfere with illness management. They may find meaning in the illness together, or they may work to identify and manage controllable aspects of the illness while actively accepting the uncontrollable aspects for what they are. This type of overt negotiation based in the underlying values and priorities of the patient and family helps reduce a sense of futility and helps increase support for living around the illness. Clinical engagement and intervention with couples and families has been shown to improve coping and self-management of serious and chronic illness (Rosland et al., 2012). Helping the patient and their closest supports cocreate a shared approach toward the illness experience has been associated with lower levels of illness-related distress (Berg & Upchurch, 2007). Those interventions that include family members in chronic disease management efforts are associated with small but meaningful benefits over individual approaches (Martire et al., 2010).

Team-Based Care Strategies to Engage Family Members and Social Supports

Myriad techniques exist to engage social supports, ranging from routinely inviting partners to engage in prenatal care to asking family members to strategize ways to support health behavior change, acute illness care, or chronic disease management (Carek et al., 2017). Teams can implement multifamily support groups in the healthcare setting, the community, or online to help the patient and family connect with others facing similar challenges (Petrie & Jones, 2019). Some practices offer group medical appointments cofacilitated by medical and behavioral health clinicians. These groups bring together people with similar clinical issues for their medical care to reduce isolation, offer models of self-management, facilitate health education, and help patients experience how others who face similar challenges cope and manage daily life (Kirsh et al., 2017).

Practice Strategies to Instill and Balance Agency and Communion

The sense of futility and "illness fatigue" people with medical issues experience reflects, in part, a low sense of agency. The sense of powerlessness may contribute to a cycle of passivity that may be reinforced by the healthcare system and the patient or illness role. The integrated care team can work collectively to help develop small, simple family rituals to maintain a sense of normalcy and identify ways to lessen the impact of the illness on daily life. This approach might include strategies to "put the illness in its place" by ensuring it does not take over every conversation, decision, and aspect of the relationship (Gonzalez et al., 1989). The team can provide consistent psychoeducation that sets realistic expectations (J. D. Smith, Berkel, et al., 2018). Anticipating and understanding changes in function, mood, energy level, behavioral inhibition, or disinhibition related to the illness can help normalize the family's common patterns and prepare for the next illness phase.

Helping the healthcare team engage significant others in care is a powerful way to instill a sense of communion. At the very time the patient most needs a community around them, they may find support difficult to access. Family members may be frustrated or uncertain how to be helpful or truly not understand the patient's experience. Inviting family to brief healthcare encounters creates a venue for these concerns to be explored. Furthermore, the focus on setting goals and completing key tasks in these encounters can help family members have more clarity about how they can be of assistance in a way the patient has validated. Even in brief encounters, the patient and their supports can discuss treatment plan options and implementation. This dialogue can reveal and address knowledge gaps to ensure decisions reflect truly informed consent regarding different treatment options, including sometimes rejecting treatment.

Manage Conflict

At times the patient and family may experience conflict or frustration with the medical team. In these situations, the behavioral health clinician may use their expertise in communication and interpersonal process to moderate disagreements. Many requests for behavioral health services in healthcare are secondary to issues around medical regimen management. Medical clinicians may not recognize when nonadherence is an attempt to gain a sense of agency or control. Emphasizing the impermanence of treatment decisions— that people can change their minds as they adjust to new information—can enhance willingness to try a suggestion or reconsider hardline decisions. The goal is to help people have the information and dialogue they need to choose a path of truly informed decision making that aligns with their wishes and values.

Conflictual or particularly complex patient situations may be best managed via a joint appointment that includes the patient, their support network, and the various clinicians involved in their care (Ruddy et al., 2008). This creates a venue to address questions and concerns and formalize a plan that clarifies roles, strategies, and goals for everyone involved. It is particularly important to include the team when problematic patterns develop between the family and the treatment team. These meetings can inform the health-care team about the individual's and family's coping and how the team can improve the care of this patient and family. These meetings also are an opportunity for mutual support, connection, and collaboration among the clinicians as they seek to be of service in challenging situations.

Help the Family and the Clinical Team Manage Uncertainty

Up to two thirds of clinical presentations in primary care—and a significant number in specialty care—do not align with a medical diagnosis or explanation (Steinbrecher et al., 2011). Families facing medically unexplained symptoms often struggle to have a sense of agency in the face of such uncertainty. The treatment team can validate how vexing it is to live with an illness that defies diagnosis and has no clear prognosis or treatment plan. Brief symptom management strategies (e.g., relaxation techniques, mindfulness) can be helpful to improve daily functioning. Involving the family can address blame, confusion, and frustration as patients, families, and medical professionals can become embroiled in these emotions.

Medical teams also struggle with medically unexplained symptoms. The behavioral health clinician can help the team avoid bifurcated conceptualizations or care that labels symptoms as exclusively psychosocial or "stress-related." In addition, an integrated care clinician can help the team cope with their own as well as the family's frustrations in a productive way. Clinicians and patients benefit from a family-oriented, team-based approach when struggling to manage frustration and fear related to the inherent uncertainty of complex, vague, and unclear diagnostic presentations (McDaniel, Doherty, & Hepworth, 2014; Van Houtven et al., 2019).

SUMMARY

In the sometimes overwhelming world of healthcare, it can seem, on the surface, as if dealing with just the person in the exam room is more than enough to handle. Clinicians who are not familiar with the interplay of family dynamics and illness may be tempted to focus on the individual. Yet research increasingly shows the importance of relational and other social effects on health and illness. Systemic integrated care garners these supports and engages family, in whatever way the patient defines it, to make the work of primary and specialty healthcare much more rewarding, efficient, and effective. To do so, medical and behavioral clinicians must make a mental shift to include family members as partners in care, considering how family affects the health condition and how the health condition affects the family. Clinicians can use many assessment and brief intervention strategies to bring the family into the room (literally or figuratively). In so doing, they utilize the power of family and social support networks to facilitate change, improve coping, and improve chronic disease self-management.

TAKEAWAY POINTS

- Family therapy techniques can be adapted to focus on helping a patient and family cope with a medical condition; these techniques can be adapted for application in integrated care environments.

- Individual and family developmental issues at any point in the life cycle interact with an illness and its psychosocial demands and are usefully taken into account for effective treatment planning.

- A systemic lens facilitates reflective practice to help the care team work together effectively and to understand the patient's experiences and behaviors in the context of their family, community, and culture.

- Engaging the family in care facilitates many care processes, including assessment, measurement-based care, care planning, enhancing social supports, and understanding the interplay of the family and care.

8 THE DEVELOPING EVIDENCE BASE FOR SYSTEMIC INTERVENTIONS

In this chapter, we turn our attention to the research literature regarding families and health. We first provide a high-level review of the impact of social connections on health, with a specific focus on families. We then shift to the relationship between family functioning and health condition management and outcomes. This discussion highlights how family characteristics affect the group's ability to cope with the inevitable adaptations needed in the context of illness. Finally, we examine the effect of involving family members in care on health, mental health, and relational outcomes. In this section of this chapter, we rely on systematic and strategic literature reviews to provide a broad review of the empirical evidence for the role of families in healthcare. Specifically, how do family-oriented (rather than individual) interventions impact families living with a broad array of health conditions? In later chapters, we present individual studies that examine the impact of family interventions with specific health issues.

https://doi.org/10.1037/0000381-009
A Systemic Approach to Behavioral Healthcare Integration: Context Matters, by
N. B. Ruddy and S. H. McDaniel

THE INTERSECTIONALITY OF FAMILIES AND HEALTH: A BRIEF REVIEW OF THE RESEARCH LITERATURE

Families have enormous influence on health behaviors, adherence, and caregiving. Therefore, the literature on families and health forms an important context that can inform programmatic and direct clinical service designs. Although an exhaustive review of the families and health literature is beyond the scope of this chapter, we provide a broad-brushstroke review of how social connection, baseline family function, and the family's ability to adapt to medical issues are related to health outcomes.

Social Connection

Research underscores the centrality of social connection in health. As we better understand the deleterious health impacts of social isolation and loneliness (Moieni & Eisenberger, 2020), public health efforts increasingly focus on how to best create human connection. For example, in response to almost half of older adults reporting loneliness (Jovicic & McPherson, 2020), the United Kingdom National Health Service established a "Loneliness Minister for loneliness" whose focus is reducing the ubiquity and impact of loneliness on the general U.K. public (Tatz, 2019). U.S. health officials, recognizing how the COVID-19 pandemic exacerbated loneliness, recommended screening for high-risk individuals and connecting those who report loneliness to social service and social engagement organizations (National Academies of Sciences, Engineering, and Medicine, 2020).

At the direct clinical service level, systemic integrated care clinicians routinely assess social support and normalize difficulties in maintaining social connection, particularly as people age. Some have suggested that clinicians "prescribe" outreach and connection to social groups as part of the negotiated treatment plan (Trad et al., 2020). Group interventions can help patients create connection and reduce the sense of isolation ill health can exacerbate (O'Rourke et al., 2018). Systemic therapy strategies to assess and enhance family functioning also serve to increase social connection and social support.

Family Functioning and Overall Health and Wellness

Empirical evidence suggests that general family functioning has important health consequences. García-Huidobro and colleagues (2012) found that people in high-functioning families were less likely to have chronic health conditions than were people in low-functioning families. This study was correlational, so we cannot conclude that high-functioning family life results in fewer health problems, only that the two co-occur. Even so, these researchers cite a public health opportunity to address family functioning in health prevention efforts.

In a subsequent article, García-Huidobro and Mendenhall (2015) outlined health pathways associated with family factors, such as family structure (e.g., whether two adults live in the home with children), communication (e.g., whether there are effective ways to resolve conflict), and social support. They noted the interrelationship of these factors with other biopsychosocial factors (e.g., genetics, socioeconomic status), health behaviors, illness self-management, and mental health. This model emphasizes the need for a systemic lens to understand the recursive and interdependent nature of all these factors as they affect overall health and wellness, as well as formal assessment of and intervention to address issues in family functioning.

THE ROLE OF FAMILY FUNCTIONING IN MANAGING HEALTH CONDITIONS

In a 2020 systematic review, Woods and colleagues noted that much of the research that examines family factors and outcomes for health conditions in adults analyzes only the impact of the dyadic relationship between the patient and their caregiver (Woods et al., 2020). They stated, "We continue to assert that family relationships, other than the marital relationship, are understudied and underutilized in adult health research and practice" (p. 1619). Despite these limitations, they cite research that links high family conflict (e.g., critical comments) to stress reactions that have a well-established link to poor health outcomes (e.g., Ha & Granger, 2016; Priest et al., 2019). This research also supports linkages between family functioning and shifting health behaviors such as diet, smoking, and sedentary lifestyle (K. Li et al., 2012; S. Li & Delva, 2012). In this context, research shows that engaging the patient's support system in lifestyle adaptations increases the likelihood of positive change (Greaves et al., 2011).

The degree to which the family focuses on health and wellness also may form a subtext for disease management. Individuals from families with high levels of interest in and communication about health issues may be more likely to seek health information and be more actively engaged in their own healthcare (V. M. Rodríguez et al., 2016; Yang et al., 2017). Family relationship factors also correlate with disease self-management. One study conducted in Nigeria found a significant correlation between good glycemic control and positive family functioning indices for individuals with type 2 diabetes (Abdulsalam et al., 2019). Negative family factors seem to also have a significant impact on health. For example, critical, overprotective, controlling, and distracting behaviors from family members have been associated with less effective self-management and negative patient outcomes (Rosland et al., 2012).

The U.S. healthcare system increasingly recognizes the opportunities and benefits of engaging families as partners in care for adults, particularly older adults. Jennifer Moye, then editor in chief of the journal *Clinical Gerontologist*, titled her summative 2019 editorial "Healthcare Systems Meet Family Systems: Improving Healthcare for Older Adults and Their Families" in recognition of this critical link and the need for more research.

Although there is much to be learned about the intersection of family relationships and adult health, research on pediatric populations tends to be more systemically focused, recognizing the child's broader context, including family relationships, siblings, schools, and myriad social factors (Woods et al., 2020). In multiple studies, family functioning correlated with physical and mental health outcomes as well as to quality of life in pediatric cancer (e.g., Moscato et al., 2022; Van Schoors et al., 2017), chronic illnesses (e.g., Popp et al., 2014), type 1 diabetes (Luo et al., 2019), and adaptation to the COVID pandemic (Prime et al., 2020).

The intersection of families and health is multidirectional. Research offers evidence that the intrusion of serious illness at any point in the family life cycle tests the family's functioning and ability to adapt. Dalteg and colleagues (2011) found five disease-specific themes for families living with serious cardiac disease: overprotection, communication deficiency, sexual concerns, changes in domestic roles, and adjustment to illness, noting that some concerns about these themes were nearly universal. For people living with chronic obstructive pulmonary disease, Ek and colleagues (2011) used qualitative analysis to reveal relational impacts. Their analyses revealed an overarching theme, "living with the disease and one's spouse in a new and changeable life rhythm," and three underlying themes, "living with uncertainty," "living in a changed intimate relationship," and "finding new ways of living together." Clearly, the patient is not the only person who must adapt to a health condition. Attending to this reality can guide clinical intervention that recognizes common family and relational challenges.

THE ROLE OF FAMILY FUNCTIONING IN CAREGIVING

A great deal of research exists on the impact of family factors on caregiver burden, caregiver quality of care, and health outcomes for caregivers. Our review outlines common themes and takeaways that inform the provision of systemic integrated care.

First, caregiver burden is a complex phenomenon related to the type of illness experienced by the family member and their associated care needs, the relationship between the caregiver and patient (e.g., parent, partner, adult child), and the baseline and ongoing health of the caregiver. In sum, providing caregiving for an individual with an illness with a high care burden (e.g., greater functional impairment and/or complex treatment regimens) is correlated with greater caregiver struggle (e.g., Bom et al., 2019; Schulz et al., 2020; Tramonti et al., 2019). Social support and sociocultural factors mediate the impact of caregiving, with higher education, positive family functioning, and social support mitigating caregiver stress (Toledano-Toledano & Domínguez-Guadea, 2019). Finally, the relational role of the patient and caregiver (parent/child, partners, adult child/parent) and the gender of the caregiver are important. Women tend to feel more responsible for caregiving and to be more involved in caregiving tasks (e.g., Friedemann & Buckwalter, 2014). Perhaps in part because it requires a role reversal, adult child caregivers of a parent tend to be more stressed by the caregiver role than do spousal caregivers, even though spousal caregivers tend to devote more time to the role (Fenton et al., 2022). When the patient is a child, mothers tend to be more involved in caregiving tasks than do fathers, with the impact on their health more pronounced. Caring for a child also, at times, can have a deleterious impact on the couple relationship and overall family functioning, although the relationship is a complex intersection of illness demands, family, and sociocultural factors (Pinquart, 2018). Couple-based interventions are effective in improving communication, reducing caregiver distress, and improving relationship functioning (Regan et al., 2012).

However, Ferrell and Wittenberg (2017) focused on quality of life and noted that caregiver support is linked to improved caregiver quality of life. They suggested that clinicians include a family assessment as part of new patient diagnoses, assess caregivers for their own health and mental health problems, and assess communication issues between couples or dyads. They commented that all of these issues point to the need for an interprofessional, integrated approach to cancer care.

Interventions to support caregivers typically focus on psychoeducation and skill-building as well as shoring up social support (Ferrell & Wittenberg, 2017). However, results of these studies on interventions to support caregivers have mixed results. A Cochrane review of psychosocial interventions for caregivers of cancer patients noted that most were psychoeducational; only two of the 19 trials met criteria as psychotherapy (Treanor et al., 2019). These authors concluded that psychoeducational interventions with this population had minimal impact on both caregivers' and patients' psychological and physical outcomes.

Research continues to investigate the range of factors that can enhance coping with the stresses of caregiving (Palacio G. et al., 2020). Beyond psycho-educational studies, there are not yet sufficient studies to determine if systemically oriented psychotherapeutic intervention is associated with meaningful and lasting improvement for caregivers. Clearly, more research is needed to determine the best psychosocial practices to support caregivers coping with stressful, challenging illnesses.

FAMILY-FOCUSED AND MEDICAL FAMILY THERAPY INTERVENTIONS: CURRENT EVIDENCE

Multiple publications over the past decade have reported the results of literature reviews on family therapy interventions for families living with various health conditions. Some articles reported findings across multiple health conditions, whereas others focused on only one health condition (e.g., diabetes) or a class of health conditions (e.g., cardiovascular disease).

The high level of variation in the level of family inclusion across studies complicates interpretation and application. Therefore we differentiate between family-oriented and systemic relational interventions, based on Pratt and Sonney's 2020 rubric to evaluate the level of family inclusion as follows:

- Low family inclusion research involves only the patient and a targeted family member, with outcomes that focus on the patient's medical outcome or the family member's perception of the medical outcome.

- Moderate family inclusion research includes one or more family members and the patient, with outcomes of interest focused on the family members' perceived roles in the patient's health outcome as well as the patient outcomes themselves.

- High family inclusion research involves the patient and one or more family members as well, but the outcome of interest reflects relational functioning in addition to patient health outcomes.

We combine studies with low and medium levels of family inclusion under the label "family-oriented" because they do not target relational change specifically. Here, we review systematic and strategic reviews of this literature. This overview is organized chronologically.

2012: Family-Oriented Interventions in Multiple Health Conditions

Shields and colleagues (2012) reviewed studies published between 2002 and 2010 that were randomized clinical trials of family interventions for common neurological and cardiac diseases, diabetes, and cancer. They found that most research conducted during this time period evaluated family interventions that were primarily psychoeducational rather than focused on systemic relational factors.

Studies that examined family-oriented interventions included many different types of medical conditions. Their summary included evidence of positive impacts on patients and caregivers in traumatic brain injury and spinal cord injury, with mixed results for families coping with the consequences of a stroke. Studies on family-oriented treatments for cardiac conditions were inconclusive. Results of dyadic interventions to improve cancer coping and outcomes also were mixed; however, evidence supported the use of family interventions at the end of life to improve coping and communication.

Those studies that did evaluate systemic relational interventions and outcomes generally focused on distressed families of children with type 1 diabetes. Multisystemic therapy was found to improve treatment adherence, reducing utilization of emergency services for families with an adolescent with poor glycemic control at baseline. Behavioral family systems therapy was associated with improved glycemic control, improved family cohesion, and decreased conflict around diabetes management when compared with psychoeducation only or no intervention in adolescents with poor glycemic control. These interventions focused specifically on developing a sense of teamwork between adolescents and their parents. A series of these studies published by D. A. Ellis and colleagues (e.g., Ellis et al., 2005a, 2005b, 2007, 2012), yielded similar results and included high proportions of minority children that increased study generalizability. In sum, Shields and colleagues (2012) emphasized the clinical significance of targeting parental involvement for improving diabetes management, particularly for children with poor glycemic control.

Overall, Shields and colleagues (2012) described the state of the research on family interventions for health programs as "developmental." In general, they noted that more research is needed to understand the impact of family-oriented interventions, recognizing especially a relative paucity of research on systemic psychotherapeutic intervention.

2013: A Review of Family-Oriented Interventions for Type 2 Diabetes

Lister et al. (2013) focused exclusively on the impact of dyadic interventions in diabetes management in adults. They did not review studies that examined family therapy interventions per se, so the results reflect the impact of family-oriented interventions. They noted that dyadic educational interventions improved health behaviors (exercise and medication adherence) and enhanced weight loss. Lister and associates argued that including partners in diabetes care and research offered multiple benefits. These include the ability to assess and manage the impact of the nondiabetic partner's behavior on coping and disease management, as well as a greater understanding of how relational factors affect the emotional well-being of both the patient and the partner.

2014: A Review of Cost-Effectiveness of Family and Relational Interventions

Crane and Christenson's 2014 review of family therapy in healthcare focused on the cost-effectiveness of family and relational interventions. They compared the outcomes of family-oriented therapies and systemic relational therapies with individually oriented therapies and control groups that received little to no intervention. Their primary endpoint was the correlation between family psychotherapies and healthcare utilization and costs. From a review of 21 studies, they concluded that family-focused interventions were associated with reduced healthcare utilization, especially for patients who were considered high utilizers of care. They noted: "The evidence presented here supports the argument that family therapy (as a distinct treatment modality) is a cost-effective means of delivering quality services to patients" (Crane & Christenson, 2014, p. 431). However, the review did not establish superiority of relational and systemic therapies' cost-effectiveness over individual treatment modalities.

2014: The Impact of Family Systems Nursing

Östlund and Persson (2014) reviewed how a family systems approach to nursing care impacted health outcomes. This approach to nursing care parallels the approach of family systems therapists, recognizing the family as the unit of care and focusing on relational outcomes. Family systems nursing specifically emphasizes offering families support and health education. Their review revealed that family-oriented educational interventions enhanced understanding of the illness, disease management skills, and overall coping. Family support was correlated with improved family and individual well-being as well as enhanced family functioning, as indicated by improved interactions and higher levels of perceived connection and caring between family members.

2016: Empirically Supported Treatments in Couples and Family Therapy on Health Conditions

A special issue of *Family Process* (Lebow, 2016) reviewed the empirical evidence for various models of family therapy. Here we review those articles that specifically addressed evidence for the efficacy of a given family therapy model in helping families cope with health conditions and the impact of these interventions on health outcomes.

Fischer et al. (2016) reviewed the empirical evidence for cognitive behavior couple therapy (CBCT). They found that CBCT was as effective as individual cognitive behavior therapy for psychological issues, with the added benefit of improved relational functioning. However, they found more variable results when focusing on the impact of CBCT for couples coping with health conditions. They noted a high volume of research that examines the impact of dyadic interventions for couples facing cancer, most focused on psychoeducation for the partner and enhancing the sense of "team" for the couple. The authors stated that couples-based interventions "have positive effects on individual and couples functioning. It is not clear whether, and for which couples, there are unique added [health] benefits" (p. 434). Fischer and colleagues summarized the literature on CBCT for couples living with cardiac disease as showing benefits in successful lifestyle changes and couples functioning. Regarding chronic pain, diabetes, and HIV, the authors noted some areas of promise regarding chronic disease management (including medication adherence) and improved couples coping, acknowledging that the research was still in a developmental phase.

In the same issue, Wiebe and Johnson (2016) reported on the empirical evidence for emotionally focused therapy (EFT) for couples. This research focused on helping couples cope with cancer in a child, with positive effects on the couple's relationships as compared with controls. These benefits may transcend the type of childhood illness, as subsequent research found that EFT for couples with a child with a chronic illness had similar benefits, still evident at 5-year follow-up. Finally, they noted that multiple studies of couples with relationship distress prior to a cancer diagnosis support the use of EFT as more effective than couples' psychoeducational interventions.

Henggeler and Schaeffer (2016) reviewed research that supports the use of multisystemic therapy with couples facing health conditions. They also reviewed research on families living with various pediatric medical conditions. Results correlated multisystemic family therapy with reductions in childhood obesity, improved medication adherence in HIV-positive youth, improved glycemic control in children with type 1 diabetes, and improved asthma control in adolescents.

2019: Couples Interventions for Cancer Survivors and Caregivers

Badr and colleagues (2019) reviewed interventions for cancer survivors and caregivers. They noted that dyadic interventions tend to either engage the partner/caregiver as a "coach" to enhance education and coping for the person with cancer or address dyadic functioning more directly in an attempt to address the needs and concerns of both partners. They summarized the outcome literature as showing small to moderate effects for the impact of dyadic interventions on survivor and caregiver emotional functioning. However, they noted less robust impacts on dyadic relational functioning, with limited information regarding the durability of any positive effects. They also described the impact of these interventions on physical health outcomes as small. Importantly, they recognized that the effect sizes may reflect the seriousness of the disease, especially for patients living with metastatic cancer. They also noted that they were unable to determine what effect sizes reflect clinically meaningful impacts. As did others, they called for research that more specifically addresses clinical significance of systemic relationally oriented therapies.

2019: A Review of Systemic Reviews Regarding Family Involvement in Chronic Disease Care

Gilliss and colleagues (2019) conducted a systematic review of systematic reviews regarding the impact of family involvement in adult chronic disease care. They used rigorous inclusion criteria that winnowed 364 systemic reviews down to 10 reviews that focused on either diabetes (1), coronary disease (1), poststroke management (1), cancer (4), and varied chronic physical illnesses (3). As did other reviewers, they noted overall low levels of family involvement in clinical interventions with family members primarily involved to support medical treatment regimens at home. The studies gave little attention to the impact of interventions on family relationships and dynamics, focusing more on helping the family member provide care. Their general summary stated:

> The evidence for the *added value of family intervention* over *intervention with a single individual* has generally not demonstrated added value for the family [itself]. In contrast, the majority of these studies do show some benefit [of family involvement] to the identified patient. In all likelihood, this stems from a common approach to interventions in which family members or other informal care partners are employed as surrogates for formal healthcare providers. (p. 24)

2020: Family Interventions for Childhood Obesity

J. D. Smith et al. (2020) reviewed the literature on the prevention and management of childhood obesity. As noted earlier, there is significant evidence that home environment and family functioning play a role in weight issues for children. However, little research has evaluated systemic relational interventions to reduce overweight. Smith and colleagues (2020) described a significant increase in family-oriented interventions for childhood obesity over the past 2 decades. Their review of the evidence for family-oriented childhood-obesity management interventions noted that many interventions actively engage parents as change agents to address underlying environmental and behavioral issues associated with childhood obesity (Sung-Chen et al., 2013). Most studies used randomized controlled trial methodology, but interventions tended to be short-term, occurring only in one environment (e.g., school vs. home vs. community), with parental involvement decreasing as the child matured. They cited Kothandan's 2014 summation that family-based interventions were effective for prepubescent (under 12 years old) children, whereas school-based interventions appeared to be most effective for ages 12 and up. These interventions target psychoeducation, establishment of rules and boundaries, family communication, and dynamics, with a focus on physical activity and dietary habit change. The evidence for these interventions is robust, with research now shifting toward specifying which elements work best with which populations under what circumstances.

The authors noted that there is much to be learned regarding childhood-obesity interventions across cultures and suggested a focus on how existing interventions can be adapted to families from various cultures, socioeconomic status, and backgrounds. They highlighted a program known as the Family Check-Up4 Health being tested in pediatric primary care (J. D. Smith et al., 2018) and in community settings (Berkel et al., 2019) in low-income diverse neighborhoods with high rates of childhood obesity.

A subsequent systematic review and meta-analysis by St. George and colleagues (2022) that focused specifically on childhood obesity in Hispanic populations noted overall small effect sizes. They highlighted how policy and dissemination could ensure these programs are implemented at the population level to maximize impact. St. George and associates also emphasized the need for more research to direct care for culturally diverse populations.

2022: Review of Family Interventions in Common High-Mortality Conditions

Lamson and colleagues (2022) conducted a strategic review of 87 couple and family health-focused interventions published between 2010 and 2019. They noted that the review was defined as "strategic" rather than "systematic" because the study selection process included multiple people as secondary coders, rather than one consistent coder. Although influenced by the review conducted by Shields and colleagues in 2012, their methodology was quite different in that they focused only on research findings for high-morbidity conditions across the lifespan rather than on disease states that have been studied extensively. The high-morbidity disease states selected for this review were based on Centers for Disease Control and Prevention data, as follows:

- ages 0–4: Congenital malformations, deformations and chromosomal anomalies, and accidents/unintentional injuries;

- ages 5–14: Accidents/unintentional injuries and cancer;

- ages 15–24: Accidents/unintentional injuries; and

- ages 25–end of life: Heart disease, cancer, accidents/unintentional injuries, chronic lower respiratory diseases, stroke, Alzheimer's disease, diabetes, kidney disease, and obesity (Lamson et al., 2022).

The reviewers used Pratt and Sonney's (2020) levels of family inclusion and Southam-Gerow and Prinstein's level of efficacy (2014) to guide the review. Notably, less than 1% of studies that examined some aspect of family inclusion and intervention with health conditions met strategic review inclusion requirements. Many of the studies had low to moderate levels of family inclusion. Overall, the authors stated, "The evidence presented in this strategic review suggests that there has been little movement in the development of well-established couple and family interventions (in context of health) since the previous review by Shields et al. (2012)" (Lamson et al., 2022, p. 331).

However, the authors noted that the review highlights the enhanced efficacy of interventions that include family members in the management of health conditions, particularly changes in health behaviors. Lamson et al. (2022) also stated that the lack of strong evidence regarding systemic relational interventions is due largely to a paucity of research that includes family members in health-focused or related relational interventions, with a specific dearth of studies examining the impact of systemic interventions on relational functioning and family dynamics.

WHAT IS NEEDED NOW?

As our review illustrates, we are in an early stage of understanding the intersection of family variables and health, including the most effective ways to help families successfully manage health conditions. We are in particular need of intervention research to guide clinicians in the practice of medical family therapy. Until relatively recently, research was focused on the impact of simply including family members in care processes, and outcome measures of interest were generally medical, rather than relational. In the past few years researchers have started to investigate the impact of family inclusion on the wellness of not just the patient but also other family members, family relationships, and functioning. We also need research that examines specific systemic relational interventions on disease management success, relational functioning, and mitigation of potential negative impacts of health conditions on the family as a unit.

As a caveat, we also want to acknowledge the inherent problems in an umbrella review such as this. Although this type of overview does serve the purpose of describing the lay of the land, it also reduces attention to nuance and does not outline study characteristics that might enable the reader to apply the results to a specific disease state, population, or situation. As Gilliss and colleagues (2019) stated regarding their review: "The heterogeneity of diseases, samples, treatment content, dosage, delivery methods, and outcome measures complicate meaningful data synthesis across these family studies" (p. 22). In recognition of this reality, in Chapters 9, 10, and 11 on adult, pediatric, and women's health settings, we review specific studies that evaluated systemic relational interventions (high family inclusion, in Pratt and Sonney's nomenclature).

SUMMARY

This summary of literature reviews highlights the degree to which our current knowledge regarding the intersection of families and health is incomplete. Some evidence does support involving families in management of conditions that require significant lifestyle adjustment because family involvement may facilitate these adjustments. In addition, there is evidence that patients and partners experience reduced distress and enhanced coping when partners are included in care, particularly if the couple was distressed prior to the illness onset or the disease is particularly intrusive on daily functioning. The impact of systemic interventions on family relational functioning is less clear. Overall, when researchers include family functioning outcome measures, there have been some positive results. We might conclude, as Shields and colleagues did in 2012, that "the existing literature shows that there is potential for family interventions to reduce patient and caregiver distress, to improve patient functioning through greater adherence to medical regimens, and to strengthen family and couple relationships" (p. 273). Yet many of the same methodological and conceptual problems continue to be reflected in ongoing research, despite calls for shifts to address these challenges. The struggle continues to capture the complexity of systemic relational interventions, use outcomes that measure relational impacts, use diverse sample populations, and ensure interventions meet criteria for relational psychotherapy and high family inclusion.

In some ways, the status of research evaluating the metaframework of medical family therapy parallels that of the research that examines the impact of integrated behavioral health as a model of care. Just as integrated behavioral health takes many forms, medical family therapy integrates many individual and relational therapeutic strategies. While this complexity matches the human experience, it is not easily studied. We seek to understand complex, heterogeneous phenomena that are ill-suited to randomized controlled trials.

TAKEAWAY POINTS

- There is evidence that including family members in care for medical conditions can enhance outcomes, particularly when the condition impairs functioning or management requires substantial lifestyle modification.

- The vast majority of studies researching the intersection of families and health have focused on dyads, with few evaluating interventions that align with systemic family therapy.

- Research evidence on the impact of the metaframework of medical family therapy is still in a developmental stage, perhaps secondary to the challenges inherent in capturing complex processes and outcomes.

9

ADULT HEALTHCARE

Many integrated care concepts and clinical strategies have focused on caring for adults as individuals, largely removed from their family and social context. Yet social support and healthy family functioning are crucial to overall health and wellness. The patient's interface with larger system structures, the healthcare system itself, and sociocultural factors are also key. In this chapter, we make the case for a systemic lens for adult healthcare services, with a focus on chronic disease management.

About half of the general adult population has at least one chronic condition (B. W. Ward et al., 2014). The Milken Institute (Waters & Graf, 2018) used data from 2016 to estimate the cost of healthcare for chronic disease in the United States to be approximately $1.1 trillion, with indirect costs (e.g., lost productivity, family caregiving) of $3.7 trillion. They noted the six most common chronic conditions are poorly regulated cholesterol, hypertension, arthritis, type 2 diabetes, chronic back pain, and asthma.

Health behaviors form the most common, changeable risk factors for chronic disease. The Milken Institute (Waters & Graf, 2018) reported that obesity is the most common risk factor, followed by smoking and excessive

https://doi.org/10.1037/0000381-010
A Systemic Approach to Behavioral Healthcare Integration: Context Matters, by
N. B. Ruddy and S. H. McDaniel

drinking. Increased family and social support is correlated with successful health behavior change (Pietromonaco & Collins, 2017). However, the specifics of how to engage families in successful behavioral change are still unclear (e.g., Hubbard et al., 2016). Some evidence supports that involving families in behavior change related to a specific illness may improve adherence. For example, in cardiac disease management, dyadic interventions improved adherence to an exercise regimen and medication adherence (Sher et al., 2014). Similar improvements in adherence to regimen have been found in diabetes such that treatment guidelines recommend involving the family in medical care (Young-Hyman et al., 2016) and supportive educational programs for people with diabetes (Powers et al., 2020).

In the United States, people who live with chronic illnesses must maneuver through a challenging healthcare system and often contend with access challenges. In addition, many chronic diseases are expensive to treat, and people must manage the complex reimbursement system to get services and medications (Sav et al., 2015).

On a population level, people from marginalized groups have significantly worse outcomes in most chronic disease categories (e.g., James et al., 2017). These outcomes reflect access to care problems, the impact of socioeconomic disadvantage, and well-documented issues in the healthcare system vis-à-vis care for minorities and the poor. Recent research draws a direct line between the impact of the chronic stress of systemic racism and heteronormativity and chronic inflammatory processes and immunosuppression, possibly another link between these systemic factors and health outcomes (Brody et al., 2020; Flentje et al., 2020). This research emphasizes the importance of ensuring family-based interventions are culturally adjusted to enhance effectiveness (McEwen et al., 2017, 2019).

Involving families in care may also support primary prevention. One promising area focuses on the use of the Marriage (or Couples) Checkup (Cordova, 2009, 2014) adapted for use in primary care. The Air Force is currently evaluating the checkup, which typically occurs across three 30-minute sessions with an integrated behavioral health clinician. The clinician provides psychoeducation regarding common stressors in military couples and relationship-building strategies to mitigate these stressors (Cordova et al., 2017). This couples intervention has been shown to be efficacious in military primary care settings with positive outcomes related to relationship satisfaction, depression symptoms, and work stress (Cigrang et al., 2022).

In Chapters 7 and 8, we focused on the interface of health and families in broad brushstrokes, with a focus on systemic interventions for individuals and families living with a health condition. Here, in Chapter 9, we revisit

Woods and colleagues' (2020) systematic review of the literature on family systems and adult health. They described the following 10 themes in the relationship between families and health that inform integrated services for adults, particularly those living with a chronic medical condition:

- The impact of positive family relationships and support: "Life satisfaction" is associated with better health and better outcomes for people with health issues. However, research outcomes were not always specific to family satisfaction, making interpretation of these results somewhat difficult.

- The impact of family conflict: Studies show that family conflict over time is associated with level of somatic symptoms and worse outcomes in older adults. Overall, family conflict is negatively correlated with self-reported health status and health-related quality of life (e.g., Widmer et al., 2018).

- Family composition: Multiple studies noted that fewer women in the home is related to poorer health outcomes (e.g., Mondesire et al., 2016).

- Role of psychophysiological mediators in health: Stress and, to a lesser degree, family stress have been associated with inflammation and increased activity in the hypothalamic–pituitary–adrenal and sympathetic nervous systems, both associated with chronic conditions (e.g., Priest et al., 2019).

- Health behaviors: Health behaviors and family functioning are closely related.

- Communication: Communication about health within the family was positively associated with family members seeking health information (Yang et al., 2017). In contrast, avoiding discussion of health issues (cancer, in particular) was associated with worse physical and mental health outcomes (Shin et al., 2016).

- Attendance at healthcare appointments: In general, family member attendance at healthcare visits is associated with better understanding of visit content and improved self-care (e.g., Cené, 2015).

- Family interventions to improve self-care: Most research has focused on families living with diabetes, finding positive impact for family interventions that improve social support and help the patient improve self-care (e.g., Baig et al., 2015).

- Impact of caregiving on health: As we described in Chapter 8, the impact of caregiving on health is complex. Substantial evidence relates caregiving to the onset of health issues as well as poor outcomes in existing health issues, particularly with high caregiving burden and lack of reciprocal relationship (such as when caring for a person with dementia). Woods and colleagues (2020) called for research to identify protective interventions for adult caregivers of a partner or child, as they appear to experience more adverse effects than do adult children caring for aging parents.

- Family relationships and health in later life: For older adults, living situations appear to align with health status (e.g., people with more health conditions were more likely to live with offspring). Positive relationships earlier in the family's development were associated with greater elder health, whereas stepfamily structures were associated with earlier placement for elders with serious illness and functional impairment. Of note, most of this research was completed in China, where caregiving relationships may be very different than in the West.

Given the ubiquity of chronic disease in healthcare, we now shift to focus on the management of chronic conditions in integrated care. We first discuss chronic disease management. We then present common reactions to chronic illness and coping strategies. Often, individuals within the family respond differently, and relational patterns can support or impair chronic disease self-management. Whereas self-management implies management by an individual, with any health or illness issue, relationships are usually part of that process. So, to be clear, in systemic integrated care we use the prevalent term *self-management* to reflect the ways both the individual patient and their family work to manage the chronic illness itself as well as the impact the chronic illness has on their lives. In this context, we discuss strategies to help families adjust to the illness over time and ways to address problematic relational patterns. Finally, we review how healthcare teams can engage family members and other social supports in their communities to help patients successfully self-manage their illness.

Here we focus on integrating families into care for chronic conditions in a manner consistent with the chronic care model's emphasis on supporting self-care (Wagner et al., 1996). The chronic care model recognizes that all care occurs in the context of the broader healthcare system, which may not engender an experience of empowerment. In a systemic review seeking to identify the effectiveness of model elements, Davy and colleagues (2015) concluded,

> Several factors including supporting reflective healthcare practice, sending clear messages about the importance of chronic disease care and ensuring that leaders support the implementation and sustainability of interventions, may have been just as important as a chronic care model's elements in contributing to the improvements in healthcare practice or health outcomes for people living with chronic disease. (p. 1)

A critical element in supporting families living with chronic conditions is to create patient-centric, empowering care systems as discussed in Part II of this book.

CHRONIC DISEASE MANAGEMENT WITH COUPLES AND FAMILIES

As noted earlier, the families and health research tends to focus primarily on the partner or marriage relationship. Our focus here is on family-based interventions for specific conditions. We review studies that examine specific family therapy interventions and provide information regarding the impact of the intervention on couples functioning.

Cancer

For couples facing cancer, engaging partners via supportive encounters and psychoeducation has been found to reduce patient and caregiver distress (Badr et al., 2019; Northouse et al., 2012). Manne and colleagues (2014, 2019) found that intimacy-enhancing couples therapy improved relationship satisfaction for couples facing breast and prostate cancer but had a less clear effect on the impact of the illness itself. Their summary stated, "Helping couples consider ways they can maintain normalcy and quality during the cancer experience, framing coping with cancer as a [team] effort may facilitate better communication and ultimately enhance relationship intimacy" (p. 314). Cognitive–existential couples therapy for couples living with prostate cancer also improved coping and lowered cancer distress for partners (Couper et al., 2015). Emotion-focused couples therapy helped families cope with advanced cancer. Finally, family-focused therapy during palliative care reduced the severity of complicated grief and the likelihood of a prolonged grief disorder for high-risk families (Kissane et al., 2016).

Cardiovascular and Pulmonary Conditions

Compared with cancer, less research has been conducted on family therapy interventions for cardiovascular and pulmonary conditions. Evidence exists that including families in pulmonary rehabilitation programs for patients with chronic obstructive pulmonary disease reduces patient distress, but the impact on the dyadic relationship and distress in caregivers is less clear (Figueiredo et al., 2016; Marques et al., 2015). Dyadic intervention in cardiac disease management improves self-management and couples functioning

(Sher et al., 2014). Furthermore, the dyadic intervention helped couples with initial poor marital satisfaction improve, whereas low-satisfaction couples who did not receive the dyadic intervention experienced further decline in relationship quality. For poststroke patients, Robinson-Smith and colleagues (2016) found that dyadic intervention helped reduce depressive symptoms and improved quality of life for patients. In general, these couples interventions appear to have some disease management benefits, improve disease coping, and improve or protect the quality of the couple's relationship.

Diabetes

A great deal of research has focused on involving family members to enhance adherence to the many lifestyle adaptations necessary to manage diabetes. Surprisingly few have examined how family interventions affect family functioning and relational health for adults living with diabetes (Baig et al., 2015). Further research is needed on family variables in type 2 diabetes, given the studies that correlate poor glycemic control with negative family behaviors such as stigmatizing the illness and self-care behaviors, blaming the patient for diabetes onset, and sabotaging self-care efforts (Mayberry & Osborn, 2014). In addition, survey data indicate that families experience significant distress and treatment burden related to diabetes in a family member (Kovacs Burns et al., 2013). The potential of family involvement to improve health, psychological, and relational outcomes in type 2 diabetes is recognized, but current research offers little guidance as to best practices in systemic relational interventions (Pamungkas et al., 2017).

Facilitating Family-Based Chronic Disease Management

Sturhahn and colleagues (2017) recommended a three-step model to create a practice structure that engages families and achieves family-centered healthcare:

- Step 1: Inclusion of family members from the "front desk to the exam room,"
- Step 2: Education for family members regarding mental health and medical concerns, and
- Step 3: Targeted therapy for families with relational or systemic concerns.

They noted that psychosocial assessment that includes family factors can enhance care and help clinicians understand the patient's context and risk factors. They also recommended routinely obtaining consent to involve family members early in care, rather than waiting for an issue to arise. In this model, family-centered care is part of the DNA of the practice that engages all staff and clinicians to include relational elements in their patient interactions and conceptualizations of issues and solutions.

Implementing integrated behavioral health is, in and of itself, one of the most effective ways a healthcare practice can improve chronic disease management. Broadly, interprofessional, team-based care has been shown to improve chronic disease outcomes (Pascucci et al., 2021). For example, the Collaborative Care Model (CoCM) of integrated care improved chronic disease management for those patients who have concomitant chronic disease and serious mental health issues (Katon et al., 2010). Given that mental health issues are approximately twice as likely in people with chronic disease and that outcomes are worse and costs higher, those with both mental health issues and chronic medical conditions are an important target for prevention (Rossom et al., 2017).

To be effective, an integrated behavioral health service must have processes to identify patients struggling with self-management and offer outreach and ongoing support. In parallel, medical clinicians should be made aware of research findings that indicate behavioral health involvement with patients improves chronic disease self-management.

As medical reimbursement in the United States begins to shift toward value-based pay-for-performance, medical practices are under increased pressure to produce better health outcomes. Unfortunately, when patients struggle with self-care, medical clinicians may feel as if they are being held accountable for something over which they have little control. This response can easily spiral into frustration, even patient-blaming. Integrated care can interrupt this cycle. The behavioral health clinician can coach the medical clinician, offering clinical tools as well as support. Empathizing and acknowledging the effort staff and clinicians have expended in care provision can avoid a negative spiral of criticism among the patient, medical clinician, and behavioral health clinician (McDaniel, Doherty, & Hepworth, 2014). As McDaniel and colleagues (2014) stated, "Ultimately, the medical family therapist tries to promote agency and communion for all involved: the patient, the family, the provider and provider team, and oneself" (p. 148).

Other practice-level interventions to improve a sense of agency and communion for patients include joint appointments with multiple members of the care team, group medical appointments, and psychoeducational and support groups. Systemically oriented practices often include family members and other key supports in these groups, along with psychoeducation about the impact of chronic disease on family relationships and the impact of family relationships on chronic disease (Hodgson et al., 2018). These groups expose patients and families to others' experience managing ill health and may normalize the inevitable distress. They also enable conversations regarding cultural and family beliefs about health and illness, such as how one should act when ill, the meaning of various illnesses (sometimes based in beliefs about the origin of an illness), and what types of treatments are appropriate and acceptable (Rolland, 2018). Hearing how other families manage issues can allow members to consider alternative viewpoints both within and outside their own family.

In terms of health behavior change, behavioral health clinicians are often guided by two rubrics—SBIRT and the "5 A's" model. Both can facilitate assessment, intervention, and collaborative treatment planning for behavior related to chronic disease management (Glasgow et al., 2006), as well as for mental health and substance misuse issues (Babor et al., 2007; Hargraves et al., 2017). SBIRT stands for screening, brief intervention, refer to treatment. In this model, a patient who screens positive for a given issue receives a brief behavioral health intervention. If these interventions alleviate the symptoms, the patient returns to routine care with some additional monitoring to address any recurrence. If brief interventions are not successful, the team refers the patient to specialty mental health or substance misuse treatment. The patient then is to return to routine care when specialty intervention is no longer warranted.

In parallel, the "5 A's" process guides clinicians to *assess* patient's (and family's) current behaviors, beliefs, and motivations regarding a specific issue. Systemic management of chronic disease includes eliciting the patient's and family's key concerns, readiness to change, and desired endpoints. The clinician can then *advise* patients as to the best path forward based on their personal health risk, ensuring the patient and family *agree* on a realistic set of goals. The clinician then *assists* the patient and family to anticipate barriers to follow-up in this plan and then *arrange* follow-up support. A review of potential referral barriers and assistance in overcoming them is important to successful referral and follow-up (Glasgow, Goldstein, et al., 2004). The "5 A's" approach tailors decision making and action planning to the patient and family, helping families use resources and establish a good relationship with the care team (Suleman et al., 2021). Each of the '5 A's" has been shown to support self-care (P. Ryan & Sawin, 2009), encompassing self-management elements such as medical and emotional management of the chronic condition (Lorig et al., 2001).

Individually focused strategies for self-care include motivational interviewing, cognitive behavior therapy (Barrett et al., 2018), psychoeducation, and supportive interventions (Allegrante et al., 2019). Each can be implemented at the family systems level as well (Gance-Cleveland, 2005). With couples, cognitive behavior and skills-building interventions have been found to be particularly helpful with chronic medical conditions (Berry et al., 2017).

Family-oriented clinicians focus on how a particular chronic illness affects daily family life. Rolland's (2018) typology[1] described common concerns related to specific illnesses, which then can help elicit additional concerns from the family. Inquiring about common concerns normalizes inevitable struggles and can initiate discussions about challenges they might otherwise not acknowledge or feel they can discuss. In addition, the clinician must assess the quality of family involvement in chronic disease management. Obstructive behaviors by family (e.g., nagging, interfering with self-care) should be addressed as they are associated with poor self-management, poor outcomes (Mayberry & Osborn, 2014), and relationship problems.

CONTINUA RELEVANT TO SYSTEMIC CHRONIC CARE SELF-MANAGEMENT

The quality of family coping with chronic illness falls along a series of continua, illustrated in Figure 9.1. Assessing each family member's place on these continua helps to identify polarized areas at risk for conflict about illness management. Ideally, differing perspectives are normalized as the clinician helps the family communicate and accept and evolve in their differing positions. This process must be completed with care to ensure that the clinician's own beliefs are not presented as "correct" or superior to other opinions. Humility and respect for the family's knowledge of their own situation are key. Over time acceptance helps families negotiate a way forward that is acceptable to all. Understanding these continua can also help clinicians with assessment, setting their own expectations in recognition of the patient's and family's differing levels of motivation, readiness to change, and acceptance of/agreement with the stated treatment plan.

In Chapters 9, 10, and 11, we discuss common presentations associated with chronic disease coping. We also offer systemic strategies to address self-management issues related to these continua.

---

[1] Rolland's illness typology is described in detail in Chapter 7.

FIGURE 9.1. Continua of Family Coping With Chronic Illness

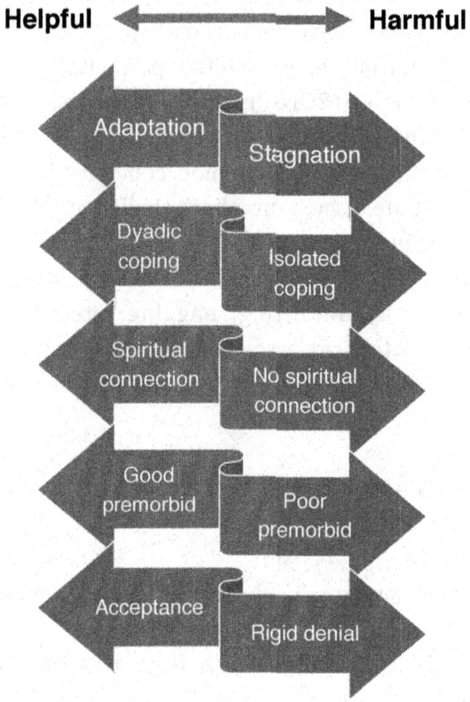

Helpful ⟵⟶ Harmful

Adaptation — Stagnation

Dyadic coping — Isolated coping

Spiritual connection — No spiritual connection

Good premorbid — Poor premorbid

Acceptance — Rigid denial

Continuum 1: Acceptance and Denial of Illness Chronicity

To help patients mitigate the impact of chronic diseases with effective self-management, they must realize that the condition is not, or is no longer, acute. Many people struggle to accept the reality that a symptom or health condition is not going to go away. Furthermore, different members of the family may fall at different points on this continuum, and polarized opinions can spark conflict. Eliciting each person's perspective regarding the illness can highlight the normal, inevitable differences, which can be explored and sometimes resolved. In some circumstances, overt discussion can raise awareness of differences in perspective and opinion as they relate to these continua. Ultimately, recognizing that the illness and its impact are not going to disappear sets the stage for the individual and family to realize they need to make adaptations and seek a new normal. It also allows the patient and family to manage the symptom or condition, rather than focusing on finding a cure. This refocus is particularly important when the symptom in question is very troubling or intrusive on daily life, such as moderate to severe pain (Thompson & McCracken, 2011).

It is also helpful to consider where each member of the family is on the acceptance and denial continuum. Each individual's level of acceptance and denial is dynamic over time and circumstances. Conflict can ensue when there is great variation, and the family may need assistance in recognizing, accepting, and managing these differences. Issues related to acceptance and denial are illustrated by Fran's[2] situation, in which her belief about her symptoms denied their severity, while her children hoped that her physician would help their mother accept her chronic illness:

Fran was diagnosed with chronic obstructive pulmonary disorder (COPD) when she was 48, after years of heavy smoking. Fran lived alone but maintained a close relationship with three of her four adult children and their families, all of whom worried that Fran was more sick than she acknowledged. She met with Dr. Thompson, the behavioral health clinician, a few times shortly after her diagnosis. Her medical clinician, Ms. Young, was frustrated with Fran because she took her medications only when she was having symptoms; she did not seem to understand that her symptoms reflected an underlying disease process. Dr. Thompson explored Fran's understanding of her symptoms. Fran said that her father "had a cough" for the last 20 years of his life, but it "was nothing." Fran believed that she had the same cough. She was adamant that coughing was her only issue and denied being short of breath at other times, even though her pulmonary function tests showed ongoing decline.

Systemic Integrated Care Strategies to Address the Acceptance–Denial Continuum

Recognize and name each family member's level of acceptance or denial of the illness. Where needed, help the family accept these differences. Where possible, work through any conflicts that may arise secondary to these differences. Medical and behavioral health clinicians can provide psychoeducation about the illness, overtly discussing with patients and families the emotional and mental shifts they must make when a symptom or condition becomes chronic. They can help the patient and family understand how to mitigate symptoms or flares while also recognizing the losses inherent in a chronic condition. A consistent message from the entire team can help the family begin to accept new realities and necessary changes.

Dr. Thompson quickly realized that Fran was not ready to accept a diagnosis of a chronic illness, let alone engage in self-management and

---

[2]The case description aligns with common presentations in healthcare but does not reflect a real person or specific situation.

make important behavioral changes such as smoking cessation. She consulted with Ms. Young to share Fran's low readiness and motivation for change and encouraged a focus on relationship development. The treatment team discussed the likelihood that Fran might not address her breathing issues until she experienced a critical incident that sharply affected her functioning. A couple of months later, Dr. Thompson asked Fran if she would be willing to have her children come to a medical appointment with Ms. Young to answer any questions they might have. Fran agreed. Two of Fran's children, Amelia and Joanne, attended an appointment with Ms. Young and Dr. Thompson. Amelia and Joanne were quite concerned about their mother and expressed a great deal of frustration that she was unwilling to cut down on her smoking. They confronted Fran with examples of how her breathing issues affected her functioning and reminded Fran that her father had become more incapacitated by "the cough" over time. They encouraged Fran to work with the treatment team to help her stay healthy as long as possible, expressing their love for her and desire to have her be part of her grandchildren's lives.

Continuum 2: Level of Adaptation to a "New Normal" and Willingness to Make Ongoing Adaptations

Adapting to a new normal requires patients and families to take charge of what can be changed and accepting what cannot. The degree of adaptation depends on the illness's characteristics. Regardless, behavioral health clinicians can help families find an acceptable new normal that aligns with their goals and values, as seen with Fran and her family.

> Fran loved being "Grandma" and was the primary caregiver of her daughter Amelia's three young children 2 days each week. Initially Fran had no problem taking care of the kids, but 3 years into her diagnosis, she had a serious flare-up that adversely affected her energy and daily functioning. Fran's other daughter, Joanne, came with her to a medical appointment and reported that the caregiving role was "too much" for Fran but that Fran refused to talk to Amelia about the issue.

Systemic Integrated Care Strategies to Address Adaptation/Stagnation Continuum Challenges

At times, the concept of a new normal can be a helpful starting point for dialogue. Even in a brief encounter, clinicians can differentiate the perfect outcome from an acceptable outcome. Clinicians can help the patient and family recognize where progress may continue and where the current plateau is unlikely to change significantly. Family psychoeducation illuminates available options. Support groups not only increase social support but also provide models for adaptation to living with a given condition.

> Ms. Young heard Joanne's concerns and asked Fran for her perspective. Fran acknowledged that caring for her grandchildren was getting to be too much, leaving her exhausted for much of the rest of the week. Yet Fran felt guilty for "letting Amelia down" and expressed concern she wouldn't see her grandchildren as much if she did not continue to care for them. Ms. Young asked if they would like to meet briefly with Dr. Thompson to chart a path forward. They agreed. Dr. Thompson asked them what they thought Amelia would say if she were there. Joanne said that Amelia was actually quite worried about Fran but had been hesitant to bring it up. Dr. Thompson helped Fran plan a conversation with Amelia. They discussed how Fran's role didn't need to be "all or nothing" and how she could maintain a close connection to her beloved grandchildren.
>
> Fran had a medical appointment about a month later. Dr. Thompson met with her briefly as she was waiting for Ms. Young. Dr. Thompson and Fran discussed Amelia's positive reaction to Fran's concerns and how she was helping Fran maintain contact with her grandchildren without becoming overwhelmed. Fran also completed a depression inventory because Dr. Thompson knew that declines in functioning are often accompanied by mood changes. Through the screen, Fran did report symptoms consistent with moderate depression and acknowledged that her reduced capacity was troubling to her. They agreed that Dr. Thompson would check in with her at each appointment. He and Fran then talked with Ms. Young for a few minutes to alert her to Fran's struggles and share the plan. Ms. Young introduced the idea of psychotropic medication, but Fran was not willing to consider taking antidepressants.

Part of adapting to a new normal is integrating necessary disease management behaviors and lifestyle changes into daily life. Self-management involves monitoring symptoms, taking medications as prescribed, attending medical appointments, and making necessary lifestyle changes (Martire & Helgeson, 2017). Conditions that require a great deal of lifestyle change or those with a high disease burden (e.g., requiring resources such as time and money to manage) can be particularly challenging (Heckman et al.,

2015). Research indicates that health behaviors often are shared among family members, particularly partners or spouses (Jeong & Cho, 2018; K. K. Li et al., 2013). Not surprisingly, then, improvement in one partner has been found to predict improvement in the other (Jackson et al., 2015).

A systematic review of family interventions found evidence they improve adherence to prescribed medical regimens (Shields et al., 2012). However, if family members do not see a need to change health behaviors or continue to engage in behaviors inconsistent with the treatment plan, the patient as well is unlikely to make and sustain changes. For example, patients who do not have family support are less likely to be adherent to prescribed medications (T. A. Miller & DiMatteo, 2013).

> Fran had been a heavy smoker since her teens and "loved" smoking. Dr. Thompson and Ms. Young checked in with Fran regularly about her readiness to address her smoking habit, with the check-in becoming a shorthand of "So, about the smoking, how ready are you today?" Fran's consistent response was a resolute "Zero!"

Individual strategies often center on consistently asking the patient about their motivation to change and belief in their ability to accomplish that change. As with Fran's response about readiness to quit smoking, scaling questions (on a scale from 1 to 10) not only delineate the degree of motivation but also set the stage to use motivational interviewing strategies with multiple members of the family. For example, when asked about their motivation for their mother to quit smoking, Fran's daughters would likely select a different number than Fran's own response of "zero." The clinician can then ask each family member the reasons behind their motivation level and those factors that push them toward, or away from, change. These dialogues offer an opportunity to ease any tension and frame family assistance with chronic disease management as a way to show caring and concern.

People with chronic illnesses such as COPD often blame themselves for their illness (Plaufcan et al., 2012), so ensuring the family's conversation is supportive, rather than blaming, is key. The behavioral health clinician can play a key role in helping the patient and family address feelings of guilt and blame as well as how these feelings relate to the family's relational history.

> As Fran's functioning declined, she began to beat herself up about her smoking and her failure to heed warnings earlier. She felt incredibly guilty about the impact the illness had on her family, particularly the

reality that they now cared for her, rather than her caring for them. Ms. Young normalized this guilt and worked with Fran to identify ways to forgive herself. Fran eventually became active with an anti-smoking education group, using her story to deter young people from starting to smoke. This work brought her some peace and a sense of meaning in her own struggle.

Fran's children had a very difficult time moving past their feelings of anger and blame. They wanted to be present and supportive of their mother but had strong residual feelings about Fran's inability to quit smoking earlier. It became clear over time that their anger about her smoking also reflected anger about other ways Fran and their father had let them down. Dr. Thompson helped the children realize they were funneling all of their disappointment into the smoking issue and begin to work on healing old wounds in their own therapy. She also helped them talk to Fran about some of their painful memories and supported Fran in hearing them. Dr. Thompson reframed this process as a way the illness gave the family an opportunity to have needed discussions—discussions many children and parents never have. The family acknowledged they likely never would have talked about these issues if not for Fran's illness. Fran's openness to her children's concerns helped smooth over some painful memories for her children, who then were able to be more present to support her as her illness progressed.

Scaling questions regarding belief in one's ability to change spur conversations about perceived barriers to change. Awareness creates an opportunity to problem-solve with the patient and family. The conversation also may reveal barriers that the care team did not know. Even highly motivated people struggle with chronic disease management over time, experiencing a reduced impact of any interventions over time. They have *management fatigue*, a term that describes how patients often simply run out of steam. These issues can interfere with coping and maintaining gains (Heckman et al., 2015; Park et al., 2019). Reminding the treatment team, patient, and family of these realities and normalizing how challenging they can be helps to set the stage to expect occasional relapses that can be overcome. These discussions also contribute to a collaborative rather than contentious relationship between the care team, patient, and family.

Issues with adherence to the medical plan may also reflect a disconnect between the family and the primary or specialty care team. Sometimes clinicians believe there is resistance to, as opposed to disagreement about, the plan. Patients and families are often reluctant to express disagreement unless clinicians encourage them directly to express their concerns. Clinicians can diminish adherence problems by aligning their recommendations with the patient's and family's readiness to change, matching their recommendations to their level of motivation (Prochaska et al., 2013).

> About 3 years after her diagnosis, Fran had an upper respiratory infection that took months to resolve. She felt miserable all the time and had to withdraw from friends and family because she had no energy. As the infection started to clear, Ms. Young ended an appointment as usual with "So, how ready are you today?" To her surprise, Fran said, "Eight! Yep. Today's the day. I don't want to live like this anymore." Ms. Young practically ran down the hall to get Dr. Thompson, who met with Fran for about 15 minutes to generate a quit-smoking plan. Fran agreed to come back to follow up.
>
> At the next appointment, Dr. Thompson asked Fran who could best help her be successful with the quit plan. Fran said that her son, John, had quit smoking a few years before, and she hoped he might help her. John wasn't able to come to an appointment, but Fran talked with him about her plan and he agreed to work with her. Furthermore, he offered strategies that had helped him quit, some of which Fran found very helpful. She and John had become a bit distant because he was very busy, and Fran was very touched that John put aside other commitments to help her reduce her smoking.

Continuum 3: Degree of Dyadic Coping

Dyadic coping refers to the degree to which the partners or family view ownership of the illness in the individual versus in the couple or family. Dyadic coping refers to the nature of the couple's involvement in illness management (Martire & Helgeson, 2017). Berg and Upchurch (2007) argued that illness management is facilitated by a shared illness appraisal in which family members view the illness as a family matter. They also noted that collaborative behaviors among family members are most likely to support successful disease self-management.

Couples research delves deeper into various dyadic coping behaviors and their relationship to disease self-management and health outcomes. Falconier and Kuhn (2019) identified dyadic coping dimensions including how the couple communicates about their experience of stress, positive dyadic coping in one versus both partners, and negative dyadic coping in one versus both partners. Positive dyadic coping includes behaviors such as empathic responding and active engagement, whereas negative dyadic coping includes overprotection, disengaged avoidance, hostility, and ambivalence. These results validate earlier research that associates positive dyadic coping with better disease management. Negative dyadic coping or pressure such as nagging or generating guilt for the patient has been associated with poorer illness management in a variety of conditions (Fekete et al., 2009; Martire & Helgeson, 2017).

Systemic Integrated Care Strategies to Improve Dyadic Coping

Offering psychoeducation and normalizing worry or frustration that may underlie controlling behavior by family members may help some family members interact differently with the patient.

> In a routine appointment, Fran told Ms. Young that she felt her children were trying to run her life. Ms. Young asked Dr. Thompson to reach out to Fran to discuss her concerns. They had a brief phone conversation in which Dr. Thompson helped Fran differentiate what felt intrusive and controlling from what felt supportive. They also discussed how her children might be trying to obtain a sense of control as they watched their mother struggle more over time, reframing the behaviors Fran found intrusive as an expression of their caring. Dr. Thompson encouraged Fran to consider this perspective when she experienced her children's help as intrusive, while also setting clear limits with them when their assistance was troubling to her.

Reinforcing positive dyadic coping in all encounters can also be helpful, recognizing that these behaviors may be dynamic over time. Suggesting a partner-assisted approach, in which other family members partner with the patient to engage in the healthier behaviors, can spark change (Baucom et al., 2012).

When family members are not willing or able to support the patient's self-management, clinicians can coach the patient regarding how to manage family members' unhelpful behaviors. For example, family members may encourage the patient to eat or drink more than they want. The clinician can role-play with the patient how to decline offers of alcohol or unhealthy foods at a family or social event. Clinicians must also mind their own emotional reactions to the problems and how this reaction affects their ability to engage productively with all the family members. When some family members are not supportive or able to be of assistance, the clinician can help the patient identify family and other supports who will assist them in staying the course on healthy lifestyle changes and medical regimen adherence.

> Nine years after her diagnosis, Fran experienced a series of setbacks. She ultimately became oxygen dependent and largely homebound. Initially, Amelia took on the bulk of the caregiving responsibilities, which caused stress with her romantic partner. Ms. Young became concerned about Amelia after she appeared stressed and tired at one of Fran's appointments. Ms. Young asked Dr. Thompson to check in at the next appointment.
>
> At the next appointment, Dr. Thompson met with Amelia alone (with Fran's permission). Dr. Thompson asked how Amelia was managing the stress of taking care of her mother. Amelia broke down and said she wasn't sure she could keep going. She expressed frustration with John and Joanne, feeling they did not help enough. She was also frustrated with Fran, because she felt Fran should be the one to ask them to help more. Dr. Thompson normalized how frustrated Amelia felt and noted that many families struggle to negotiate caregiving duties as they increase over time. Amelia did not want to have a family meeting, as she felt this might be too confrontational, and she worried Fran would be upset if she knew that Amelia was so overwhelmed. Dr. Thompson reviewed some strategies Amelia might use to engage her siblings in caregiving, such as creating a caregiving calendar, overtly asking for breaks, and asking her siblings to take Fran to various appointments. Amelia felt she could do this on her own and admitted she had not actually asked for help. Dr. Thompson also asked Amelia if she had seen her primary care clinician recently regarding her own health. Amelia acknowledged she had been neglecting her own health and agreed to schedule a checkup as she left that day. Dr. Thompson promised to check in with Amelia when she returned for her physical.

Continuum 4: Level of Spirituality and Connection to a Spiritual Tradition

One important cultural touchstone for health is about meaning and the family's spiritual beliefs about illness and level of spiritual life in general. Robust evidence supports a relationship between strong faith, coping with health conditions, and improving health-related quality of life (Stewart & Yuen, 2011). These studies support the importance of the systemic integrated care team exploring the meaning of the illness or condition to the patient and family. Sometimes the meaning has humanistic, spiritual, or religious underpinnings, other times scientific or superstitious, and sometimes a mix of these.

Rolland (2018) noted that spiritual resources may mean very different things to different people, including "prayer, meditation, or sacred rituals; belief in a higher power, a faith community; and/or involvement in nature, the creative arts or social activism" (p. 135). The patient's and family's meanings can lead the team to craft an intervention in the language that supports the patient. For some clinicians, discussing specific meanings or spiritual beliefs about illness and health may not be part of their typical approach, so consultation or additional training can help to develop these skills (Keith & Rogers, 2017).

> Fran's condition continued to deteriorate. She moved in with Amelia and became confined to her bedroom in Amelia's home. Her pulmonary function tests and her daily functioning showed that she was in end-stage disease. Because Ms. Young had an established relationship with the family, she was able to discuss Fran's condition frankly with them so they understood she was reaching the end of her life. Ms. Young consulted with Dr. Thompson about how to talk to Fran and her children about her advance directive and end-of-life wishes. The goal was to enable Fran and her children to make truly informed decisions that aligned with their beliefs and values. Dr. Thompson also coached Ms. Young to inquire about Fran's "missing" son, who had never been involved in her care, and the possibility of hosting a meeting with the family and the care team to address some of these issues.

Systemic Integrated Care Strategies to Explore the Spiritual Dimension

Rolland (2018) offered guidelines for inquiring about the spiritual beliefs and lives of patients and families that can be applied to healthcare. First, simply exploring the role of spiritual beliefs and religion sends the message that these topics are valued and an appropriate part of the conversation, if the patient and family desire. Rolland described this exploration as part of a larger conversation about different ways the patient and family view illness and suffering, including psychological and social aspects. For patients and families from minoritized cultures, respectful curiosity regarding spiritual beliefs can be integrated into a larger discussion of culture—how it affects their experience of the illness and of the healthcare system. This can convey respect and support for culturally based coping strategies that facilitate health.

Ms. Young talked to Fran about her personal wishes for end-of-life care, and Fran expressed a desire to engage with home-based hospice, for herself and because she wanted Amelia to have more support. She was ready to forgo "heroic measures" at the time when she declines further. Fran agreed to express these wishes to her children directly in a family meeting. When Ms. Young asked about her "missing" son, Fran shared that Paul had serious issues with addiction but had recently reached out as he was working toward sobriety. Ms. Young hosted a virtual family meeting, enabling all of Fran's children to attend. Amelia, John, and Joanne were at peace with their mother's wishes, as they had watched her decline and did not want her to suffer. Paul was silent for some time after Fran expressed her desire to go on hospice. He became tearful and expressed his anger at himself for not being there for his family or his mother. He noted it was very hard to come into her care as she approached the end of life. With Ms. Young's assistance, Fran, Amelia, Joanne, and John agreed that this situation was an opportunity for Paul to reconnect just in time. Paul started to visit Fran regularly and help with her care. When Fran died 6 months later, Ms. Young and Dr. Thompson attended her visiting hours, and the family expressed their gratitude for their assistance.

Continuum 5: Level of Premorbid Individual and Relational Functioning

Family functioning has been variously defined in the families and health literature. A conceptual analysis of family variables in the context of an adult illness found that the key concepts related to family functioning are the family's ability to maintain cohesive relationships, fulfill family roles, cope with problems, adjust family routines, and communicate effectively (Çuhadar et al., 2015; Y. Zhang, 2018).

The family resilience literature is helpful in considering how to approach families with a history of struggle or stress even before a chronic illness enters their lives. Not surprisingly, many of the concepts that align with resilience are the very same as those that help families adjust to, cope with, and even thrive when facing illness. Walsh (2015) described three foundational factors in resilient families. The first involves family belief systems. Resilient families tend to make meaning out of adversity and approach the challenge from a place of hope and spiritual grounding. The second described organizational processes within the family, including their ability to adapt and provide mutual support and have social and economic resources. The third are communication factors, ensuring there is clear information exchange, including sharing emotional responses and collaborative problem solving. In addition to being foundational factors of resilience in families, these same processes are also hallmarks of family-centered care, the medical home, and team-based, patient-centered care.

> Amelia was also a patient of the practice, and her primary care clinician, Dr. Reynolds, reached out to Dr. Thompson when Amelia came in for an appointment a few months after Fran passed away. He expressed concern that Amelia seemed lost without her caregiving duties. He said that Amelia reported the siblings were not getting along after their mother's death. Dr. Thompson met with Amelia and learned that there were deep schisms in the siblings' relationships due to long-standing resentments. Amelia and Joanne had extreme enmity toward Paul because of troubles during the throes of his addiction. Amelia said they had put aside these issues when Fran was sick because they didn't want to cause her stress. Amelia expressed a sense of failure, feeling she let her mother down by expressing her negative feelings about Paul. Amelia also acknowledged she was feeling depressed and stuck in grief for her mother. She agreed to attend a few sessions of more intensive, traditional psychotherapy with Dr. Thompson to help her resolve her grief and determine if she could repair her relationship with Paul. This then led to some medical family therapy to work through the schisms that were caused by addiction and grief.

Systemic Integrated Care Strategies to Address the Impact of Premorbid Functioning

The systemic behavioral health clinician actively assesses the family's history and ability to tolerate and manage previous stressors, including illness and loss. In eliciting the current illness story, it is important to understand the context in which the symptoms and illness emerged to understand both the family's level of stress at the outset and how stress may be relevant to the illness itself. This struggle can be normalized. The clinician can recognize patient and family strengths and help care team members take a strengths-based approach, actively reminding others that pathologizing individuals and families is not productive or helpful. They can manage the illness rather than letting the illness manage them.

The systemic clinician is mindful of potential parallel processes between the family and the care team and the importance of maintaining and modeling positive relational dynamics. For example, the care team might experience conflict among themselves when working with a particularly conflictual family, or communication on the team might diminish when working with a family that tends to be less disclosing to one another. Naming these patterns and working to resolve them can benefit both the clinical team and the family.

> Dr. Thompson met with Amelia for four psychotherapy sessions. She provided psychoeducation about grief and encouraged Amelia to engage with a support group for caregivers who are grieving. Amelia was not willing during this period to have a joint appointment with any of her siblings, feeling that she wanted this space for herself. A key moment in the grief work occurred when Dr. Thompson asked Amelia about her understanding of why her family had experienced these challenges. Amelia grew tearful and expressed her belief that her mother's illness gave the siblings a chance to know what being close felt like. She noted that their shared mission of caring for their mother helped them put aside their conflicts for a time. She wondered aloud if that experience was what would ultimately motivate them to deal with the issues that caused the rifts. In a subsequent session, she told Dr. Thompson she had shared this insight with Joanne, who agreed they never would have even tried to repair relationships without Fran's illness. Joanne and Amelia agreed to reach out to John and Paul to try to repair those relationships. Upon Amelia's request, she referred the siblings to a well-respected medical family therapist with experience dealing with family issues that are revealed as a result of illness and can be resolved as the crisis eases. The family therapist worked with the siblings over a number of months to resolve issues and improve their connection to one another.

SUMMARY

Team-based, patient-centered adult healthcare is strengthened by including the family as part of the team. Insights from the family therapy and family resilience literature can guide assessment and intervention of chronic disease management. Couples and family therapy processes can be adapted usefully for the healthcare environment by taking the long view and using medical family therapy strategies to help families adapt to and thrive within a new normal of living well with a chronic illness.

TAKEAWAY POINTS

- Expanding the purview of care from the individual patient to the family system enables the clinical team to access support, understand family dynamics that affect care, and help the patient and family adapt and manage the illness.

- A systemic lens for adult healthcare also acknowledges the role of the healthcare system at every level. The lens can be particularly helpful in noting how larger system factors affect patient and family management of the illness and in helping the care team function optimally.

- Family adjustment to chronic disease includes many elements that fall across a series of five continua: acceptance and denial, adaptation and stagnation, coping with others and coping alone, having a spiritual connection and having none, and good premorbid functioning and bad premorbid functioning. Attending to variations in family members' adjustment levels and coping styles can facilitate care.

10 PEDIATRICS

Pediatrics set the ball rolling for integrated primary care by embracing the concept of team-based care and developing the idea of a Patient Centered Medical Home. The concepts initially grew out of a recognition of the need for shared records and coordinated care for children with complex special care needs (American Academy of Pediatrics Council on Pediatric Practice, 1967; Stancin & Perrin, 2014). Behavioral health and social services have been well-integrated into specialty pediatric care (e.g., cystic fibrosis, cancer) for some time, reflecting the challenges children and families with serious medical illness and disability face (Samsel et al., 2017). Although we briefly review literature regarding family interventions in specialty pediatric care, we primarily focus on clinical strategies to facilitate integrated pediatric behavioral health services with a systemic lens into primary care for children.

In addition to the discipline of pediatrics, family medicine also provides clinical services to children as part of "cradle to grave" care. Family-medicine-trained clinicians, both physicians and nurse practitioners, follow the American Academy of Pediatrics guidelines discussed in this chapter. One key difference

https://doi.org/10.1037/0000381-011
A Systemic Approach to Behavioral Healthcare Integration: Context Matters, by
N. B. Ruddy and S. H. McDaniel

is that a family medicine clinician may have also provided prenatal care to the mother and her partner and delivered the child because some family physicians practice maternity care as part of comprehensive, full-spectrum primary care. Both pediatricians and family physicians may provide care to the children and family across generations, bearing witness to the family's story over time.

FAMILY-CENTERED CARE IN PEDIATRICS

Pediatrics and family medicine have long recognized that children are most likely to be healthy in the context of a healthy family situation and that traumatic experiences are particularly harmful to the health and development of young children (Bethell et al., 2017). A nurturing home environment with good family communication is particularly important when a child has a chronic illness (Helgeson & Palladino, 2012). Ideally, pediatric medical clinicians approach care from a "two generations" model, considering the needs of parents and caregivers as well as of the children (Zuckerman, 2016). They assess family functioning and parental stress, helping parents and caregivers access assistance as needed. From a systemic perspective, they also seek to understand the impact of family issues on the child and offer support for parenting figures as well as helpful resources.

Endorsed by the American Academy of Pediatrics, family-centered care occurs in a healthcare environment of respect, honoring differences of opinion within the family and between the family and the care team. Clinicians work collaboratively with family members, using information-sharing and treatment negotiation strategies to help the children (Kuo et al., 2012). The goal is to establish a partnership with families and provide care that incorporates the family perspective at all levels. Although this model has been evaluated primarily in hospital settings, family-centered care has been cited as a critical component of the pediatric Patient-Centered Medical Home (Lichstein et al., 2018).

Family-centered care ensures that treatment plans align with family goals and values, recognizing how the family's challenges and the limitations of the healthcare system affect care planning and implementation (Kuo et al., 2012). In primary care, clinicians work to develop a solid relationship, a partnership, with the family, prioritizing parental concerns particularly during well visits. Focusing on what matters to the family during collaborative treatment planning sets the stage for improved follow-through.

Research has shown a positive relationship between family-centered care and adherence to prescribed medical treatments. Research also demonstrates an association between improved medical adherence and lower family conflict, greater family cohesion, greater family flexibility, more positive communication, and better family problem solving (Psihogios et al., 2019).

A DEVELOPMENTAL, PREVENTION-ORIENTED FRAMEWORK FOR PEDIATRIC CARE

A developmental focus is also foundational to pediatrics, with medical clinicians tracking children's development over time by using well-child visits as periodic checkpoints. The focus of well-child visits shifts over time to align with common issues or needs across the developmental trajectory. The American Academy of Pediatrics regularly updates guidance for "health supervision" as part of the Bright Futures project. The 2017 guide suggested more frequent well-child checks during infancy and toddlerhood, with encounters initially just weeks apart (Hagan et al., 2017). Eventually the appointments occur once a year. Early appointments track development, shifting from physical development to achievement of milestones, with increasing focus on social and cognitive development as the child matures. During preschool and elementary school, pediatric medical clinicians focus on the child's relationships with peers and family, stress levels and mental health, and academic functioning. During early adolescence, well-child checks focus on the impact of hormonal changes, social relationships, school functioning, mental health, and prevention of risk-taking behaviors. As children become young adults, the pediatric medical clinician uses the well-child check to continue to monitor socioemotional development, transition to adulthood, prevention and management of risk behaviors, family and relational stress, and mental health (Pratt et al., 2018).

Well-child encounters help clinicians develop a longitudinal relationship with families that supports engagement if physical, mental, or social issues arise. The well-child check can serve an early warning function when clinicians take a biopsychosocial approach, eliciting psychosocial concerns and offering follow-up to more deeply assess and manage emerging issues. Calls to revise the delivery of well-child care focus on use of technology, groups, and team-based services (Coker et al., 2013; DeLago et al., 2018). Throughout the developmental process, embedding behavioral health expertise into well-child care is recommended (Zimmermann et al., 2020).

Well-care visits are but one approach to prevention and early intervention in pediatric integrated care. Research has facilitated the development of programmatic prevention efforts focused on very young children to support healthy development, such as the Healthy Steps program (Kaplan-Sanoff & Briggs, 2016). Other such programs focus on supporting parents and families who exhibit signs of struggle, such as the Positive Parenting Program (also known as Triple P; Prinz et al., 2009). A systematic review concluded that preventive behavioral health programs in primary care offer significant benefits over usual primary care (Brown et al., 2018). Ongoing research seeks to understand which interventions are most effective and for whom. For example, researchers found the Healthy Steps program was particularly effective with mothers who experienced significant adverse childhood events (Briggs et al., 2014).

Early prevention programs tend to have five core elements (Oppenheim et al., 2016):

- developmental and behavioral screening,
- mental health consultation and psychoeducation in early care,
- targeted home visits that focus on social and emotional development,
- family strengthening and parent support, and
- integration of behavioral health services into primary care.

Integrated behavioral health is important as a support for the other elements of programmatic prevention initiatives. The other elements are difficult to achieve without a team-based care structure that includes behavioral health expertise.

Engaging families in efforts to establish and maintain healthy habits offers another important prevention opportunity. Well-care encounters typically include discussion of healthy diet, exercise, and safety behaviors such as appropriate use of car seats, seat belts, and helmets. The literature is clear that engaging parents and social supports is a key element for success because parents serve as role models for health behaviors in their children (Natale et al., 2014).

A number of programs focus on engaging families to help children with obesity (e.g., Janicke et al., 2014). These programs, separated from typical care, have proven difficult to embed in typical practices, such that uptake is far from optimal (Guo et al., 2017). If establishing separate programs for obesity management is not feasible, integrated behavioral health clinicians can help pediatric clinicians adopt a systemic lens to health promotion and prevention. In addition, they can facilitate communication that honors the family's cultural influences, health beliefs, health habits, and family history.

FAMILY SYSTEMS INTERVENTIONS FOR FAMILIES FACING CHILDHOOD ILLNESS

Pediatric clinical presentations cover the full spectrum of health, mental health, and developmental issues from minor, subclinical concerns to crises. As with adult health conditions, few studies have examined the application of family systems interventions on health outcomes or family functioning. However, systematic reviews and research on specific childhood illnesses have slowly shifted to focus more on family functioning, family interventions, and health outcomes. A systematic review and meta-analysis conducted in 2014 (Law et al., 2014) and a large review of the literature on family engagement in pediatric health conditions in 2017 (Knafl et al., 2017) both noted a paucity of research. In their review of family interventions and chronic pediatric health conditions, Knafl and colleagues (2017) did note that targeting healthy family functioning or structural elements (e.g., roles, rules) was associated with improved disease self-management and child well-being in 89% of the studies reviewed.

A 2019 meta-analysis of the impact of systemic therapies indicated that family therapy strategies offer benefits in a variety of childhood behavioral health and developmental issues as well as chronic disease management (A. Carr, 2019). A. Carr (2019) noted that evidence supports systemic therapies for behavioral issues throughout the developmental arc, from feeding and sleeping issues in very young children to conduct issues, school avoidance and dropout, and high-risk behaviors such as substance misuse in adolescents. Furthermore, systemic therapies with high-risk mother–child dyads improved attachment issues in very young children and helped children recover from child abuse and neglect while improving family functioning. The review also supported the use of systemic interventions for emotional difficulties of childhood, including depression, anxiety, obsessive–compulsive disorder, and bipolar disorder. The evidence for systemic therapy for eating disorders is particularly strong.

For our review, the following findings from A. Carr's (2019) meta-analysis of research on pediatric somatic problems are of particular interest. The analysis found that family-based interventions augment established behavioral and medical treatments for enuresis and encopresis. Cognitive behavior and family therapy shows efficacy in alleviating recurrent functional abdominal pain with unknown medical etiology. Carr noted that systemic therapies that engage family members show benefit over individual approaches in both asthma and diabetes. These therapies tend to align with cognitive behavior and multisystemic models of family therapy and focus on psychoeducation, chronic disease management strategies, relaxation training, and cognitive and narrative interventions to improve coping. Of note, studies have shown these interventions to be particularly important for adolescents with health conditions as they navigate individuation and move toward managing the illness more independently.

It should be noted that A. Carr's (2019) review focused on family therapy programs and protocols that are consistent with specialty mental health services. Although some of the therapies reviewed focused on brief engagements, all were offered in either a programmatic format or traditional psychotherapy format that would not be consistent with integrated services in healthcare settings. However, the review highlighted how family involvement may be key in helping families navigate many of the issues commonly presented in healthcare settings, particularly emotional and somatic concerns.

A similar trend can be seen in research on the impact of family variables and family interventions for specific pediatric illnesses. The research on family-oriented interventions for pediatric cancer patients and their families is particularly robust (e.g., Bidstrup et al., 2023). Moscato and colleagues (2022) conducted a systematic review examining the impact of family characteristics on children's psychological functioning and quality of life after treatment for a brain tumor. They found strong support for improved psychological outcomes for children in families with higher cohesion and adaptability, more effective communication, and lower conflict. Given these findings, the authors recommended that family assessment and inclusion be normative in cancer care (Moscato et al., 2022).

In fact, standards of pediatric cancer care emphasize including family members to reduce any potential long-term, negative psychological impact on the patient, parents, and siblings (Wiener et al., 2015). However, a review of care at multiple pediatric cancer centers noted a significant gap between these standards and care delivery. Of note, the authors reported that pediatric cancer centers with integrated behavioral health services were more successful in meeting these standards. In addition, the literature calls for treatment centers to routinely assess family functioning using a validated tool such as the Psychosocial Assessment Tool (Crosby et al., 2016; Kazak et al., 2015; Nemours Children's Health Center for Healthcare Delivery Services, 2023). Systemic family interventions may be particularly helpful for adolescents with terminal cancer (Lyon et al., 2013) and for preschool children (Yu et al., 2014).

Treatment standards for the care of children with type 1 diabetes also call for significant family involvement in care and the integration of behavioral health professionals into the care team (Delamater et al., 2018). A systematic review of the literature by Feldman and colleagues (2018) noted that family-based interventions do appear to improve family functioning, with mixed impact on glycemic control. They noted that clarity regarding treatment elements that impact glycemic control has yet to emerge, as reflected in mixed outcomes. Common elements of impactful intervention include family-based strategies such as communication skills training, cognitive restructuring to address harmful family beliefs, family psychoeducation, role clarification, parent training in chronic disease management, and promotion of positive interactions.

Wysocki and colleagues (2006) developed a model of family-centered diabetes care based in behavioral family systems therapy (BFST-D). BFST-D combines structural family therapy, problem-solving and communication training, cognitive restructuring, and diabetes-specific behavioral components. Randomized controlled trials (RCTs) showed improvement in treatment adherence and glycemic control in adolescents, with treatment effects evident at follow-up over a year later (Wysocki et al., 2007). The intervention also reduced negative communication by adolescents, as measured in a family task to discuss a conflict around diabetes management (Wysocki et al., 2008).

Multisystemic family therapy (MST) has been studied extensively by D. A. Ellis and colleagues. MST attends to multiple contextual factors and utilizes strategies from cognitive behavior therapy and parent training as well as family systems elements. It also has been shown to positively impact treatment adherence and glycemic control and reduce hospital admission and diabetes distress for adolescents with chronically poor diabetes management (D. A. Ellis et al., 2005a, 2005b). Subsequent research evidenced sustained treatment effects (D. A. Ellis et al., 2007). Though MST is an intensive intervention, research supported its efficacy when delivered as a telephone intervention (D. A. Ellis et al., 2012), reducing the treatment burden on the system as well as the family.

Other types of childhood medical conditions have less robust evidence but do support the inclusion of systemic interventions to help families cope. For example, systemic interventions for families coping with a congenital cardiac condition in a child also appear to reduce maternal distress (McCusker et al., 2009) and improve family functioning (McCusker et al., 2012).

Pratt and colleagues (2020) reviewed systemically oriented strategies for families with a chronically ill child. They highlighted the importance of family-oriented goal setting, with a focus on perceived costs and benefits of different treatment options. They also emphasized how supporting collaboration between the care team, child, and parents also can improve chronic disease self-management and adherence to the care plan, particularly as the child matures.

INTEGRATION EFFORTS IN PEDIATRICS: CHALLENGES AND PROGRESS

Whether for well-child checks or management of a serious illness, it is clear that systemically oriented behavioral health services add value for pediatric patients. Yet integrated care in pediatric practice, particularly primary care, is far from normative. The focus on prevention in pediatric primary care aligns well with the integrated care model, but it is significantly more challenging to clearly establish preventive benefits and obtain reimbursement. The Centers for Medicare and Medicaid Services does offer Medicaid coverage for early and periodic screening, with diagnosis and treatment codes intended to facilitate reimbursement for these services. However, a Milbank report noted that the process of receiving reimbursement for these services was challenging for pediatric practices and did not create the hoped-for increases in these services (Tyler et al., 2017).

Research may move pediatric integration efforts forward. A large meta-analysis focused on mental health issues in pediatrics indicated that integrated care improves both access and mental health outcomes (Burkhart et al., 2020). Asarnow and colleagues (2015) found that 66% of youth who received integrated care showed improved outcomes over usual care, particularly when the interventions targeted mental health issues and aligned with the PCBH model. A systematic review of integrated behavioral health services with Collaborative Care Model (CoCM) interventions for adolescents and young adults also found improved depression outcomes (Richardson et al., 2017). Data from a 5-year study of 13 pediatric primary care practices serving more than 100,000 patients found that integrated services by embedded behavioral health clinicians and remote child and adolescent psychiatry consultations improved access to care. The rate of services increased from 11 psychotherapy visits per 1,000 patients in typical care to 230 visits per 1,000 patients in integrated care. The number of patients seen in specialty mental healthcare did not change, indicating an increased reach of the primary-care-based services. Both behavioral health and medical clinicians felt integrated services improved care, enabling them to manage mild to moderate behavioral health issues in the primary care setting. Of note, the new services did not add substantial cost to overall care (Walter et al., 2019). Similarly, Tennessee's Cherokee Health Systems found that embedding a behavioral health clinician into a pediatric practice enabled each medical clinician to complete an additional primary care encounter each day. The resulting income more than covered the cost of the behavioral health clinician (Khatri et al., 2017).

Given these data, a groundswell of support has emerged for integrating behavioral health into pediatrics. The American Academy of Pediatrics facilitates networking between integrated care practices via their website to facilitate dissemination. As of 2023, more than 500 mental health integration initiatives across the United States are listed on the website, with program descriptions, location, and contact information for each (American Academy of Pediatrics, 2021).

HELPING FAMILIES MANAGE NEURODEVELOPMENTAL ISSUES

Reviewing systemically oriented assessment and intervention strategies for the wide range of possible presentations in pediatrics is beyond the scope of this chapter. Rather, we use care for families of children with neurodevelopmental issues as an exemplar of integrated systemic strategies. We chose these disorders because of their ubiquity and the many adaptations required of families to successfully navigate these challenges. As with many areas in family therapy, clear data on the impact of systemic, relational therapies are limited. For example, a recent Cochrane review regarding the impact of family therapy interventions for families with child with autism was not conclusive due to a lack of randomized controlled trial evidence (Spain et al., 2017).

Neurodevelopmental disorders cover a variety of clinical presentations, including autism spectrum disorders, intellectual disabilities, communication disorders, specific learning issues, and executive function issues such as attention-deficit/hyperactivity disorder (ADHD). In this discussion we acknowledge that the use of the term *disorder* in this context can be problematic. Increasingly, language is shifting toward the term *neurodivergent* in recognition of the full spectrum of developmental pathways and the many strengths of individuals whose development diverges from the typical path (Dyck & Russell, 2020). Yet this divergence often is challenging for both the individual and family, requiring adaptations of all. The degree of family adaptation depends on severity and degree of functional impairment. Key elements include protracted and difficult diagnostic processes, often with lifelong implications; a need for early intervention to mitigate impact; the effect on the entire family system; and increased caregiving needs (Craig et al., 2016). In addition, families often must interface with many systems (medical, educational, social services) to manage issues optimally, creating a need for an expanded systemic lens.

The full range of developmental divergences often is detected and addressed first in pediatric primary care. Severe developmental issues or those related to metabolic disorders are managed long-term by pediatric subspecialists. However, pediatric primary care practices help to manage a wide variety of mild to moderate developmental issues, with a focus on early intervention. Although the challenges inherent in neurodivergence often improve over time, they typically do not disappear. In fact, families may struggle more over time when a child's development increasingly diverges from typical development.

Behavioral health clinicians in pediatrics play a significant role in developmental assessment. They have a unique position from which to approach families living with neurodevelopmental issues. As with most complex clinical presentations, these families need assistance from professionals with multiple types of expertise, necessitating a team-based approach.

CLINICAL STRATEGIES TO ASSIST FAMILIES LIVING WITH NEURODIVERSE CHILDREN

Here we outline management strategies based on a developmental, systemic approach. Ramisch and Poland (2020) provided an outline of systemic approaches to these challenges; we offer adaptations to align with the primary care pediatrics setting. These strategies may not be necessary or appropriate for all families. We illustrate the strategies based on the experiences of the Warren family and their son, Emmett.[1]

> The Warren family had three children, ages 7, 10, and 12. They had been patients of the practice since their eldest was born and had a positive relationship with their pediatrician, Dr. Morse. The two eldest children did well in school and never posed any behavioral issues. Their youngest child, Emmett, had been a tough toddler, behaviorally. Multiple times he would seem to be lagging behind developmentally, only to catch up just as Dr. Morse thought about referring for an evaluation.
>
> As Emmett entered first grade, his teacher called a conference with the parents to suggest Emmett receive extra help with reading. The teacher also expressed concerns about Emmett's ability to focus in class, noting he often seemed distracted, had difficulty completing tasks, and sometimes disrupted the class. The teacher suggested they talk to his pediatrician about getting "an evaluation" but was vague beyond that.

---

[1]The case description aligns with common presentations in healthcare but does not reflect a real person or specific situation.

Mrs. Warren brought Emmett to Dr. Morse to get his opinion of what to do next. The family was one of only a few African American families in the school district, and Mrs. Warren expressed some concern that Emmett was singled out because of his race. At the same time, she had always worried a bit about Emmett; he had been very different from her other children.

Strategy #1: Facilitate diagnosis to establish eligibility for appropriate services and accommodations. When families first come to a pediatrician's office seeking advice, they are often confused, concerned, and upset. Facilitating diagnostic processes may require deft handling of relational issues about willingness to see the problem, seek evaluation, and trust in the health and mental healthcare system and management of the challenges inherent in obtaining evaluation.

Family members often experience a wide range of emotional reactions during the diagnostic process. Families with a child who struggles with a neuro-developmental disorder often must cope with chronic uncertainty about the child's future capabilities and challenges (Piland Springer et al., 2018). Behavioral health clinicians can help caregivers develop skills to manage the necessary ambiguity during the diagnostic process. These behavioral health interventions can help manage stress in the short term and also prepare the family for potentially high levels of ambiguity going forward.

Strategy #2: Elicit the degree to which family and other social supports are concerned about the issue and believe some level of intervention is warranted. The concern index can be mapped onto a continuum to acknowledge the differences of opinion and generate discussion about how to proceed given these differences. This information is also very helpful to medical clinicians as it provides diagnostic data and informs treatment in working to generate and implement a treatment plan with the family.

Dr. Morse asked if Mrs. Warren would be comfortable including the practice's psychologist, Dr. Ryan, in their conversation, because Dr. Ryan helped so many of his patients and their families. Mrs. Warren agreed, and Dr. Ryan stopped by to hear her concerns. Dr. Ryan asked Mrs. Warren if she and her husband could come back for a follow-up visit because her time was limited that day, and Mrs. Warren agreed. Dr. Ryan gave Mrs. Warren a number of behavioral checklists to be filled out by her, her husband, and Emmett's teachers. The forms were completed prior to the appointment, allowing Dr. Ryan to see a strong pattern of issues with attention, self-control, and difficulty with schoolwork reported by all three people.

After hearing Mr. and Mrs. Warren's perspective on Emmett, Dr. Ryan reviewed the behavioral checklists with them. They were not surprised at the outcome and, upon talking to friends and family, felt that Emmett definitely struggled in a number of contexts. They expressed a desire to ensure that Emmett received appropriate services in a way that did not make him feel singled out. They felt, as one of few minority children in his school, he already had too many experiences of feeling different from his peers. Dr. Ryan provided them with the names of two clinicians who specialized in evaluating attention and learning issues and coached them how to secure an evaluation.

Mr. and Mrs. Warren followed up with Dr. Morse a month later and reported they had an evaluation appointment in 4 months. Although they were frustrated with the delay, they felt that completing the checklists had helped them consider how Emmett struggled. This put them on a course to collaborate with school personnel on a plan to help Emmett while they waited for the more thorough evaluation. They were not open to discussing medication for attention issues until the full evaluation was complete.

Strategy #3: Facilitate building a multidisciplinary team to meet care needs. Primary care serves a care coordination role in all manner of health and emotional challenges, including neurodevelopmental issues. The family may need help to determine what types of assistance they hope to receive and to understand the often byzantine rules regarding eligibility for services via public health early intervention programs, school-based programs, and reimbursement for private programs. As the care team grows, it is important to attend to systemic issues within the team to ensure excellent communication, a shared understanding of the impact on the family system, and close service coordination. Coordination with the education system is especially important.

In a primary care setting, ensure that the professional support team is listed in the electronic health record, including current contact information and a brief description of each member's role. It is also essential to obtain release-of-information forms for all professionals and the school to facilitate communication and place them in the electronic health record. Documenting a global treatment plan to be disseminated to all professionals can facilitate dialogue when there is disagreement within the team or between the team and family members. These processes can be completed by a care manager or by the behavioral health clinician if care management is not available. Often, PCBH clinicians can serve as liaisons between the neurodevelopmental team and the primary care medical clinician and team to ensure each team has the necessary information to provide optimal care.

Emmett's evaluation revealed some minor attentional issues but significant language-based learning issues. Despite a rich home environment, Emmett struggled to put sounds to letters. Despite extra help in reading at school, Emmett was not making progress commensurate with his high IQ. The Warrens returned to Dr. Morse because they were not sure how to help Emmett most effectively.

Dr. Morse asked Dr. Ryan to join the appointment ahead of time, so they had a full 20 minutes to work with the family together. The Warrens were open to Dr. Ryan's participation, asking her to review the report and explain it to them. They agreed Dr. Morse could move on with his schedule, and Dr. Ryan spent about half an hour reviewing the report and answering their questions. Familiar with the school's supportive services, Dr. Ryan offered to have a virtual joint appointment with Emmett's parents and his teacher and case manager at school to create a care plan. At the joint appointment, the family agreed that Emmett would benefit from an outside tutor to augment the school's interventions and help track Emmett's progress. Dr. Ryan took this information back to Dr. Morse and suggested he meet with the family regularly to track progress and offer support, given their strong relationship. The Warrens agreed to meet with Dr. Morse every other month and voiced appreciation for his support. They signed all necessary releases of information and expressed gratitude that the pediatric team would be helping them advocate for Emmett's educational needs.

Strategy #4: Provide family psychoeducation to help families understand their child's diagnosis and its implications and medical/mental health management and treatment options. Including extended family in some conversations can help them understand the developmental issues, which may facilitate family support. These discussions also may facilitate conversations about caregiving needs and help the family openly discuss distributing or augmenting caregiving needs to avoid overwhelming any one person or part of the family (McDaniel & Pisani, 2012). Psychoeducation can give family members helpful information through which to understand their child's behaviors as well as management strategies to mitigate the impact on daily life.

Group medical appointments for patients with ADHD or specific learning issues that have developmentally appropriate psychoeducational components for children, siblings, and adult caregivers can provide psychoeducation, normalize struggles, and offer support. Well-child checks can be framed as a normative venue for the behavioral health clinician check-in to assess individual and family coping and provide psychoeducation and other supports as indicated. Finally, pediatric practices can offer nondirect service practice interventions as well. For example, they can ensure availability of health-literate educational resources that recognize children's challenges as well as their individual and family resilience factors.

It was extremely important to the Warrens that Emmett understand his learning differences to allay frustration and reduce any negative impact on his self-esteem. Emmett hated being pulled out of class and had started to resist going to the tutor. Also, Mrs. Warren reported that her mother-in-law expressed surprise that Emmett was getting extra help. Mrs. Warren was frustrated that Emmett's grandmother didn't understand the concerns. Emmett frequently saw his grandmother, so Mrs. Warren was concerned that he might pick up on their disagreements.

Emmett really liked Dr. Morse and never complained about meeting with him. Dr. Ryan suggested that Dr. Morse could provide psycho-education to Emmett, emphasizing his many strengths, and helping Emmett understand how out-of-class support and tutoring could help him reach his potential. Dr. Morse found a children's book that talked about learning differences in a positive light and gave the book to Emmett. Dr. Ryan also suggested readings on learning issues for Mr. and Mrs. Warren, which they shared with their extended family.

As Emmett learned more about why he struggled to read (and that he was far from alone in this issue), he became more cooperative with supportive services and started to put more effort into applying the techniques he learned there. The Warrens purchased multiple copies of the materials on learning issues and gifted them back to the practice. They found the materials very helpful and wanted to increase awareness of these issues. Mr. Warren told Dr. Morse, "Emmett's situation would have been so much easier if we understood earlier; maybe this will help other people understand." As Emmett progressed with his reading, the Warrens agreed to participate in a podcast with Dr. Ryan that was available to patients on the practice portal.

The practice did not offer a group for ADHD. Rather, Dr. Ryan guided the Warren family to online resources and support groups. The family felt this was more realistic for them than in-person meetings, given their busy family schedule. Mrs. Warren connected with a woman whose son was about 5 years older than Emmett, who offered her support and strategies that Mrs. Warren found very helpful.

Strategy #5: Explore the family's history with developmental issues, including family scripts about diagnoses or beliefs about the origin of issues. Many parents and family members experience a sense of shame or guilt about developmental issues and often benefit from discussing these emotions. Some cultures have strong beliefs about the genesis of developmental issues, and parents may worry they have caused the problem (Cascio, 2015). Acknowledging these beliefs, creating a place for family members to discuss their concerns, and providing information can be beneficial.

It is almost always useful to assess family lore about the diagnosis, including narratives about family members who, in retrospect, may have struggled in similar ways. If the family narrative is negative regarding cause or trajectory, use narrative therapy techniques to help the family differentiate the current issue from past problems and explore more positive narratives for their child (Lambie & Milsom, 2010). It can be helpful to ask if the child is like someone else in the family and learn more about that person's trajectory. Narrative strategies can also elicit and adapt the meaning the family has ascribed to the illness. Because of the time constraints in primary care, narrative elements are delivered over time in small increments. Clinicians and staff work toward incremental change by using language that aligns with a more balanced or positive view of the child and the developmental issue itself. Narrative approaches can help the family rewrite the script for the child.

The Warrens shared the psychoeducational materials with their extended family because they experienced some pushback about the diagnosis and their decision to get special services for Emmett. Their family shared the parents' earlier worries that Emmett was singled out as the only Black child in his class and thought the family had been pressured into accepting these services. Simply sharing the materials helped some, but sharing the podcast with their extended family was a watershed moment. Emmet's grandmother apologized to Mrs. Warren, acknowledging that she had doubted their decisions until she heard the whole story. She stated that, in retrospect, she wondered if Mr. Warren's brother had struggled in similar ways and noted that he never got help, ultimately was not successful in college, and struggled with self-esteem related to feeling different from others in his high-achieving family.

Mrs. Warren told Dr. Morse that the whole process of Emmett's diagnosis had been painful, and she would "do anything" for him not to struggle with learning issues. She noted that she felt very close to Emmett after naming the learning issue and managing them proactively. She also noted his diagnosis had spurred important conversations in the family and that she had a new appreciation for the struggles experienced by Mr. Warren's brother. Mr. Warren said that once he made the connection between Emmett's and his brother's struggles, "a lot made sense," and he felt good that he and his wife had been able to help Emmett avoid some of these difficulties.

Strategy #6: Manage behavioral issues to reduce conflict, daily challenges, and family stress. Many developmental issues are associated with challenging behaviors. The degree of problematic behavior is highly predictive of family stress and can have a detrimental impact on family members. In fact, although caregivers tend to rate hyperactivity, inattention, and peer issues as more severe, "it is the children's worries, fearfulness, and general unhappiness that is most impactful on the family's ability to maintain their social, financial, and personal wellbeing" (Gardiner et al., 2018, p. 895).

Pediatric integrated care clinicians can ask caregivers about challenging behaviors and normalize how intrusive these behaviors are in daily family life. Specifically asking about the child's emotional well-being and offering developmentally appropriate resources to help with coping as part of routine pediatric care recognizes the ubiquity of these struggles in neurodiverse individuals. Providing support and parenting resources, ideally via parent training or a support group that exists in the pediatric practice or the community, recognizes that parents often are stymied in addressing these behavioral issues; these resources offer them new strategies. These strategies often focus on helping caregivers provide a consistent environment, with consequences for challenging behaviors. Of course, problematic behaviors and emotional struggles may be best managed in specialty mental healthcare, so referral to specialty mental health should be considered if behavioral issues do not resolve with integrated care services. Serial use of behavioral checklists and other tools that track behavior over time from the perspective of multiple caregivers can facilitate stepped care, shifting the treatment plan or referring for specialty services if progress is not evident.

> Emmett came to understand that needing special help and having to learn differently did not mean he was stupid. But he reported still feeling embarrassed about getting special help. He sometimes would become frustrated with assignments that required a lot of reading and then refuse to do the reading homework assigned by the tutor.
>
> Dr. Morse asked about Emmett's functioning every time he met with Mr. and Mrs. Warren for their own health issues. Every few months he asked the couple and Emmett's teachers to complete behavioral checklists to track progress. He coached them to set firm but supportive limits with Emmett about his schoolwork. He encouraged them to let the school counselor know that Emmett's self-esteem was affected. The school counselor really liked Emmett and worked with teachers in

his strong subjects to ensure his successes were emphasized and celebrated. She encouraged Emmett to join the school band and chorus, where he thrived as he discovered strong musical talent. Emmett also benefited from knowing that the school counselor's door was always open to him, and he regularly stopped by to talk to her, even when he wasn't struggling.

Strategy #7: Managing caregiving stress enables the support system to provide care over time and reduces overall family stress. Pediatric integrated care team members can regularly assess caregiver burden and stress, providing support as needed and communicating with other team members about family stress levels.

Families often need specific strategies to increase social support and to access natural supports within the family to share caregiving burden. In addition, the integrated care team can help the family find and accept outside assistance as needed to reduce caregiving burden. The team can consider offering respite care, which often requires a referral from a medical clinician. Increased respite care has been associated with reduced caregiver stress and improved couple functioning (Harper et al., 2013). Emotional and practical support via peer mentoring also can be helpful (Dykens et al., 2014). A well-constructed natural and professional support team can significantly reduce caregiver burden and enhance coping.

Strategy #8: Seek a balanced picture of the child. Professional caregivers must balance promoting the child's strengths with acknowledging their deficits in order to successfully secure services. Regarding advocacy in the educational system, Ramisch and Poland (2020) stated, "It is important for providers to . . . be sensitive to the family's atypical experience of raising a child with a disability, as a minority within a normative setting where the general classroom structure is designed to teach the typical student" (p. 386).

Family members may struggle with the need to simultaneously advocate for services and avoid pathologizing (Acevedo & Nusbaum, 2020). The team can encourage the family to educate themselves about their child's educational rights and provide resources to facilitate advocacy.

Strategy #9: Recognize shifts in patients' and families' needs over the developmental arc. Children and family need different types of assistance at different times during the developmental trajectory. Relationship continuity in pediatric primary care facilitates ongoing dialogue and care plan adjustment as needed. In addition, team-based integrated care helps families access the kind of care they need when they need it.

A developmental approach may be particularly important with older adolescent and young adult patients with neurodevelopmental disorders. Research indicates a significant disconnect between parents' and their adolescent's or young adult's perceived needs in families with a child with Asperger's or ADHD (Eklund et al., 2018). Parents' primary concerns focused on issues related to independent living, such as managing a home, food, and money and preventing exploitation. Children's perceived needs focused on mental and physical health and safety of others (ability to maintain a safe home environment.). The authors noted that children may not overtly acknowledge their fears so that parents are not aware of them. Parents and children also viewed differently the amount of assistance parents provided. Parents indicated they gave significant support in areas necessary for independent living, but children did not recognize the help. Eklund and associates posited that children may be unaware that their parents are providing them with support in these areas because they have no other benchmark. This disconnect might underlie the child's relative lack of concern regarding independent living skills (Eklund et al., 2018).

Pediatric clinicians often work with families to help children with various health and mental health issues as they transition into the adult care system. Team-based care that elicits and addresses the concerns of family members regarding the transition to adulthood can be part of this process. The team can normalize differences of opinion and help the family collaboratively generate a plan to transition to independent living when appropriate. This plan may address pragmatic issues such as managing emergencies, level of parental engagement, and management of disagreements regarding the child's needs. Because the young adult patient may have specific, unnamed concerns about mental and physical health, the team can query these areas and normalize these concerns. The family and care team can create a pragmatic plan for managing the mental or physical health issues that may emerge.

If the child is aging out of a pediatric practice (which doesn't happen in family medicine), the team can help the family find an adult primary care integrated practice and manage the transition to adult care (Holderle et al., 2022). In addition, it can be helpful for the adult child and parents to have an overt agreement regarding the parents' roles in their child's healthcare and what a parent should do if they are concerned about their child.

> Over time, the Warrens reduced their visits to the pediatric practice, feeling they had the situation under control. When Emmett hit adolescence, he started to express his frustration more overtly and once again seemed to be very stressed by schoolwork. Emmett no longer had access to the guidance counselor at the elementary school and had not connected with anyone at the middle school in the same way. He also was less open with Dr. Morse. Mrs. Warren talked to Dr. Morse

about her growing frustration with Emmett and her concerns about how his brooding hostility might affect his relationships with friends, schoolmates, and the family.

The team worked with the family to ramp up support. The Warrens started to bring Emmett to see Dr. Morse regularly again. With more regular contact, Emmett started to open up to Dr. Morse about the various issues troubling him. Emmett expressed increasing frustration with how hard he had to work in school to get by, especially in relation to his siblings, who just seemed to sail through. Dr. Morse normalized Emmett's frustration and helped him express this to his parents.

Mrs. Warren agreed to meet with Dr. Ryan for a couple of sessions to discuss how she might support Emmett in expressing his frustrations more effectively. She worried that Emmett would be written off as an "angry young Black man" and noted that the middle school teachers were less empathetic regarding his struggles. Dr. Ryan agreed that it was important for his frustration not to be dismissed and coached Mrs. Warren on connecting with the school. She also acknowledged her frustration at how much time and effort it took to get teachers to understand why Emmett struggled and provide him with appropriate accommodations. Mrs. Warren acknowledged a general fatigue in helping Emmett directly and advocating for him at the school. When Dr. Morse pointed out the parallel process—that Mrs. Warren's fatigue likely was similar to how Emmett felt about having to work so hard—Mrs. Warren's stance toward Emmett softened. Dr. Morse also helped Mrs. Warren prioritize self-care, emphasizing that only by maintaining her own wellness could she continue to help Emmett.

Strategy #10: Recognize the experience of ambiguous loss and grief and facilitate meaning making. Families with children with a neurodevelopmental disorder respond along a long continuum, with many families evidencing great resilience (Leone et al., 2016). One theory regarding the variable reaction focuses on the impact of ambiguous loss on parents and family members (O'Brien, 2007). Ambiguous loss refers to the need for family members to adapt to the reality that "the child they thought they had is not the child they must learn to live with" (O'Brien, 2007, p. 135). Family members must cope with many ambiguities, including how the child will develop and function in the future and the impact of the disability on daily life.

For some, there is a need to grieve the loss of the dreamed-for child. Many need assistance in integrating, accepting, and celebrating the reality of who their child is. Ambiguous loss may also underlie asynchronous responses within the family, which can be challenging. Disagreement about the meaning or even the very existence of the child's issue within the family can result in conflict and distress. Systemic therapists help the family seek meaning in the experience to help the family overtly discuss this process (Springer et al., 2017). The process of acceptance and coping is dynamic over time, and the challenges and joys families face often evolve as they progress through the family life cycle (McDaniel & Pisani, 2012).

Ideally, the care team avoids making assumptions about the family's level of distress or struggle regarding their child's diagnosis and functioning, especially because distress levels can be very dynamic. Creating a safe space for exploring challenging feelings and normalizing appropriate feelings of grief and sadness can enable family members to speak the unspeakable. Toward these ends, behavioral health clinicians can check in with the family regularly to assess stress levels. One way to conveniently achieve this is to include the behavioral health clinician in well-child checks for children with developmental issues. Routine contact that does not require the family to name a presenting problem to access behavioral healthcare facilitates relationship development and creates a venue to elicit the family's struggles and successes during routine care.

> Emmett ultimately adjusted to middle school. However, he never was able to get As in classes, often earning a low B or C. Emmett continued to read very slowly and struggle to follow classroom presentations. He acknowledged there were times he didn't give his best effort, expressing how much "trying so hard every day just makes me tired." As the Warrens approached decisions regarding which high school Emmett should attend, they initially assumed he would attend the same highly competitive high school where his siblings had excelled. They knew his grades were not great but hoped the admissions office would focus on the classes where he did excel and recognize how his learning issues explained his lower grades. Hence, they were taken aback when the guidance counselor suggested he apply to the general public high school as a backup. They were even more distressed when his only acceptance was at the general high school.
>
> When Emmett came in for a sports physical, Mrs. Warren asked to talk to Dr. Morse privately. She told him about Emmett's lack of choice for high school and became tearful as she discussed the situation. Dr. Morse listened and asked her a bit more about why the situation was so troubling to her. Mrs. Warren paused and responded, "I guess I just hadn't let myself think about what may not be possible for Emmett. And it's hard because it was all so effortless for my other kids. They just excelled. And I guess I'm just now realizing that

Emmett doesn't have the same abilities—the same choices—they have." Dr. Morse asked Mrs. Warren if she and her husband had talked about this, and Mrs. Warren acknowledged they kind of avoided the topic. He encouraged her to talk to her husband more and suggested that a couples appointment with Dr. Ryan might be helpful.

Dr. Morse updated Dr. Ryan, so Dr. Ryan was not surprised when Mrs. Warren called a few weeks later asking if she and her husband could come in to talk about the situation. Dr. Ryan had two half-hour sessions with the Warrens, helping them explore their sadness about Emmett's difficulties. While normalizing their feelings, she also encouraged them to consider all of the wonderful futures that could be ahead for Emmett, given his many strengths. They admitted they bought into the idea that an elite education set the stage for a good life and refocused on Emmett's musical talents and general happiness.

Strategy #11: Address challenging family patterns in order to reduce overall family stress and mitigate the impact on other family members. Family patterns may include the impact of the neurodevelopmental problems on the marriage or partnership, the siblings, the grandparents, and other close family members.

The stress of having a child with a neurodevelopmental issue can cause family conflict in many ways. A systematic review of research on families who have a child diagnosed with ADHD showed significantly higher patterns of family distress and relational disruptions (Deault, 2010). Although raising a child with a developmental disability can be stressful, research regarding marital satisfaction in couples with disabled children has been mixed, with results ranging from divorce and a negative effect on marital satisfaction to no or positive effect (Moore et al., 2023).

Attending to relationship skews may help families cope with a neurodevelopmental issue (Rolland, 2018). Ideally, outside of a crisis, the family doesn't allow the child's issues to become the central organizing force in the family or neglect the needs of other family members. When the family views the child from a deficit lens, clinicians can elicit the family's views of the child's strengths and remind them to acknowledge the child's successes and strengths. The clinician can help the family recognize where there are imbalances in relationships and work to balance the scales to create reciprocal, self-sustaining relationships.

The primary care pediatrics team can help the family explore nonillness identities in subtle ways, such as overtly emphasizing their strengths and discussing aspects of family life that are not centered on the developmental issue. The pediatric team is in a unique position to elicit sibling issues and offer support because the sibling may not be actively involved in treatment elsewhere. When appropriate, the behavioral health clinician also can offer support and may advise specialty family therapy when it appears family functioning or sibling wellness is significantly adversely affected. Eliciting specific relational patterns can help the family recognize places they feel stuck. These patterns can be addressed in brief encounters via solution-oriented therapy strategies such as finding exceptions to any typical, problem-saturated pattern. In general, solution-focused therapy techniques are helpful in primary care because they can be delivered in brief encounters, focus on the present and future, and address patient concerns in a pragmatic way (Franklin et al., 2019).

Social isolation can reflect another problematic family pattern. Families often struggle to maintain outside social relationships and support. Many parents report feeling stigmatized or othered by their social network and other community supports (Corcoran et al., 2015). Again, the degree of variation from typical development and the visibility of the developmental differences affect the level of stigma the family might experience. Paradoxically, "invisible issues" can be challenging because others are unaware or dubious that there is a developmental issue. Behavioral issues also can exacerbate social connection difficulties for both the child and the family.

> During the sessions with Dr. Ryan, Mrs. Warren discussed how much extra energy and time it had taken to help Emmett get as far as he had. She acknowledged that some of her sadness was a sense of failure—despite her best efforts, Emmett was not going to achieve academically like the other children did. She also discussed how her focus on Emmett had affected her career and that at times she felt Mr. Warren did not understand how difficult this had been for her.
>
> During the subsequent conversation with Dr. Ryan, Mr. Warren acknowledged he had let his wife "do the heavy lifting" in helping Emmett. He expressed his gratitude to her for all she had done for Emmett and the family and in support of his successful career. Dr. Ryan asked the Warrens about any benefits they had experienced as a result of Emmett's challenges. At first they struggled, but they eventually acknowledged that they had a closeness with Emmett different from their other children, in part because of all of the extra time he needed. They also noted that refocusing on different definitions of "success"—away from only academic achievement and material success—made them reevaluate the pressure they had put on their other children. They discussed how they hoped high achievement would somehow protect their children from systemic racism. Yet subsequent

conversations with Emmett's siblings revealed how the pressure to succeed had been very difficult for them.

SUMMARY

As this case illustration suggests, the primary care pediatric team can play an important role in helping families cope with a neurodevelopmental issue in a child. Although most primary care encounters are relatively brief, the pediatric practice provides care across time and can help families connect with additional resources. When behavioral health clinicians in pediatrics are not able to help the family manage all aspects of their child's care, they can coordinate care, offer support and strategies along the way, and refer for more intensive therapy when needed. Pediatric practices can choose to implement more intensive services, such as support or parent training groups, medical family therapy in specialty mental healthcare, and assistance with care coordination and advocacy. Across the board, the goal is to help families secure services when needed, develop helpful routines, and balance the needs of a child with neurodevelopmental issues with other normative family functions.

TAKEAWAY POINTS

- Although pediatrics was an early innovator in integrated care, implementation in primary care pediatrics lags behind.

- Pediatric health issues stress families in unique ways, resulting in patterns of both struggle and resilience.

- Research literature supports the need for behavioral health services in pediatrics and the need for these services to be family-focused.

- Systemic assessment and interventions strategies have been found to be efficacious with these families and can be adapted to an integrated care setting.

11
WOMEN'S HEALTH

Although there are many parallels to adult and child primary care settings, behavioral health clinicians working in women's health sometimes assist with clinical presentations unique to that setting. Rather than offering a comprehensive review, we describe some common, illustrative presenting concerns and how behavioral health clinicians can approach these issues using a systemic, relational lens for care. In addition to brief descriptions of clinical strategies for these issues, we delve deeper into care for women and families who experience pregnancy loss.

Women's healthcare in obstetrics and gynecology (Ob/Gyn) has not always been considered part of primary care[1]. However, some women obtain care almost exclusively in these sites; an annual gynecologic check may be their only contact with the medical system (D. Cohen & Coco, 2014). A recent survey of women indicated that approximately 20% considered their OB-GYN as their primary medical clinician (Mazzoni et al., 2017).

---

[1] While "women's health" is still the most commonly used term, because of the recognition of nonbinary identities, some Ob/Gyn clinics are using alternative terms like Gender Wellness.

https://doi.org/10.1037/0000381-012
A Systemic Approach to Behavioral Healthcare Integration: Context Matters, by N. B. Ruddy and S. H. McDaniel

Family medicine clinicians also provide women's health services and receive training in well-woman care, prenatal and postnatal care, and obstetrics. Although most family physicians provide well-woman and acute and chronic illness care for women, some also provide pre- and postnatal care, and a minority provide comprehensive obstetrics services.

The range of services in women's health includes annual gynecologic checkups and routine screenings (e.g., cervical cancer, sexually transmitted infections), contraception, prenatal and postnatal care, abortion care, and management of various conditions and symptoms related to women's reproductive organs. Common presenting concerns with significant behavioral and emotional health impact include issues with breast health, menstruation, fertility, family planning, menopause, libido, sexual difficulties, and pelvic pain related to endometriosis or other causes. Behavioral health and mental health issues, such as depression, posttraumatic stress disorder (PTSD), and anxiety, are also common in women's health. Yet research suggests that although the need has been acknowledged for some time (Coons et al., 2004; Gallant et al., 1994), women's mental health issues have long been under-identified and undertreated in Ob/Gyn settings (Goodman & Tyer-Viola, 2010).

As of 2023, integrated behavioral health services are not yet normative in primary care women's health, but the model is becoming more common. A systematic review of integrated health solutions for perinatal depression concluded that "integrating depression care into obstetric practice is feasible, effective, and acceptable" (Moore Simas et al., 2018). Parallel to other primary care settings, the roles for behavioral health clinicians in women's health include implementation and management of behavioral health screening processes, brief interventions, consultation with medical clinicians, and direct clinical service to facilitate symptom and chronic disease management (Coons et al., 2004; Poleshuck & Woods, 2014).

Expanding services into women's health settings is exceedingly important, given that women are more likely than men to seek help for mental health issues (Tedstone Doherty & Kartalova-O'Doherty, 2010). The American College of Obstetricians and Gynecologists (ACOG) recommends depression screening as part of well-woman care and during the perinatal period (ACOG, 2016). Depression is a significant risk factor for poor pregnancy outcomes; women who suffer from depression are 1.5 times more likely to have a preterm birth and almost twice as likely to have an infant with low birthweight than are their nondepressed counterparts. The impact of depression on birth outcomes is even more stark among African American women with depression, who are 2.3 times as likely to have a preterm birth and almost 2.5 times more likely to deliver a low-birthweight infant, as compared with rates in White women (Simonovich et al., 2021). Women in general are at particularly high risk for a serious mental health problem after giving birth, with suicide and overdose the leading causes of death during this period (Griffen et al., 2021).

Behavioral health clinicians in women's healthcare are in a unique position to address women's experiences of trauma and violence. Women are more likely than men to experience domestic and sexual violence (Ades et al., 2019) and may view their women's health setting as a safe place to disclose. In this context, ACOG recommends routine screening and counseling regarding issues of interpersonal violence at preventive health visits (ACOG's Committee on Healthcare for Underserved Women, 2012). The U.S. Preventive Services Task Force recommended interpersonal violence screening in healthcare settings (Curry et al., 2018). However, the best processes and tools for screening continue to be a matter of debate (Chisholm et al., 2017). Survey data do indicate that fewer than half of women's health practices screen for interpersonal violence at routine preventive visits (Jones et al., 2020).

Medical clinicians in women's health recognize the impact of sexual trauma on reproductive health, yet they report struggling to address these issues. These clinicians identified a need for increased training and acknowledged that support from an integrated behavioral health clinician could assist them in providing care to this population (Sycz et al., 2021).

Trauma-informed integrated behavioral health services have potential benefits in addressing patient needs related to sexual assault, molestation, and interpersonal violence (Lutgendorf, 2019; Striepe & Coons, 2002). Behavioral health clinicians can raise awareness of the impact of female victimization and support adherence to trauma-informed care guidelines (Gerber, 2019). They can provide training to their medical colleagues regarding best practices in treating women with a trauma history. Ades and colleagues (2019) described their EMPOWER (engage, motivate, protect, organize, self-worth, educate, respect) model of care used in a continuity clinic for women with a history of sexual violence or sex trafficking. They emphasized the importance of a team-based, trauma-informed care environment that addresses the ongoing health and mental health sequelae for women who have survived sexual violence. Overall, a behavioral health presence in women's health settings offers the opportunity to improve health behaviors and outcomes, access to mental healthcare, and team-based management of patients with traumatic experiences (Ades et al., 2019).

Another area of evolution in women's health is the increasing attention to the experiences of sexual and gender identity minorities (e.g., Everett et al., 2019; Lynch, 2019). The reality that the gendered label "women's health" is not inclusive of transgender and nonbinary people who have sexual and reproductive medical needs has sparked ongoing dialogue (Moseson et al., 2020). As the field seeks to meet the needs of the continua of gender and sexual identities, behavioral health clinicians can raise awareness of strategies to enhance care for noncisgender patients. In addition, they can highlight the specific health and mental health risk factors and health disparities these individuals may face (Pharr, 2021; Warren et al., 2016).

Some patients may initially seek assistance to begin the process of gender affirmation (e.g., hormone therapy) in primary care women's health. As our society becomes more aware of the needs of the transgender community, healthcare professionals should seek appropriate training, such as that offered by the Department of Veterans Affair's transgender e-consult service (Hashemi et al., 2018) and the National LGBTQIA+ Health Education Center. Their learning modules are available at https://www.lgbtqiahealtheducation.org/resources/in/transgender-health.

ROLES FOR THE BEHAVIORAL HEALTH CLINICIAN IN WOMEN'S HEALTH

As in other primary care settings, aspects of the behavioral health clinician's role in women's healthcare align with the setting's specific health presentations and clinical challenges. Some of the more common roles are described in this section.

Preparation for Invasive Procedures

Coons and colleagues (2004) noted that behavioral health clinicians can help to prepare women for invasive or unpleasant diagnostic and treatment procedures, including routine pelvic exams. This preparation may include the option of having a chaperone (a family member, friend, or clinic staff), psychoeducation regarding the procedure, relaxation techniques, guided imagery, biofeedback, systematic desensitization, or hypnosis. It can be critical to offer these supports to patients with a history of sexual trauma who may find these procedures particularly distressing.

Behavioral health clinicians also play a significant role in designing and implementing trauma-informed protocols for invasive procedures. The goal is to help the woman feel in control of the process, set appropriate expectations for the procedure, and provide coping strategies should the patient become distressed during the procedure. The impact of these strategies for invasive procedures has not been evaluated. Even so, gynecologic surgery guidelines recommend preoperative counseling with many of these elements (G. Nelson et al., 2019).

Managing Symptoms of Menopause

Menopause is a significant life transition that can stress women during an already challenging life stage in which many women care for both children and aging parents. About 1 in 10 women experience increased psychological symptoms during menopause, such as depressed mood or anxiety (Almeida et al., 2016). Intrusive somatic symptoms are common, such as vasomotor symptoms (hot flashes, night sweats), sleep disturbance, and vaginal changes (Santoro et al., 2015). Many women find vasomotor symptoms (such as hot flashes) negatively impact quality of life, including disrupting sleep. Behavioral health clinicians can collaborate with other women's health clinicians and help women cope with these symptoms.

Cognitive behavior therapy (CBT) is an important tool in managing troubling symptoms related to menopause (M. S. Hunter & Chilcot, 2021). Research indicates that cognitive appraisal of symptoms is an important mediator of how vasomotor symptoms affect quality of life and help-seeking (M. S. Hunter et al., 2019). A randomized controlled trial of a CBT protocol specific to vasomotor symptoms of menopause (CBT-Meno) showed significant reduction in the degree to which women experienced depressive symptoms, sleep difficulties, and sexual concerns and the degree to which they reported symptoms "bothered" them (S. M. Green et al., 2019). Similarly, studies show that CBT-Insomnia helps women with significant sleep disruption during menopause (Caretto et al., 2019). While there is little research on couple or family interventions to help with menopausal symptoms, there is some evidence that an intimate partner's views on menopause may affect a woman's experience of menopausal symptoms and the impact of menopause on the relationship. Although this research is developmental, the authors noted that a man's view of menopause importance and severity and the value of treatment for symptoms may impact his partner's perceptions as well (X. Zhang et al., 2020). The reality that men also experience midlife changes (andropause) further supports the contention that issues arising from negotiating these transitions may benefit from a biopsychosocial, systemic approach to the dyadic experience (Jannini & Nappi, 2018).

Facilitating Sexual Health

Issues with sexual function and enjoyment also are common in gynecology practices. These complaints affect approximately 40% of women at some point during their reproductive years (McCool-Myers et al., 2018). Issues typically center on desire, arousal, orgasm, or pain (ACOG's Committee on Practice Bulletins–Gynecology, 2019). They are underreported, as women often do not recognize or disclose sexual issues unless sexual functioning is overtly assessed. A biopsychosocial lens highlights the intersection of biological, emotional, relational, and cultural factors that often underlie sexual issues (McCool-Myers et al., 2018). It is helpful to address attitudes and knowledge about sexuality, clarify gender role expectations, and help women learn to communicate their needs to their partner (Coons et al., 2004). Some evidence exists for the effectiveness of dyadic intervention based on the EIS (empathy, intimacy, and sexual satisfaction) model, a manualized couples therapy to help couples coping with unsatisfactory sexual functioning. This approach improves marital satisfaction and intimacy as well as sexual function for women (Konzen et al., 2018).

Behavioral health clinicians may also work with couples coping with genito-pelvic pain or penetration disorders. Vaginismus, a condition in which the vaginal muscles contract to prevent penetration and/or cause extremely painful intercourse, is one of the more commonly studied issues. However, most of the research focuses on medical and psychological care for women with vaginismus, rather than on the dyadic relationship (McEvoy et al., 2021).

Preventing and Managing Sexually Transmitted Infections

Approximately one in five people in the United States have a sexually transmitted infection (STI), and almost half of these infections occur in individuals between the ages of 15 to 24 (Centers for Disease Control and Prevention [CDC], 2020b). Patients who have experienced a STI report the diagnosis was very troubling to them, secondary to associated stigma and the need to restrict sexual activities and report the STI to sexual partners (Newton & McCabe, 2008). Some respondents indicated that concerns about disclosure affected their willingness and ability to inform partners, negatively affecting measures to reduce transmission. Furthermore, they reported that the diagnosis caused significant relational stress.

Behavioral health clinicians can facilitate prevention efforts via psychoeducation and ensure the practice makes information about STIs available to all patients (Lamson et al., 2018). When a patient receives an STI diagnosis, behavioral health clinicians may help the patient cope with the news and manage relational issues related to the diagnosis. This role may be especially relevant when the diagnosis of an STI reveals a previously unknown sexual relationship outside the primary relationship.

Supporting Women and Couples Who Seek Induced Abortion

A high proportion of pregnancies are unintended. Globally between 2010 and 2014, there were an estimated 121 million unintended pregnancies each year. Abortion rates range between approximately 40% and 60% of unintended pregnancies, depending on a variety of sociocultural factors (Altshuler & Whaley, 2018; Bearak et al., 2018), including access and stigma (Cockrill et al., 2013). After much debate and research, it appears that having an abortion is not causally linked to mental health issues in the long term (Biggs et al., 2017); in fact, many women report "relief" as the primary emotion they associate with having an abortion (Rocca et al., 2020). However, the literature also indicates that a small proportion of women who seek abortion do experience emotional difficulty after the procedure. Women with preexisting mental health issues are more vulnerable to postabortion adjustment issues (Reardon, 2018). Behavioral health clinicians can offer decision support, connection to resources where appropriate, and psychotherapeutic support after the procedure.

Helping Couples Cope With Infertility

Fertility challenges are also common in women's health. Using data from 2015 to 2017, the CDC reported that approximately 13% of all women in the United States used some form of fertility service during their lifetime, with approximately 9% of women experiencing infertility (as compared with 12% of men; Lotti & Maggi, 2018). An additional 16% of married women did not pursue fertility treatment but did report "impaired fecundity," which is defined as physical difficulty becoming pregnant or carrying a pregnancy to live birth (CDC, 2020a).

In vitro fertilization (IVF) has become much more common but is not readily available to many. IVF access and IVF success rates vary across ethnicities and socioeconomic status such that people of lower socioeconomic status and people of color are less likely to have access to IVF and less likely to have IVF that results in a live birth (Quinn & Fujimoto, 2016). Even those who have access to IVF are not assured a positive outcome, as IVF success rates vary greatly based on age, process used, and other factors (CDC, 2019a).

The IVF process and other fertility treatments are physically and emotionally arduous. A significant percentage of women undergoing fertility treatment report symptoms of depression and anxiety (Patel et al., 2018). In one study, 39% of people who had insurance coverage for more IVF cycles did not pursue further treatment. They cited stress as the primary factor, feeling that the negative impact on their relationship and emotional health was too high to continue (Domar et al., 2010). A systematic review of factors that resulted in discontinuation of IVF found that about 20% of couples cited physical and psychological burden (Gameiro et al., 2012) as the primary factor.

Behavioral health clinicians can help the couple deal with relational conflict in part by acknowledging the stress of infertility (Read et al., 2014) and the unique challenges it poses for conflict resolution. Couples' responses to infertility are variable; there is some evidence that shared coping styles and attitudes toward the treatment can be protective (Pasch & Sullivan, 2017). Therefore, interventions should focus on understanding and aligning coping and attitudes and address differences. Research supports this focus, as couples therapy based on the Common Fate Model, which specifically targets helping the couple view infertility as a shared issue and developing shared coping mechanisms, showed positive effects on increasing dyadic quality of life and decreasing dyadic stress (Donarelli et al., 2019). Multicouple support groups also appear to help improve coping (Chow et al., 2016). Of note, most of the research investigating the impact of clinical interventions focuses on interventions for the woman only (Bach, 2018).

Couples who decide to pursue fertility treatments generally transfer to specialty care rather than remaining in primary care or general women's health setting. However, primary care clinicians may help the couple accept the need for treatment and determine next steps. If the fertility clinic does not have embedded behavioral health clinicians, the women's behavioral health clinician may stay involved even after referral, especially if there is an established relationship. Furthermore, primary-care-based behavioral health services may help patients prior to seeking fertility treatment and after they conceive, as research indicates women struggle during these stages of the process as well (Patel et al., 2018). Treatments often center on helping couples cope with communication and the stressors and decision making that are inherent in the process, with a focus on the impact on the relationship.

Providing Family Planning and Prenatal Care

For couples who are able to conceive with or without assistance or those who have unanticipated pregnancies, behavioral health clinicians facilitate biopsychosocial family planning and prenatal care (Coons et al., 2004). These services can address the relatively high rates of depression and anxiety women experience during pregnancy (Fairbrother et al., 2015), both of which are associated with poor outcomes (Dunkel Schetter & Tanner, 2012).

Unfortunately, sharp health disparities continue in family planning, prenatal care, and birth outcomes (Parekh et al., 2018). Embedding behavioral health services and utilizing partners or other social supports in prenatal care have been shown to reduce these disparities (Lu et al., 2010). Behavioral health clinicians may help run group prenatal appointments and routinely meet with pregnant women early in the pregnancy to assess needs for ongoing support and follow-up. In addition, some women's health and pediatric practices offer specific programs aimed at preventing postpartum depression, with increasing calls for these initiatives to be normative (Lewis Johnson et al., 2020).

An impending birth is a family affair, with implications for every member of the family. Family-oriented prenatal care strategies include engaging the partner or other social supports in prenatal care, exploring family functioning, assessing psychosocial risk factors and strengths, and discussing the impact of the pregnancy on all family members and relationships (McDaniel et al., 2005). The dialogue can help the family plan who will attend the delivery, when permitted, and define each person's role. The family can be engaged after the baby's birth by inviting siblings to well-baby checks and conducting a home visit. Among the many stressors of the COVID-19 pandemic was the restrictions on direct family involvement in healthcare, leaving many women who delivered babies in the hospital isolated from their usual sources of support (Sanders & Blaylock, 2021).

Postpartum engagement with a behavioral health clinician aids screening and management of a broad array of postpartum emotional challenges, including postpartum depression and anxiety. Stressful life events, poor social support, and poor family relationship quality all are strong predictors of postpartum depression (Yim et al., 2015). Research regarding the effect of integrated behavioral health service on postpartum adjustment is still to be done. However, it seems likely that an established relationship with a behavioral health clinician during pregnancy may be protective or, at a minimum, facilitate meaningful engagement in behavioral healthcare if needed.

SUPPORTING FAMILIES AFTER MISCARRIAGE

Miscarriage is extremely common; it is challenging to measure accurately because many miscarriages go unreported. Between 1991 and 2011 the risk of pregnancy loss overall was 19.7%, with early pregnancy loss representing the bulk at 13.5% (Rossen et al., 2018). A survey of more than 50,000 women who gave birth indicated that more than 40% of women reported having one or more prior first trimester miscarriages, with 18.5% having had a miscarriage before their first live birth. Sixteen percent of women reported multiple miscarriages (Cohain et al., 2017).

Miscarriage is associated with feelings of sadness and grief that can last for months and increased rates of depression. The emotional impact of a miscarriage tends to be more challenging for women than men, especially for women who miscarry a first pregnancy, suffer multiple miscarriages, and/or had infertility issues prior to miscarriage (Volgsten et al., 2018). Systemic integrated behavioral health clinicians can be of assistance during this time, using the following strategies.

Acknowledge Stress and Loss

Many reproductive losses are invisible to the outside world. If a woman's pregnancy was not physically obvious, such as in a first trimester miscarriage, others know of the loss only if she or the family tells them. It is helpful to assist couples in a mindful process of choosing whom they tell. Behavioral health clinicians also can help the family overtly acknowledge the loss. Many families choose to engage in a ritual or ceremony to memorialize the lost life and lost hopes. In addition, some couples find attending a support group to be helpful to share the loss with others who have had similar experiences (Simon, 2013).

Provide Psychoeducation

Although people experience and express loss in a variety of ways, there are common individual and relational patterns. Behavioral health clinicians should ask about prior losses—how the family experienced and honored their grief, what strategies were useful, and what individual and relational strengths promoted their resilience. It is important to highlight how multiple losses tend to increase distress exponentially. It may help couples to recognize the miscarriage as a dyadic stressor that may be viewed differently by each member of the couple (Chachamovich et al., 2010), highlighting common gender differences in reaction to pregnancy loss (Péloquin et al., 2018). Couples may need assistance in recognizing their emotional triggers and understanding the link between the trigger and intense emotional reactions. Common triggers include learning of another person's pregnancy or new child, anniversaries of the loss itself, the passing of the lost baby's due date, others' baby showers, and seeing infants or infant-related items.

Process the Emotions

Explore the meaning and emotions associated with the loss, listening for feelings of guilt, ambivalence about the pregnancy, and worries about causing the miscarriage. These reactions are associated with increased emotional distress and protracted grieving (Kersting & Wagner, 2012). Many women experience reproductive loss as an affront to their identity and value (Greil et al., 2010). Behavioral health clinicians can address and normalize feelings of inadequacy, inquire how the issues and treatment affect daily life, and build on strengths and approaches that recognize the loss while also supporting resilience. Couples who experience pregnancy loss, particularly those who terminate a pregnancy secondary to fetal abnormality, are at risk for complicated grief reactions. This protracted and intrusive experience of grief is most likely when the couple has poor social support, has preexisting relationship issues, or is childless (Kersting & Wagner, 2012).

Encourage a Return to Normalcy on the Family's Timeline

Families may need encouragement to focus on other areas of life and allow normalcy to return. For example, psychoeducation can normalize how all-consuming the grief can be, while encouraging a return to previous hobbies and other enjoyable activities. For many couples the spiritual element of the biopsychosocial model helps the family cope and find a sense of meaning in the experience to help them move forward.

At the practice level, medical clinicians can ensure that behavioral health clinicians are aware when a patient has suffered a pregnancy loss. Ideally, practices develop a standard workflow that engages a team to ensure families get support at this critical time. The behavioral health clinician can offer outreach and a clinical encounter when appropriate, ideally in the first weeks after the miscarriage (Brier, 1999). All clinicians should check in on the emotional and relational function of the couple and address common patterns.

Behavioral health clinicians can facilitate education regarding the impact of pregnancy loss. They can implement training for staff that includes teaching supportive strategies and creating space to help the staff process emotions about these challenging circumstances. They also can work with colleagues to identify or develop psychoeducational materials for patients and make them available throughout the practice.

Some practices implement a professional or peer patient navigator program for families who have experienced pregnancy loss, similar to navigator programs used with many serious illnesses. Peer navigators are people who have experienced similar challenges. They can offer support and help patients find the information and services they need, especially because some patients and families will prefer to seek supports outside of their OB-GYN practice after a loss (McKenney et al., 2018). The following clinical situation illustrates some of these points:

> Kiara and Sam[2] were expecting their first child. Just as Kiara finished the first trimester, she experienced bleeding and cramping. Her OB-GYN, Dr. Matthews, explained that she was likely having a miscarriage. She ultimately needed to have a dilation and curettage (D&C) procedure. Sam was visiting family abroad during this time and was unable to return. Dr. Matthews told Kiara about Dr. Koplar, the psychologist on his team, saying Dr. Koplar was helpful to many of his patients like her.
>
> Prior to the D&C, Dr. Koplar briefly met with Kiara. She expressed her condolences for Kiara and Sam's loss and comforted Kiara. She ensured that Kiara understood what was going to happen during the procedure. Because Kiera's partner was away, both Dr. Koplar and Dr. Matthews called her the next day to check in. Though she was very sad and very tired, she expressed her gratitude for their care.
>
> When Sam returned from his trip, he apologized to Kiara for not being able to be with her at this time of loss and sadness for both of them. After that brief conversation, he avoided talking to Kiara about the miscarriage. When she tried to talk about it, Sam was kind and comforting but then consistently changed the subject.
>
> When Kiara came in for a follow-up appointment a few weeks after the miscarriage, Dr. Matthews checked in to see how she was doing. Kiara told him that Sam's reaction and avoidance was troubling her. Dr. Matthews suggested she meet again with Dr. Koplar, who wondered if his avoidance might be rooted in a fear of saying the wrong things or in guilt. Dr. Koplar suggested it is common for partners to cope with loss in very different ways. She offered Kiara strategies to approach Sam, assuming positive intent such as a belief that it might be best for them to move on. Dr. Koplar also offered to see them together, but Kiara declined. At a subsequent appointment, Kiara told Dr. Koplar that her conversation with Sam had gone well, and they were communicating much better. Sam had been worried that sharing his own feelings would burden his wife further.
>
> A few months later Kiara brought Sam with her for her appointment with Dr. Matthews to discuss trying again to have a baby. Sam asked

---

[2] The case descriptions align with common presentations in healthcare but do not reflect a real person or specific situation.

why the miscarriage occurred and how they could prevent another from happening. Dr. Matthews reassured them that they had not caused the miscarriage and that a first miscarriage does not necessarily predict future outcomes.

HELPING FAMILIES FACING AND RECOVERING FROM THIRD TRIMESTER LOSS (STILLBIRTH)

Losing a pregnancy during the third trimester is tragic. Each year approximately 24,000 stillbirths occur in the United States (CDC, 2020a). Approximately six out of every 1,000 pregnancies result in fetal demise in utero (FDIU) after 20 weeks of gestation, with much higher rates for non-Hispanic Blacks at approximately 10 out of every 1,000 pregnancies (Gregory et al., 2014).

Late-term pregnancy loss represents one of the most challenging issues in women's behavioral health. After stillbirth, women experience high rates of depression, anxiety, posttraumatic stress, suicidal ideation, panic, and phobia (Burden et al., 2016). The negative impact of this loss on the couple's emotional and physical wellness and functioning is well-documented (Cacciatore et al., 2013; Galvão et al., 2020), and significant impact on other family members is assumed. Almost 90% of women in one sample met criteria or reported subclinical yet troubling symptoms of PTSD (Chung & Reed, 2017). It is telling that couples who experience a late-term pregnancy loss are significantly more likely to separate (K. J. Gold et al., 2010), making immediate involvement of an embedded systemic behavioral health clinician very important to any threatened or actual pregnancy loss.

BIOPSYCHOSOCIAL SYSTEMIC MANAGEMENT OF STILLBIRTH

The first signs of trouble may occur in a routine outpatient visit when a heartbeat cannot be detected, after which the tragedy typically unfolds in a hospital setting. Sensitive management of the situation is critical to mitigating the impact of the stillbirth on the mother and family, but research reveals great variability in the quality of biopsychosocial care delivered during this difficult time (Mills et al., 2016). Ideally, patients have input in as many decisions as possible (e.g., autopsy, pain control during labor) to help them feel they have some control over the process. Some hospitals and practices have memory-making processes, such as seeing and holding the stillborn baby and creating mementos such as photographs or foot- and handprints of the baby. These rituals can facilitate the mother's and family's grieving process. However, despite increased understanding and focus on the needs of women and family during stillbirth, room for improvement remains. These patients indicate they need more preparation for vaginal birth, more time to understand and consider their options, and more support and information after the loss. Approximately 30% of the respondents in the Mills and colleagues (2016) study cited a desire for "privacy not abandonment." A. Ellis and colleagues (2016) found that some patients felt that some clinicians withdraw emotionally during the stillbirth, focusing on medical tasks and avoiding a connection to the woman and her partner.

Families may benefit from a supportive review of their experiences at the time of the stillbirth to help them process the trauma and loss. Qualitative research indicates that parents need acknowledgment of their loss and of the irreplaceable individual identity of their lost child. These parents noted that they want support people and clinicians to use the baby's name and to acknowledge their role as parent of a child (Farrales et al., 2020). Unfortunately, few studies have established more comprehensive best practices to help women, couples, and families process this experience. Researchers do emphasize the importance of a broader family approach that offers ongoing support to partners, children, and grandparents, although the impact of this support has yet to be adequately studied (Bakhbakhi et al., 2017).

The behavioral health clinician should be informed at the earliest possible time when a patient experiences an FDIU in order to provide supportive counseling before and after the delivery. Proactive emotional support and emotion-focused coping strategies offered within a week of the stillbirth have been associated with improved emotional outcomes for women a year after stillbirth (Engler & Lasker, 2000).

Behavioral health clinicians function to ensure patients have access to helpful information and supportive care as needed. Clinicians can ensure that psychoeducational materials are available to families to normalize their experiences and help them recognize when further psychotherapy might be helpful (Markin, 2017). Visits with the couple or family may focus on psychoeducation, along with processing grief and mitigating—or serving as a referral person for—any complicated grief reactions. Over time, the behavioral health clinician can check in and assess the impact of the loss on the family's functioning and relationships. As with miscarriage, group interventions may be helpful. Practices may elect to offer support groups or to maintain a referral relationship with a community-based group.

The behavioral health clinician's role extends to the needs of colleagues involved in the care before, during, or after the stillbirth. Qualitative research indicates that medical clinicians also go through a grieving process after a stillbirth and often question if there was something they could have done to prevent the tragedy (Nuzum et al., 2014). Behavioral health clinicians can normalize these emotional reactions and struggles. They also can train staff and other clinicians regarding self-care and appropriate responses to pregnancy loss, subsequent grief, and trauma reactions with families. In one survey regarding training and clinical practices about stillbirth, more than 90% of clinicians indicated they would value additional training in helping families during this difficult time (Ravaldi et al., 2018).

If and when a subsequent pregnancy occurs, the behavioral health clinician is usefully involved early in the care and as part of the care team throughout the pregnancy. Women who have experienced a stillbirth and their family members are significantly more likely to experience anxiety and depression during a subsequent pregnancy (Gravensteen et al., 2018; Heazell, 2016). Pregnant women and families post-stillbirth need additional psychosocial support, an individualized care plan that addresses their specific needs (Fockler et al., 2017), and an integrated care team with a focus on the emotional and relational experience of the couple and family, as illustrated below.

Stella and Maggie endured three rounds of IVF before Stella finally became pregnant. They were beyond excited as the due date approached. They learned the baby's sex at an early ultrasound, a boy they planned to name Liam. A week before Stella was due, she realized she had not felt any fetal movement all afternoon. She called her OB-GYN, Dr. Jameson, who encouraged her to come to the fetal monitoring service that evening. Multiple clinicians tried to find heart tones, but none were to be found. The team induced labor, and Stella endured giving birth knowing Liam was dead. Dr. Jameson and Maggie were there to support her, but the couple and Dr. Jameson were devastated. The hospital provided strong support to Maggie and Stella. The staff followed the protocol for a stillbirth, giving Maggie and Stella information ahead of delivery about the process of vaginal birth, eliciting and following their wishes for care. They gave Maggie and Stella time to hold Liam, helping them save a lock of hair and foot- and handprints as memorials.

The day after the stillbirth, Dr. Jameson asked the family therapist, Ms. Votia, if she could schedule some time to talk later in the day about her own experience of this patient. Ms. Votia sat quietly as Dr. Jameson unspooled the story of Maggie, Stella, and Liam. Dr. Jameson broke down when she talked about what it was like to be in the fetal monitoring lab and unable to find Liam's heartbeat. She recounted her first

FDIU during her intern year. At the time, she felt too scared and worried her emotional reaction was unprofessional to process the impact it had on her. Losing Liam brought it all back. Ms. Votia and Dr. Jameson discussed self-care for Dr. Jameson. She also gently asked Dr. Jameson if she felt responsible for the tragic outcome or worried that she had missed something. Dr. Jameson said that she had reread the chart and thought about their last encounter. She knew intellectually there was nothing she could have done, but there was still this small kernel of doubt. Ms. Votia normalized this reaction and encouraged Dr. Jameson to talk to respected peers about the case to process both the care and her emotional reaction with others who would understand.

When Maggie and Stella came to see Dr. Jameson for follow-up, Ms. Votia provided some recommendations to Dr. Jameson and made herself available. Both Maggie and Stella were truly shell-shocked and agreed they weren't ready to meet with Ms. Votia that day. Subsequently, they scheduled a session with Ms. Votia and came in to process how they were coping with the loss. Stella expressed a sense that her loss was deeper than Maggie's because the child had been in her womb. Maggie tried to understand but also felt that her own grief wasn't being honored. Ms. Votia bore witness to their pain and empathized with their struggles to make sense of what had happened. She normalized each of their reactions, given their different physical experiences and their different ways of grieving, while honoring their common loss. They later discussed how different ways of grieving occurred with extended family members as well.

Ms. Votia met with Maggie and Stella for a number of sessions and checked in with them at subsequent appointments with Dr. Jameson. In addition to psychoeducation about pregnancy loss, she provided grief counseling and attention to their relational issues. Although some extended family members were supportive of their relationship, others had never accepted them as a couple. Maggie's grandmother even suggested that the stillbirth was a sign that they should break up and "have a normal relationship." In some ways, this adversity brought Stella and Maggie closer together. They reflected on other struggles they had overcome as a couple, and Ms. Votia noted the strength of their bond. Ms. Votia helped Stella and Maggie share their hopes and dreams for their future family. Ultimately, Stella and Maggie used the space to discuss when they might want to try to conceive and decided to start IVF cycles again for Stella. Stella conceived on the second cycle, and they had a healthy baby girl 18 months after losing Liam.

THE EVIDENCE BASE FOR SYSTEMIC INTERVENTION AFTER PREGNANCY LOSS

Appropriate intervention strategies for individuals, couples, and families after pregnancy loss have been the topic of many scholarly articles, including a special issue on the topic in *Psychotherapy* in 2017 (Markin, 2017). The various strategies outlined in this chapter align with the best practices described in these publications. However, there is little in the way of outcome research to provide empirical evidence for which strategies work with which populations and issues related to pregnancy loss. These strategies align with research that focused on best practices in helping people cope with grief and loss. They support the use of cognitive behavioral and supportive approaches, along with psychoeducation (Johannsen et al., 2019). Of interest to our focus on integrated care, McGill and colleagues (2022) found that offering supportive psychoeducation in brief contacts is viewed positively by bereaved patients, who often report enhanced well-being. However, this research did not focus on helping people cope with pregnancy loss per se. Women's health is another arena in which further research is much needed about the systemic influences, opportunities, interventions, and outcomes that affect the health of women and their families.

SUMMARY

Although integrated care is not yet normative in women's health primary or specialty care, the settings offer many clinical presentations that warrant the inclusion of a behavioral health clinician on the team. In addition to common behavioral health issues, women who struggle with menopause, sexual symptoms, pain, and fertility challenges can benefit from a team approach. An integrated care team approach is particularly important for patients, families, and the clinical team during the emotional and physical stress of miscarriage and stillbirth. Systemic behavioral health clinicians' expertise in processing trauma, loss, and grief is also extremely helpful to the team, both at the time of the loss and during any subsequent maternity care.

TAKEAWAY POINTS

- People who seek care in women's health settings can benefit from integrated behavioral health services to address symptom and chronic condition management; manage menstrual and menopausal difficulties; facilitate gender affirmation care; and address relational issues, trauma, and issues related to infertility and pregnancy loss.

- Systemic, family-oriented care may be particularly important when the presenting concern has a significant impact for other family members. Although including family in care for sexual health, menopause, infertility, and pregnancy loss seems obvious, the evidence base to guide this work is early in its development.

- Pregnancy loss challenges families and medical clinicians, potentially having long-term emotional and relational impacts. Integrated behavioral health clinicians can work with all involved to facilitate grieving and adjustment.

12 CONCLUSION

Envisioning an Integrated Healthcare Home

We started our narrative focused on the historical context that resulted in the emergence of integrated behavioral health in healthcare. As recently as the 1980s, integrated care was a novel response to the increasing fragmentation and specialization of healthcare. Integrated behavioral health, particularly the primary care behavioral health model, emerged largely independently in different types of healthcare systems. Our intent in sharing this origin story is to describe the multiple factors that led to the need for a systemic lens to help the reader understand how integrated care emerged and evolved. Knowing where we've been informs where we're going.

As we close, we focus on a different use of the word *emergence*. Systems and complexity theorists use the term as a noun. *Emergence* refers to how patterns of unanticipated behaviors arise out of interactivity among system components in the context of imbalance, complexity, and even chaos (Mihata, 1997). It reflects the process of change in complicated systems, change that sometimes occurs in unanticipated ways. Emergence occurs in everyday life, in ways large and small. The emerging pattern may be relatively unimportant, such as when each individual in a group sits in the same seat in every meeting,

https://doi.org/10.1037/0000381-013
A Systemic Approach to Behavioral Healthcare Integration: Context Matters, by
N. B. Ruddy and S. H. McDaniel

an unspoken agreement about who sits where. Other emergences are very powerful, such as human behavior that contributes to climate change. The parts of a whole create phenomena together they would not create alone. Emergence is one expression of the phrase, "a whole is greater than the sum of its parts."

Our current healthcare conundrum exemplifies the problem of unintended consequences. Challenging unintended consequences, such as our current bifurcated system, emerge even in the context of excellent intentions. Early mental health advocates fought to define, legitimize, and fund mental healthcare. The National Institute of Mental Health did not even exist until 1946. Creating a separate government entity focused on mental health was hailed as a victory. And it was a victory. It portended the recognition that mental health issues are central to health. But it also set the stage for separate and vastly unequal resources for mental health issues. It presaged our largely separate education, research, and reimbursement systems. As healthcare reform gathered steam in the late 1980s and early 1990s, mental health advocates feared increased alignment with the healthcare system. As Kiesler (1992) stated, "The mimicry of health services by mental health leads to demonstrably more expensive and less effective mental healthcare and dooms mental health policy to failure" (p. 1077). The intention to avoid overmedicalization and advocate for mental health as foundational in its own right inadvertently contributed to the fragmentation and silos between health and mental health.

The emergence of integrated care has served as a systemic counterbalance to the healthcare fragmentation that spiraled in the second half of the 20th century. Integrated care models emerged to pull in the opposite direction as the system sought homeostasis. Different parts of the system began to work together in completely new ways that were unanticipated and impossible as separate entities. In this context, behavioral health clinicians needed to create qualitatively different approaches to their work. Clinicians, administrators, and staff had to adapt and work as teams. Not surprisingly, this recalibration away from fragmentation developed in the complex adaptive system of primary care, whose prescribed function is to coordinate care and create navigational tools for people to manage health challenges.

As the biopsychosocial model reflects, human health and illness depend on a complex mix of cells, organ systems, emotions, relationships, social structures, and culture. Health reflects balance in all of these areas, and we increasingly recognize how an imbalance in any part of the system can contribute to a cascade of consequences. Our healthcare system has responded to this complexity with specialization, breaking our mind and body into its components.

The solution that fragmented our approach to health was not based in common sense or science; it was based on the sense that dealing with every aspect of health at once is overwhelming. No one person can master the overwhelming amount of knowledge or the range of skills required to manage all ills.

To manage this overwhelming field, we created false walls between different parts of the human experience as it relates to our health and wellness. We separated our understanding of the individual from their social context, culture, and relationships to focus on the experience of *one* person—the person who brings their distress. We separated our understanding of the body from the mind to focus on one or the other, depending on our status as a medical clinician or a mental health clinician. We separated the psychological from the social, focusing on intrapsychic experience rather than relationships. We separated the parts of the body into organ systems and sometimes even into parts of an organ system. We hoped a singular focus would result in deep knowledge of a small area—to master at least one element of health. But in our good intentions, we fragmented the health and the human experience into parts, without recognition that health and wellness emanate from the balance of the parts. As sometimes happens, the solution has become the problem.

We lose so much in this hyperspecialization and fragmentation. Those who managed COVID-19 isolation with jigsaw puzzles now know all too well that staring at only one or two pieces of the puzzle, no matter how intently, was not a good strategy. Only when stepping back and looking at the big picture can one see how it all fits together. Of course, there is a place for specialization in some areas—like finding the corner pieces of that puzzle or all the straight edges to create the frame. But the overall solution is in the interlocking web of the parts. The emergence of the picture requires us to acknowledge the whole is greater than the sum of its parts.

As our healthcare system and our understanding of the human condition evolve, we know that promoting health requires looking at the big picture and bringing humanity back into our medical system. The big picture truly is too much for any one person—there is too much to know, too much to attend to. We need someone to look over our shoulder, find the weird chunk of puzzle we have been missing, and put it into its place. We need to remember the value of multiple perspectives—not just of our professional team but of the patient, the family, the community. We need a collaborative team.

The move toward interprofessional teams has been and continues to be challenging in part because it swims upstream against the structure of our healthcare system. It requires medical and mental health professionals to see themselves as part of a great whole. It requires people to go outside their comfort zone, change routines, and trust others. Change takes motivation and energy—adaptive reserve. As we emerge from this pandemic, our healthcare system is running on fumes, and yet the experience has made clear both the need and the possibility for change.

From a systemic (rather than only an individual) lens, integrated care has an elegant simplicity for the patients and families we seek to serve. Integrating behavioral health enables, simply, one-stop shopping. Of course it doesn't meet every need, but it does allow people to explore multiple pathways to health. The presence of behavioral health clinicians on a healthcare team sends a clear message that we care about whole-person health. It announces that we respect the mind–body connection and realize that good care requires multiple types of expertise working in concert. It recognizes that distress can be rooted in the bio, psycho, and/or social and illustrates that the team stands ready to address these areas and their intersectionalities. Team-based care reflects an appreciation that the whole is greater than the sum of its parts.

Integrated care is a systemic manifestation of caring. We do not require the patient and family, in the midst of suffering, to identify what type of help they need. There is no wrong door because medical and mental healthcare are offered together. The necessary services are provided in real time, based on the patient's need and schedule. When we embrace the complexity of health, the *simple* truth emerges—it doesn't make sense to separate our minds, our choices, our health. Integrated care recognizes that finding the corner pieces to the puzzle is just the beginning; filling in the middle—understanding how things come together—is the science, art, and joy of practice.

Perhaps in rediscovering the core of relationships with patients and teams, the joy of practice can be rediscovered (Sinsky et al., 2013). "Joy of practice" is a phrase coined to describe that feeling of accomplishment and meaning that, sadly, has been in too short supply for many healthcare clinicians. We posit that integrated care may be a key to recapturing the lightning in a bottle that is joy of practice. Working in healthcare is hard, and most healthcare clinicians made major sacrifices to achieve their roles. People typically come into the world of healthcare out of a desire to serve others, such that being of service is its own reward. Joy of practice is based in relationship. It is based in seeing someone get better over time, in being part of another's healing. This experience gets lost when patient care is fragmented, ultimately disrupting the clinician–patient relationship and the clinician's joy of practice. The relationships that sustain joy of practice are not just those with patients but also those with one's clinical team based in a shared purpose and mission. COVID taught us what happens when people are isolated from one another. In the clinical sphere, telehealth had many benefits. But clinicians also crave connection, not only with patients but also with each other. We all need to know that we have backup—not just in clinical practice but to process the emotional impact that practice has on our own humanity.

With systemic integrated care, there is an elegant simplicity in the interwoven net of supports that brings together relevant expertise in one accessible place to provide proactive, comprehensive patient-centered care. There is an elegant simplicity in a team of professionals who support each other to provide a level of care that transcends what any one person can do.

We close with prescient words from an early pioneer in family systems medicine. In 1984, Donald Ransom, PhD, wrote

> By opening up the once-invisible doctor-patient exchange to include other persons on both sides of this relationship, both a more comprehensive approach to assessing problems and initiating change and a redistribution of control and responsibility are achieved. The family focus expands the ordinary view to identify ways health is affected by our relations with others and includes them in the process of creating change. (p. 22)

Ransom's words echo to this day, motivating us to continue our collective effort to build the healthcare system we all deserve.

EPILOGUE

The goal is clear:

> A healthcare system where everyone—
> patients, families, and clinicians alike—
> benefits from systemic, integrated care.

> Where physical and mental health professionals work together
> to provide wholistic care centered on what matters most to patients and families.

It can be that simple.

We can harness the power and effectiveness of a systemic lens to improve care for our communities. We can enhance a sense of pride and fulfillment for all healthcare professionals. We can harness the power of teams to support professional wellness.

It can be fun.

When we recognize that healthcare is multifaceted, reflecting the biopsychosocial complexity of the human experience, when we use a systemic lens to embrace integration at the clinical, educational, operational, policy and larger system levels, integrated care, like oxygen, becomes essential.

It is the air we breathe.

https://doi.org/10.1037/0000381-014
A Systemic Approach to Behavioral Healthcare Integration: Context Matters, by
N. B. Ruddy and S. H. McDaniel

References

Aarons, G. A., Hurlburt, M., & Horwitz, S. M. (2011). Advancing a conceptual model of evidence-based practice implementation in public service sectors. *Administration and Policy in Mental Health and Mental Health Services Research,* *38*(1), 4–23. https://doi.org/10.1007/s10488-010-0327-7

Abdulsalam, L. B., Pitmang, S., Sabir, A., & Olatunji, L. K. (2019). Relationship between family dynamics and glycemic control among adults with Type 2 diabetes mellitus presenting at Usmanu Danfodiyo University Teaching Hospital, Sokoto, Nigeria. *International Archives of Medicine and Medical Sciences, 1*(3), 1–7.

Accreditation Council for Graduate Medical Education. (1989). *Special requirements for residency training in family practice.*

Acevedo, S. M., & Nusbaum, E. A. (2020). Autism, neurodiversity, and inclusive education. In G. W. Noblit (Ed.), *Oxford research encyclopedia of education.* Oxford University Press. https://doi.org/10.1093/acrefore/9780190264093.013.1260

Adelman, R. D., Tmanova, L. L., Delgado, D., Dion, S., & Lachs, M. S. (2014). Caregiver burden: A clinical review. *JAMA, 311*(10), 1052–1060. https://doi.org/10.1001/jama.2014.304

Ader, J., Stille, C. J., Keller, D., Miller, B. F., Barr, M. S., & Perrin, J. M. (2015). The medical home and integrated behavioral health: Advancing the policy agenda. *Pediatrics, 135*(5), 909–917. https://doi.org/10.1542/peds.2014-3941

Ades, V., Wu, S. X., Rabinowitz, E., Chemouni Bach, S., Goddard, B., Pearson Ayala, S., & Greene, J. (2019). An integrated, trauma-informed care model for female survivors of sexual violence: The Engage, Motivate, Protect, Organize, Self-Worth, Educate, Respect (EMPOWER) clinic. *Obstetrics and Gynecology, 133*(4), 803–809. https://doi.org/10.1097/AOG.0000000000003186

Agency for Healthcare Research and Quality. (n.d.). *Defining the PCMH.* https://pcmh.ahrq.gov/page/defining-pcmh

AIMS Center. (2020, July 21). *Caseload size guidance for behavioral health care managers.* https://aims.uw.edu/sites/default/files/Behavioral%20Health%20Care%20Manager%20Caseload%20Guidelines_072120%20Final.pdf

AIMS Center. (2023a). *Behavioral health care manager*. https://aims.uw.edu/collaborative-care/team-structure/care-manager

AIMS Center. (2023b). *Measurement-based treatment to target*. https://aims.uw.edu/resource-library/measurement-based-treatment-target

AIMS Center. (2023c). *Registry tools*. https://aims.uw.edu/registry-tools

AIMS Center. (2023d). *Training and support: Behavioral health care managers*. https://aims.uw.edu/online-bhcm-modules

AIMS Center. (2023e). *Training and support: Primary care provider*. https://aims.uw.edu/training-support/online-trainings/primary-care-provider

Ali, M. K., Chwastiak, L., Poongothai, S., Emmert-Fees, K. M. F., Patel, S. A., Anjana, R. M., Sagar, R., Shankar, R., Sridhar, G. R., Kosuri, M., Sosale, A. R., Sosale, B., Rao, D., Tandon, N., Narayan, K. M. V., Mohan, V., & the INDEPENDENT Study Group. (2020). Effect of a collaborative care model on depressive symptoms and glycated hemoglobin, blood pressure, and serum cholesterol among patients with depression and diabetes in India: The INDEPENDENT randomized clinical trial. *JAMA, 324*(7), 651–662. https://doi.org/10.1001/jama.2020.11747

Allegrante, J. P., Wells, M. T., & Peterson, J. C. (2019). Interventions to support behavioral self-management of chronic diseases. *Annual Review of Public Health, 40*(1), 127–146. https://doi.org/10.1146/annurev-publhealth-040218-044008

Allen, J. A., Reiter-Palmon, R., Crowe, J., & Scott, C. (2018). Debriefs: Teams learning from doing in context. *American Psychologist, 73*(4), 504–516. https://doi.org/10.1037/amp0000246

Almeida, O. P., Marsh, K., Flicker, L., Hickey, M., Sim, M., & Ford, A. (2016). Depressive symptoms in midlife: The role of reproductive stage. *Menopause, 23*(6), 669–675. https://doi.org/10.1097/GME.0000000000000598

Altshuler, A. L., & Whaley, N. S. (2018). The patient perspective: Perceptions of the quality of the abortion experience. *Current Opinion in Obstetrics & Gynecology, 30*(6), 407–413. https://doi.org/10.1097/GCO.0000000000000492

American Academy of Family Physicians, American Academy of Pediatrics, American College of Physicians, & American Osteopathic Association. (2007). *Joint principles of the patient-centered medical home*. https://www.aafp.org/dam/AAFP/documents/practice_management/pcmh/initiatives/PCMHJoint.pdf

American Academy of Pediatrics. (2021, June 16). *Mental health initiatives*. https://www.aap.org/en-us/advocacy-and-policy/aap-health-initiatives/Mental-Health/Pages/ProgramSearch.aspx

American Academy of Pediatrics Council on Pediatric Practice. (1967). Pediatric records and a "medical home." In *Standards of Child care* (pp. 77–79). American Academy of Pediatrics.

American Association for Marriage and Family Therapy. (2018, November). *Competencies for family therapists working in healthcare settings*. https://www.aamft.org/healthcare

American College of Obstetricians and Gynecologists. (2016, Jan. 26). *ACOG statement on depression screening*. https://www.acog.org/news/news-releases/2016/01/acog-statement-on-depression-screening

American College of Obstetricians and Gynecologists' Committee on Healthcare for Underserved Women. (2012). *Committee Opinion No. 518: Intimate partner violence. Obstetrics and Gynecology, 119*(2, Pt. 1), 412–417. https://doi.org/10.1097/AOG.0b013e318249ff74

American College of Obstetricians and Gynecologists' Committee on Practice Bulletins–Gynecology. (2019). Female sexual dysfunction: ACOG practice bulletin clinical management guidelines for obstetrician–gynecologists, number 213. *Obstetrics and Gynecology, 134*(1), e1–e18. https://doi.org/10.1097/AOG.0000000000003324

American Psychological Association. (2015, February). *Standards of accreditation for health service psychology.* https://www.apa.org/ed/accreditation/about/policies/standards-of-accreditation.pdf

Anastas, T., Waddell, E. N., Howk, S., Remiker, M., Horton-Dunbar, G., & Fagnan, L. J. (2019). Building behavioral health homes: Clinician and staff perspectives on creating integrated care teams. *The Journal of Behavioral Health Services & Research, 46*(3), 475–486. https://doi.org/10.1007/s11414-018-9622-y

Andrilla, C. H. A., Patterson, D. G., Garberson, L. A., Coulthard, C., & Larson, E. H. (2018). Geographic variation in the supply of selected behavioral health providers. *American Journal of Preventive Medicine, 54*(6, Suppl. 3), S199–S207. https://doi.org/10.1016/j.amepre.2018.01.004

Angantyr, K., Rimner, A., Nordén, T., & Norlander, T. (2015). Primary care behavioral health model: Perspectives of outcome, client satisfaction, and gender. *Social Behavior and Personality, 43*(2), 287–301. https://doi.org/10.2224/sbp.2015.43.2.287

Archer, J., Bower, P., Gilbody, S., Lovell, K., Richards, D., Gask, L., Dickens, C., & Coventry, P. (2012). Collaborative care for depression and anxiety problems. *Cochrane Database of Systematic Reviews, 2012*(10), Article CD006525. https://doi.org/10.1002/14651858.CD006525.pub2

Arnaez, J. M., Krendl, A. C., McCormick, B. P., Chen, Z., & Chomistek, A. K. (2020). The association of depression stigma with barriers to seeking mental health care: A cross-sectional analysis. *Journal of Mental Health, 29*(2), 182–190. https://doi.org/10.1080/09638237.2019.1644494

Asarnow, J. R., Rozenman, M., Wiblin, J., & Zeltzer, L. (2015). Integrated medical-behavioral care compared with usual primary care for child and adolescent behavioral health: A meta-analysis. *JAMA Pediatrics, 169*(10), 929–937. https://doi.org/10.1001/jamapediatrics.2015.1141

Babor, T. F., McRee, B. G., Kassebaum, P. A., Grimaldi, P. L., Ahmed, K., & Bray, J. (2007). Screening, Brief Intervention, and Referral to Treatment (SBIRT): Toward a public health approach to the management of substance abuse. *Substance Abuse, 28*(3), 7–30. https://doi.org/10.1300/J465v28n03_03

Bach, M. (2018). Psychosocial interventions for individuals with infertility [Master's alternative plan paper, Minnesota State University, Mankato]. In *Cornerstone: A Collection of Scholarly and Creative Works for Minnesota State University, Mankato.* https://cornerstone.lib.mnsu.edu/etds/760

Baciu, A., Negussie, Y., Geller, A., Weinstein, J. N., & National Academies of Sciences, Engineering, and Medicine. (2017). The state of health disparities in the United States. In J. N. Weinstein, A. Geller, Y. Negussie, & A. Baciu (Eds.), *Communities in action: Pathways to health equity* (pp. 57–99). National Academies Press.

Badr, H., Bakhshaie, J., & Chhabria, K. (2019). Dyadic interventions for cancer survivors and caregivers: State of the science and new directions. *Seminars in Oncology Nursing, 35*(4), 337–341. https://doi.org/10.1016/j.soncn.2019.06.004

Baig, A. A., Benitez, A., Quinn, M. T., & Burnet, D. L. (2015). Family interventions to improve diabetes outcomes for adults. *Annals of the New York Academy of Sciences, 1353*(1), 89–112. https://doi.org/10.1111/nyas.12844

Baird, M., Blount, A., Brungardt, S., Dickinson, P., Dietrich, A., Epperly, T., Green, L., Henley, D., Kessler, R., Korsen, N., McDaniel, S., Miller, B., Pugno, P., Roberts, R., Schirmer, J., Seymour, D., & deGruy, F. (2014). The development of joint principles: Integrating behavioral health care into the patient-centered medical home. *Annals of Family Medicine, 12*(2), 183–185. https://doi.org/10.1370/afm.1634

Bakan, D. (1966). *The duality of human existence: Isolation and communion in western man.* Beacon Press.

Baker, G. R. (2020, May 19). *Evidence boost: A review of research highlighting how patient engagement contributes to improved care.* Canadian Foundation for Healthcare Improvement. https://www.cfhi-fcass.ca/about/news-and-stories/news-detail/2020/05/19/evidence-boost-a-review-of-research-highlighting-how-patient-engagement-contributes-to-improved-care

Baker, J. M., Grant, R. W., & Gopalan, A. (2018). A systematic review of care management interventions targeting multimorbidity and high care utilization. *BMC Health Services Research, 18*, Article 65, 1–9. https://doi.org/10.1186/s12913-018-2881-8

Bakhbakhi, D., Burden, C., Storey, C., & Siassakos, D. (2017). Care following stillbirth in high-resource settings: Latest evidence, guidelines, and best practice points. *Seminars in Fetal & Neonatal Medicine, 22*(3), 161–166. https://doi.org/10.1016/j.siny.2017.02.008

Balas, E. A., & Chapman, W. W. (2018). Road map for diffusion of innovation in health care. *Health Affairs (Project Hope), 37*(2), 198–204. https://doi.org/10.1377/hlthaff.2017.1155

Balasubramanian, B. A., Chase, S. M., Nutting, P. A., Cohen, D. J., Strickland, P. A. O., Crosson, J. C., Miller, W. L., Crabtree, B. F., & the ULTRA Study Team. (2010). Using Learning Teams for Reflective Adaptation (ULTRA): Insights from a team-based change management strategy in primary care. *Annals of Family Medicine, 8*(5), 425–432. https://doi.org/10.1370/afm.1159

Balasubramanian, B. A., Cohen, D. J., Jetelina, K. K., Dickinson, L. M., Davis, M., Gunn, R., Gowen, K., deGruy, F. V., III, Miller, B. F., & Green, L. A. (2017). Outcomes of integrated behavioral health with primary care. *Journal of the American Board of Family Medicine, 30*(2), 130–139. https://doi.org/10.3122/jabfm.2017.02.160234

Balasubramanian, B. A., Fernald, D., Dickinson, L. M., Davis, M., Gunn, R., Crabtree, B. F., Miller, B. F., & Cohen, D. J. (2015). REACH of interventions integrating primary care and behavioral health. *Journal of the American Board of Family Medicine, 28*(Suppl. 1), S73–S85. https://doi.org/10.3122/jabfm.2015.S1.150055

Bao, Y., Druss, B. G., Jung, H. Y., Chan, Y. F., & Unützer, J. (2016). Unpacking collaborative care for depression: Examining two essential tasks for implementation. *Psychiatric Services, 67*(4), 418–424. https://doi.org/10.1186/1748-5908-10-s1-a33

Barefoot, J. C., & Schroll, M. (1996). Symptoms of depression, acute myocardial infarction and total mortality in a community sample. *Circulation, 93*(11), 1976–1980.

Bareil, C., Duhamel, F., Lalonde, L., Goudreau, J., Hudon, E., Lussier, M. T., Lévesque, L., Lessard, S., Turcotte, A., & Lalonde, G. (2015). Facilitating implementation of interprofessional collaborative practices into primary care: A trilogy of driving forces. *Journal of Healthcare Management, 60*(4), 287–300. https://doi.org/10.1097/00115514-201507000-00010

Barrett, S., Begg, S., O'Halloran, P., & Kingsley, M. (2018). Integrated motivational interviewing and cognitive behaviour therapy for lifestyle mediators of overweight and obesity in community-dwelling adults: A systematic review and meta-analyses. *BMC Public Health, 18*, Article 1160. https://doi.org/10.1186/s12889-018-6062-9

Barry, D., Nordberg, S. S., & Stevens, F. L. (2020). Termination in integrated primary care behavioral health. *Psychotherapy, 57*(4), 521–530. https://doi.org/10.1037/pst0000299

Baucom, D. H., Porter, L. S., Kirby, J. S., & Hudepohl, J. (2012). Couple-based interventions for medical problems. *Behavior Therapy, 43*(1), 61–76. https://doi.org/10.1016/j.beth.2011.01.008

Bearak, J., Popinchalk, A., Alkema, L., & Sedgh, G. (2018). Global, regional, and subregional trends in unintended pregnancy and its outcomes from 1990 to 2014: Estimates from a Bayesian hierarchical model. *The Lancet. Global Health, 6*(4), e380–e389. https://doi.org/10.1016/S2214-109X(18)30029-9

Beckard, R. (1975). Strategies for large system change. *Sloan Management Review, 16*(2), 43.

Beehler, G. P., Funderburk, J. S., King, P. R., Possemato, K., Maddoux, J. A., Goldstein, W. R., & Wade, M. (2020). Validation of an expanded measure of integrated care provider fidelity: PPAQ-2. *Journal of Clinical Psychology in Medical Settings, 27*(1), 158–172. https://doi.org/10.1007/s10880-019-09628-0

Beehler, G. P., Funderburk, J. S., King, P. R., Wade, M., & Possemato, K. (2015). Using the primary care behavioral health provider adherence questionnaire (PPAQ) to identify practice patterns. *Translational Behavioral Medicine, 5*(4), 384–392. https://doi.org/10.1007/s13142-015-0325-0

Beehler, G. P., Funderburk, J. S., Possemato, K., & Vair, C. L. (2013). Developing a measure of provider adherence to improve the implementation of behavioral health services in primary care: A Delphi study. *Implementation Science, 8,* Article 19. https://doi.org/10.1186/1748-5908-8-19

Beehler, G. P., Lilienthal, K. R., Possemato, K., Johnson, E. M., King, P. R., Shepardson, R. L., Vair, C. L., Reyner, J., Funderburk, J. S., Maisto, S. A., & Wray, L. O. (2017). Narrative review of provider behavior in primary care behavioral health: How process data can inform quality improvement. *Families, Systems & Health, 35*(3), 257–270. https://doi.org/10.1037/fsh0000263

Begun, J. W., Zimmerman, B., & Dooley, K. (2003). Health care organizations as complex adaptive systems. In S. S. Mick & M. E. Wyttenbach (Eds.), *Advances in health care organization theory* (pp. 253–288). Jossey-Bass.

Bennett-Levy, J., & Thwaites, R. (2007). Self and self-reflection in the therapeutic relationship: A conceptual map and practical strategies for the training, supervision and self-supervision of interpersonal skills. In P. Gilbert & R. L. Leahy (Eds.), *The therapeutic relationship in the cognitive behavioral psychotherapies* (pp. 271–298). Routledge.

Berg, C. A., & Upchurch, R. (2007). A developmental-contextual model of couples coping with chronic illness across the adult life span. *Psychological Bulletin, 133*(6), 920–954. https://doi.org/10.1037/0033-2909.133.6.920

Berkel, C., Smith, J. D., Fu, E., Bruening, M., & Dishion, T. (2019). NP29 the Family Check-Up 4 Health: A health maintenance approach to improve nutrition and prevent early childhood obesity. *Journal of Nutrition Education and Behavior, 51*(7, Suppl.), S23. https://doi.org/10.1016/j.jneb.2019.05.353

Berry, E., Davies, M., & Dempster, M. (2017). Exploring the effectiveness of couples interventions for adults living with a chronic physical illness: A systematic review. *Patient Education and Counseling, 100*(7), 1287–1303. https://doi.org/10.1016/j.pec.2017.02.015

Berwick, D. M. (2019). Reflections on the chronic care model—23 years later. *The Milbank Quarterly, 97*(3), 665–668. https://doi.org/10.1111/1468-0009.12414

Berwick, D. M. (2002). A user's manual for the IOM's 'Quality Chasm' report. *Health Affairs (Project Hope), 21*(3), 80–90. https://doi.org/10.1377/hlthaff.21.3.80

Best, M., Butow, P., & Olver, I. (2015). Do patients want doctors to talk about spirituality? A systematic literature review. *Patient Education and Counseling, 98*(11), 1320–1328. https://doi.org/10.1016/j.pec.2015.04.017

Bethell, C. D., Solloway, M. R., Guinosso, S., Hassink, S., Srivastav, A., Ford, D., & Simpson, L. A. (2017). Prioritizing possibilities for child and family health: An agenda to address adverse childhood experiences and foster the social and emotional roots of well-being in pediatrics. *Academic Pediatrics, 17*(7, Suppl.), S36–S50. https://doi.org/10.1016/j.acap.2017.06.002

Beverly, E. A., Ritholz, M. D., Brooks, K. M., Hultgren, B. A., Lee, Y., Abrahamson, M. J., & Weinger, K. (2012). A qualitative study of perceived responsibility and self-blame in type 2 diabetes: Reflections of physicians and patients. *Journal of General Internal Medicine, 27*(9), 1180–1187. https://doi.org/10.1007/s11606-012-2070-0

Bidstrup, P. E., Salem, H., Andersen, E. W., Schmiegelow, K., Rosthøj, S., Wehner, P. S., Hasle, H., Dalton, S. O., Johansen, C., & Kazak, A. E. (2023). Effects on pediatric cancer survivors: The FAMily-Oriented Support (FAMOS) randomized controlled trial. *Journal of Pediatric Psychology, 48*(1), 29–38. https://doi.org/10.1093/jpepsy/jsac062

Biggs, M. A., Upadhyay, U. D., McCulloch, C. E., & Foster, D. G. (2017). Women's mental health and well-being 5 years after receiving or being denied an abortion: A prospective, longitudinal cohort study. *JAMA Psychiatry, 74*(2), 169–178. https://doi.org/10.1001/jamapsychiatry.2016.3478

Bloch, D. (1983). Family systems medicine: The field and the journal. *Family Systems Medicine, 1*(1), 3–11. https://doi.org/10.1037/h0090105

Bloch, D. (1988). Dr. Biomedicine and Dr. Biopsychosocial: The dual optic II. Why referral (mostly) does not work. *Family Systems Medicine, 6*(2), 131–133. https://doi.org/10.1037/h0090001

Bloch, D. (2002). Dr. Biomedicine and Dr. Psychosocial: The dual optic II: Why referral (mostly) does not work. *Families, Systems & Health, 20*(4), 338–340. https://doi.org/10.1037/h0089508

Blok, A. C., Amante, D. J., Hogan, T. P., Sadasivam, R. S., Shimada, S. L., Woods, S., Nazi, K. M., & Houston, T. K. (2021). Impact of patient access to online VA notes on healthcare utilization and clinician documentation: A retrospective cohort study. *Journal of General Internal Medicine, 36*(3), 592–599. https://doi.org/10.1007/s11606-020-06304-0

Blount, A. (1998). *Integrated primary care: The future of medical and mental health collaboration*. Norton.

Blount, A. (2019a). It takes a team. In S. B. Gold & L. A. Green (Eds.), *Integrated behavioral health in primary care: Your patients are waiting* (pp. 131–155). Springer Cham. https://doi.org/10.1007/978-3-319-98587-9_6

Blount, A. (2019b). *Patient-centered primary care: Getting from good to great*. Springer Nature. https://doi.org/10.1007/978-3-030-17645-7

Blount, F. A., & Miller, B. F. (2009). Addressing the workforce crisis in integrated primary care. *Journal of Clinical Psychology in Medical Settings, 16*(1), 113–119. https://doi.org/10.1007/s10880-008-9142-7

Bodenheimer, T., & Sinsky, C. (2014). From triple to quadruple aim: Care of the patient requires care of the provider. *Annals of Family Medicine, 12*(6), 573–576. https://doi.org/10.1370/afm.1713

Bogucki, O. E., Craner, J. R., Berg, S. L., Wolsey, M. K., Miller, S. J., Smyth, K. T., Johnson, M. W., Mack, J. D., Sedivy, S. J., Burke, L. M., Glader, M. A., Williams, M. W., Katzelnick, D. J., & Sawchuk, C. N. (2021). Cognitive behavioral therapy for anxiety disorders: Outcomes from a multi-state, multi-site primary care practice. *Journal of Anxiety Disorders, 78*, 102345. https://doi.org/10.1016/j.janxdis.2020.102345

Bom, J., Bakx, P., Schut, F., & van Doorslaer, E. (2019). The impact of informal caregiving for older adults on the health of various types of caregivers: A systematic review. *The Gerontologist, 59*(5), e629–e642. https://doi.org/10.1093/geront/gny137

Booth, C. B., & Lazar, R. (2015, July). Implementing the CLAS standards. *CLC Hub Resource Brief 2.* http://cfclinc.org/wp-content/uploads/2018/10/CLC-Research-Brief-2-DRAFT5.pdf

Bothwell, L. E., Greene, J. A., Podolsky, S. H., & Jones, D. S. (2016). Assessing the gold standard—Lessons from the history of RCTs. *The New England Journal of Medicine, 374*(22), 2175–2181. https://doi.org/10.1056/NEJMms1604593

Boyczuk, A. M., & Fletcher, P. C. (2016). The ebbs and flows: Stresses of sandwich generation caregivers. *Journal of Adult Development, 23*(1), 51–61. https://doi.org/10.1007/s10804-015-9221-6

Brandt, K. (2014). Transforming clinical practice through reflection work. In K. Brandt, B. Perry, S. Seligman, & E. Tronick (Eds.), *Infant and early childhood mental health: Core concepts and clinical practice* (pp. 293–307). American Psychiatric Association.

Brashers, V. L., Curry, C. E., Harper, D. C., McDaniel, S. H., Pawlson, G., & Ball, J. W. (2001). Interprofessional health care education: Recommendations of the National Academies of Practice expert panel on healthcare in the 21st century. *Issues in Interdisciplinary Care, 3*(1), 21–31.

Brier, N. (1999). Understanding and managing the emotional reactions to a miscarriage. *Obstetrics and Gynecology, 93*(1), 151–155.

Briggs, R. D., Silver, E. J., Krug, L. M., Mason, Z. S., Schrag, R. D., Chinitz, S., & Racine, A. D. (2014). Healthy steps as a moderator: The impact of maternal trauma on child social-emotional development. *Clinical Practice in Pediatric Psychology, 2*(2), 166–175. https://doi.org/10.1037/cpp0000060

Brody, G. H., Yu, T., Chen, E., & Miller, G. E. (2020). Persistence of skin-deep resilience in African American adults. *Health Psychology, 39*(10), 921–926. https://doi.org/10.1037/hea0000945

Brown, C. M., Raglin Bignall, W. J., & Ammerman, R. T. (2018). Preventive behavioral health programs in primary care: A systematic review. *Pediatrics, 141*(5), e20180611. https://doi.org/10.1542/peds.2018-0611

Bryan, C. J., Morrow, C., & Appolonio, K. K. (2009). Impact of behavioral health consultant interventions on patient symptoms and functioning in an integrated family medicine clinic. *Journal of Clinical Psychology, 65*(3), 281–293. https://doi.org/10.1002/jclp.20539

Buchanan, G. J. R., Piehler, T., Berge, J., Hansen, A., & Stephens, K. A. (2022). Integrated behavioral health implementation patterns in primary care using the cross-model framework: A latent class analysis. *Administration and Policy in Mental Health, 49,* 312–325. https://doi.org/10.1007/s10488-021-01165-z

Budde, K. S., Friedman, D., Alli, K., Randell, J., Kang, B., & Feuerstein, S. D. (2017). Integrating behavioral health and primary care in two New Jersey federally qualified health centers. *Psychiatric Services, 68*(11), 1095–1097. https://doi.org/10.1176/appi.ps.201700240

Burden, C., Bradley, S., Storey, C., Ellis, A., Heazell, A. E., Downe, S., Cacciatore, J., & Siassakos, D. (2016). From grief, guilt pain and stigma to hope and pride—A systematic review and meta-analysis of mixed-method research of the psychosocial impact of stillbirth. *BMC Pregnancy and Childbirth, 16*, Article 9. https://doi.org/10.1186/s12884-016-0800-8

Burkhart, K., Asogwa, K., Muzaffar, N., & Gabriel, M. (2020). Pediatric integrated care models: A systematic review. *Clinical Pediatrics, 59*(2), 148–153. https://doi.org/10.1177/0009922819890004

Butler, M., Kane, R. L., McAlpine, D., Kathol, R. G., Fu, S. S., Hagedorn, H., & Wilt, T. J. (2008). Integration of mental health/substance abuse and primary care. *Evidence Report/Technology Assessment, 173*, 1–362.

Butts, C. T., & Carley, K. M. (2007). Structural change and homeostasis in organizations: A decision-theoretic approach. *The Journal of Mathematical Sociology, 31*(4), 295–321. https://doi.org/10.1080/00222500701542517

Byrd, M., Warfield, C., Brookshire, K., & Ostarello, L. (2018). Screening for behavioral health problems in adult primary care. In M. P. Duckworth & W. T. O'Donohue (Eds.), *Behavioral medicine and integrated care* (pp. 75–87). Springer, Cham. https://doi.org/10.1007/978-3-319-93003-9_5

Cabana, M. D., & Jee, S. H. (2004). Does continuity of care improve patient outcomes? *The Journal of Family Practice, 53*(12), 974–980.

Cacciatore, J., Frøen, J., & Killian, M. (2013). Condemning self, condemning other: Blame and mental health in women suffering stillbirth. *Journal of Mental Health Counseling, 35*(4), 342–359. https://doi.org/10.17744/mehc.35.4. 15427g822442h11m

Candib, L. M. (1995). *Medicine and the family: A feminist perspective.* Basic Books.

Carek, P. J., Anim, T., Conry, C., Cullison, S., Kozakowski, S., Ostergaard, D., Potts, S., & Pugno, P. A. (2017). Residency training in family medicine: A history of innovation and program support. *Family Medicine, 49*(4), 275–281.

Carlo, A. D., Unützer, J., Ratzliff, A. D., & Cerimele, J. M. (2018). Financing for collaborative care—A narrative review. *Current Treatment Options in Psychiatry, 5*, 334–344. https://doi.org/10.1007/s40501-018-0150-4

Caretto, M., Giannini, A., & Simoncini, T. (2019). An integrated approach to diagnosing and managing sleep disorders in menopausal women. *Maturitas, 128*, 1–3. https://doi.org/10.1016/j.maturitas.2019.06.008

Carleton, K. E., Patel, U. B., Stein, D., Mou, D., Mallow, A., & Blackmore, M. A. (2020). Enhancing the scalability of the collaborative care model for depression using mobile technology. *Translational Behavioral Medicine, 10*(3), 573–579. https://doi.org/10.1093/tbm/ibz146

Carr, A. (2019). Family therapy and systemic interventions for child-focused problems: The current evidence base. *Journal of Family Therapy, 41*(2), 153–213. https://doi.org/10.1111/1467-6427.12226

Carr, D., Springer, K. W., & Williams, K. (2014). Health and families. In J. Treas, J. L. Scott, & M. Richards (Eds.), *The Wiley Blackwell companion to the sociology of families* (pp. 255–276). Wiley Blackwell. https://doi.org/10.1002/9781118374085.ch13

Cascio, M. A. (2015). Introduction. Cross-cultural autism studies, neurodiversity, and conceptualizations of autism. *Culture, Medicine and Psychiatry, 39*(2), 207–212. https://doi.org/10.1007/s11013-015-9450-y

Casellas-Grau, A., Ochoa, C., & Ruini, C. (2017). Psychological and clinical correlates of posttraumatic growth in cancer: A systematic and critical review. *Psycho-Oncology, 26*(12), 2007–2018. https://doi.org/10.1002/pon.4426

Caswell, G., Pollock, K., Harwood, R., & Porock, D. (2015). Communication between family carers and health professionals about end-of-life care for older people in the acute hospital setting: A qualitative study. *BMC Palliative Care, 14*, Article 35. https://doi.org/10.1186/s12904-015-0032-0

Celano, C. M., & Huffman, J. C. (2011). Depression and cardiac disease: A review. *Cardiology in Review, 19*(3), 130–142. https://doi.org/10.1097/CRD.0b013e31820e8106

Cené, C. W., Haymore, L. B., Lin, F. C., Laux, J., Jones, C. D., Wu, J. R., DeWalt, D., Pignone, M., & Corbie-Smith, G. (2015). Family member accompaniment to routine medical visits is associated with better self-care in heart failure patients. *Chronic Illness, 11*(1), 21–32. https://doi.org/10.1177/1742395314532142

Centers for Disease Control and Prevention. (2019a). *IVF success estimator.* https://www.cdc.gov/art/ivf-success-estimator

Centers for Disease Control and Prevention. (2020a). *From data to actions: CDC's public health surveillance of women, infants and children* (2nd ed.). https://www.cdc.gov/reproductivehealth/productspubs/data-to-action-e-book/pdf/Data-To-Action_508.pdf

Centers for Disease Control and Prevention. (2020b). *Sexually transmitted infections, prevalence, incidence, and cost estimates in the United States.* https://www.cdc.gov/std/statistics/prevalence-incidence-cost-2020.htm

Chachamovich, J. R., Chachamovich, E., Ezer, H., Fleck, M. P., Knauth, D., & Passos, E. P. (2010). Investigating quality of life and health-related quality of life in infertility: A systematic review. *Journal of Psychosomatic Obstetrics and Gynaecology, 31*(2), 101–110. https://doi.org/10.3109/0167482X.2010.481337

Chakraborti, C., Boonyasai, R. T., Wright, S. M., & Kern, D. E. (2008). A systematic review of teamwork training interventions in medical student and resident education. *Journal of General Internal Medicine, 23*(6), 846–853. https://doi.org/10.1007/s11606-008-0600-6

Chapman, S., Correa, N., Cummings, A., Van Horne, B. S., & Schwarzwald, H. (2020). Integration of behavioral health services into primary pediatric care: The behind the scenes story of a pilot study in Southeast, Texas. *The Journal of Applied Research on Children, 11*(1), 8–15.

Chisholm, C. A., Bullock, L., & Ferguson, J. E. J., II. (2017). Intimate partner violence and pregnancy: Screening and intervention. *American Journal of Obstetrics and Gynecology, 217*(2), 145–149. https://doi.org/10.1016/j.ajog.2017.05.043

Chow, K. M., Cheung, M. C., & Cheung, I. K. (2016). Psychosocial interventions for infertile couples: A critical review. *Journal of Clinical Nursing, 25*(15–16), 2101–2113. https://doi.org/10.1111/jocn.13361

Christian, E., Krall, V., Hulkower, S., & Stigleman, S. (2018). Primary care behavioral health integration: Promoting the quadruple aim. *North Carolina Medical Journal, 79*(4), 250–255. https://doi.org/10.18043/ncm.79.4.250

Christie-Seely, J. (1984). *Working with the family in primary care: A systems approach to health and illness.* Praeger.

Chung, M. C., & Reed, J. (2017). Posttraumatic stress disorder following stillbirth: Trauma characteristics, locus of control, posttraumatic cognitions. *Psychiatric Quarterly, 88*(2), 307–321. https://doi.org/10.1007/s11126-016-9446-y

Chwastiak, L. A., Jackson, S. L., Russo, J., DeKeyser, P., Kiefer, M., Belyeu, B., Mertens, K., Chew, L., & Lin, E. (2017). A collaborative care team to integrate behavioral health care and treatment of poorly-controlled Type 2 diabetes in an urban safety net primary care clinic. *General Hospital Psychiatry, 44,* 10–15. https://doi.org/10.1016/j.genhosppsych.2016.10.005

Cifuentes, M., Davis, M., Fernald, D., Gunn, R., Dickinson, P., & Cohen, D. J. (2015). Electronic health record challenges, workarounds, and solutions observed in practices integrating behavioral health and primary care. *Journal of the American Board of Family Medicine, 28*(Suppl. 1), S63–S72. https://doi.org/10.3122/jabfm.2015.S1.150133

Cigrang, J. A., Cordova, J. V., Gray, T. D., Fedynich, A. L., Maher, E., Aiehl, A. N., & Hawrilenko, M. (2022). Marriage checkup in integrated primary care: A randomized controlled trial with active-duty military couples. *Journal of Consulting and Clinical Psychology, 90*(5), 381–391. https://doi.org/10.1037/ccp0000734

Clement, S., Schauman, O., Graham, T., Maggioni, F., Evans-Lacko, S., Bezborodovs, N., Morgan, C., Rüsch, N., Brown, J. S., & Thornicroft, G. (2015). What is the impact of mental health-related stigma on help-seeking? A systematic review of quantitative and qualitative studies. *Psychological Medicine, 45*(1), 11–27. https://doi.org/10.1017/S0033291714000129

Coates, D., Coppleson, D., & Schmied, V. (2020). Integrated physical and mental healthcare: An overview of models and their evaluation findings. *International Journal of Evidence-Based Healthcare, 18*(1), 38–57. https://doi.org/10.1097/XEB.0000000000000215

Cockrill, K., Upadhyay, U. D., Turan, J., & Greene Foster, D. (2013). The stigma of having an abortion: Development of a scale and characteristics of women experiencing abortion stigma. *Perspectives on Sexual and Reproductive Health, 45*(2), 79–88. https://doi.org/10.1363/4507913

Cohain, J. S., Buxbaum, R. E., & Mankuta, D. (2017). Spontaneous first trimester miscarriage rates per woman among parous women with 1 or more pregnancies of 24 weeks or more. *BMC Pregnancy and Childbirth, 17,* Article 437. https://doi.org/10.1186/s12884-017-1620-1

Cohen, D., & Coco, A. (2014). Do physicians address other medical problems during preventive gynecologic visits? *Journal of the American Board of Family Medicine, 27*(1), 13–18. https://doi.org/10.3122/jabfm.2014.01.130045

Cohen, D. J., Balasubramanian, B. A., Davis, M., Hall, J., Gunn, R., Stange, K. C., Green, L. A., Miller, W. L., Crabtree, B. F., England, M. J., Clark, K., & Miller,

B. F. (2015). Understanding care integration from the ground up: Five organizing constructs that shape integrated practices. *Journal of the American Board of Family Medicine, 28*(Suppl. 1), S7–S20. https://doi.org/10.3122/jabfm.2015.S1.150050

Cohen, D. J., Davis, M., Balasubramanian, B. A., Gunn, R., Hall, J., deGruy, F. V., III, Peek, C. J., Green, L. A., Stange, K. C., Pallares, C., Levy, S., Pollack, D., & Miller, B. F. (2015). Integrating behavioral health and primary care: Consulting, coordinating and collaborating among professionals. *Journal of the American Board of Family Medicine, 28*(Suppl. 1), S21–S31. https://doi.org/10.3122/jabfm.2015.S1.150042

Cohen, D. J., Davis, M. M., Hall, J. D., Gilchrist, E. C., & Miller, B. F. (2015). *A guidebook of professional practices for behavioral health and primary care integration: Observations from exemplary sites*. Agency for Healthcare Research and Quality.

Coker, T. R., Windon, A., Moreno, C., Schuster, M. A., & Chung, P. J. (2013). Well-child care clinical practice redesign for young children: A systematic review of strategies and tools. *Pediatrics, 131*(Suppl. 1), S5–S25. https://doi.org/10.1542/peds.2012-1427c

Colquhoun, H. L., Squires, J. E., Kolehmainen, N., Fraser, C., & Grimshaw, J. M. (2017). Methods for designing interventions to change healthcare professionals' behaviour: A systematic review. *Implementation Science, 12*, Article 30. https://doi.org/10.1186/s13012-017-0560-5

Combrinck-Graham, L. (1985). A developmental model for family systems. *Family Process, 24*(2), 139–150. https://doi.org/10.1111/j.1545-5300.1985.00139.x

Commonwealth Fund Task Force on Payment and Delivery System Reform. (2020). *Health care delivery system reform: Six policy imperatives*. https://www.commonwealthfund.org/sites/default/files/2021-01/CMWF_DSR_TaskForce_Six_Policy_Imperatives_report_v3.pdf

Comprehensive Health Manpower Training Act of 1971, P.L. No. 92-157, 85 Stat. 431.

Conrad, D. A., Grembowski, D., Hernandez, S. E., Lau, B., & Marcus-Smith, M. (2014). Emerging lessons from regional and state innovation in value-based payment reform: Balancing collaboration and disruptive innovation. *The Milbank Quarterly, 92*(3), 568–623. https://doi.org/10.1111/1468-0009.12078

Cook, B. L., Trinh, N. H., Li, Z., Hou, S. S. Y., & Progovac, A. M. (2017). Trends in racial-ethnic disparities in access to mental health care, 2004–2012. *Psychiatric Services, 68*(1), 9–16. https://doi.org/10.1176/appi.ps.201500453

Coons, H. L., & Gabis, J. E. (2010). Contractual issues for independent psychologists practicing in health care settings: Practical tips for establishing the agreement. *Independent Practitioner, 30*(3), 181–183.

Coons, H. L., Morgenstern, D., Hoffman, E. M., Striepe, M. I., & Buch, C. (2004). Psychologists in women's primary care and obstetrics-gynecology: Consultation and treatment issues. In R. G. Frank, S. H. McDaniel, J. H. Bray, & M. Heldring (Eds.), *Primary care psychology* (pp. 209–226). American Psychological Association. https://doi.org/10.1037/10651-011

Corcoran, J., Berry, A., & Hill, S. (2015). The lived experience of US parents of children with autism spectrum disorders: A systematic review and meta-synthesis. *Journal of Intellectual Disabilities, 19*(4), 356–366. https://doi.org/10.1177/1744629515577876

Cordova, J. V. (2009). *The Marriage Checkup: A scientific program for sustaining and strengthening marital health.* Jason Aronson.

Cordova, J. V. (2014). *The marriage checkup practitioner's guide: Promoting lifelong relationship health.* American Psychological Association.

Cordova, J. V., Cigrang, J. A., Gray, T. D., Najera, E., Havrilenko, M., Pinkley, C., Nielsen, M., Tatum, J., & Redd, K. (2017). Addressing relationship health needs in primary care: Adapting the Marriage Checkup for use in medical settings with military couples. *Journal of Clinical Psychology in Medical Settings, 24*, 259–269. https://doi.org/10.1007/s10880-017-9517-8

Coronavirus Aid, Relief, and Economic Security (CARES) Act, 15 U.S.C. § 9001 *et seq.* (2021).

Corso, K. A., Hunter, C. L., Dahl, O., Kallenberg, G. A., & Manson, L. (2016). *Integrating behavioral health into the medical home: A rapid implementation guide.* Greenbranch Publishing.

Couper, J., Collins, A., Bloch, S., Street, A., Duchesne, G., Jones, T., Olver, J., & Love, A. (2015). Cognitive existential couple therapy (CECT) in men and partners facing localised prostate cancer: A randomised controlled trial. *BJU International, 115*(Suppl. 5), 35–45. https://doi.org/10.1111/bju.12991

Coventry, P. A., Hudson, J. L., Kontopantelis, E., Archer, J., Richards, D. A., Gilbody, S., Lovell, K., Dickens, C., Gask, L., Waheed, W., & Bower, P. (2014). Characteristics of effective collaborative care for treatment of depression: A systematic review and meta-regression of 74 randomised controlled trials. *PLOS ONE, 9*(9), Article e108114. https://doi.org/10.1371/journal.pone.0108114

Crabtree, B. F., Nutting, P. A., Miller, W. L., Stange, K. C., Stewart, E. E., & Jaén, C. R. (2010). Summary of the National Demonstration Project and recommendations for the patient-centered medical home. *Annals of Family Medicine, 8*(Suppl. 1), S80–S90, S92. https://doi.org/10.1370/afm.1107

Craig, F., Operto, F. F., De Giacomo, A., Margari, L., Frolli, A., Conson, M., Ivagnes, S., Monaco, M., & Margari, F. (2016). Parenting stress among parents of children with neurodevelopmental disorders. *Psychiatry Research, 242*, 121–129. https://doi.org/10.1016/j.psychres.2016.05.016

Crane, D. R., & Christenson, J. (2014). A summary report of cost-effectiveness: Recognizing the value of family therapy in health care. In J. Hodgson, A. Lamson, T. Mendenhall, & D. Crane (Eds.), *Medical family therapy* (pp. 419–436). Springer, Cham. https://doi.org/10.1007/978-3-319-03482-9_22

Cronholm, P. F., Shea, J. A., Werner, R. M., Miller-Day, M., Tufano, J., Crabtree, B. F., & Gabbay, R. (2013). The patient centered medical home: Mental models and practice culture driving the transformation process. *Journal of General Internal Medicine, 28*(9), 1195–1201. https://doi.org/10.1007/s11606-013-2415-3

Crosby, L. E., Joffe, N. E., Reynolds, N., Peugh, J. L., Manegold, E., & Pai, A. L. H. (2016). Psychometric properties of the Psychosocial Assessment Tool-General in adolescents and young adults with sickle cell disease. *Journal of Pediatric Psychology, 41*, 397–405. https://doi.org/10.1093/jpepsy/jsv073

Crowley, R. A., & Kirschner, N. (2015). The integration of care for mental health, substance abuse, and other behavioral health conditions into primary care: Executive summary of an American College of Physicians position paper. *Annals of Internal Medicine, 163*(4), 298–299. https://doi.org/10.7326/M15-0510

Crumb, L., Larkin, R., Johnson, M., Smith, J., Howard, A., & Glenn, C. T. (2018). An interprofessional internship model for training master's level social work and counseling students in higher education settings. *Journal of Human Behavior in the Social Environment, 28*(8), 1091–1096. https://doi.org/10.1080/10911359.2018.1470952

Cubic, B., Mance, J., Turgesen, J. N., & Lamanna, J. D. (2012). Interprofessional education: Preparing psychologists for success in integrated primary care. *Journal of Clinical Psychology in Medical Settings, 19*(1), 84–92. https://doi.org/10.1007/s10880-011-9291-y

Çuhadar, D., Savaş, H. A., Ünal, A., & Gökpinar, F. (2015). Family functionality and coping attitudes of patients with bipolar disorder. *Journal of Religion and Health, 54*(5), 1731–1746. https://doi.org/10.1007/s10943-014-9919-y

Curry, S. J., Krist, A. H., Owens, D. K., Barry, M. J., Caughey, A. B., Davidson, K. W., & U.S. Preventive Services Task Force. (2018). Screening for intimate partner violence, elder abuse, and abuse of vulnerable adults: U.S. Preventive Services Task Force final recommendation statement. *JAMA, 320*(16), 1678–1687. https://doi.org/10.1001/jama.2018.14741

Dalteg, T., Benzein, E., Fridlund, B., & Malm, D. (2011). Cardiac disease and its consequences on the partner relationship: A systematic review. *European Journal of Cardiovascular Nursing, 10*(3), 140–149. https://doi.org/10.1016/j.ejcnurse.2011.01.006

Daniel, H., Bornstein, S. S., & Kane, G. C. (2018). Addressing social determinants to improve patient care and promote health equity: An American College of Physicians position paper. *Annals of Internal Medicine, 168*(8), 577–578. https://doi.org/10.7326/M17-2441

Dannemiller, K. D., & Jacobs, R. W. (1992). Changing the way organizations change: A revolution of common sense. *The Journal of Applied Behavioral Science, 28*(4), 480–498. https://doi.org/10.1177/0021886392284003

Davies, S. (2012). Embracing reflective practice. *Education for Primary Care, 23*(1), 9–12.

Davis, M. M., Balasubramanian, B. A., Cifuentes, M., Hall, J., Gunn, R., Fernald, D., Gilchrist, E., Miller, B. F., deGruy, F., III, & Cohen, D. J. (2015). Clinician staffing, scheduling, and engagement strategies among primary care practices delivering integrated care. *Journal of the American Board of Family Medicine, 28*(Suppl. 1), S32–S40. https://doi.org/10.3122/jabfm.2015.S1.150087

Davis, M. M., Gunn, R., Cifuentes, M., Khatri, P., Hall, J., Gilchrist, E., Peek, C. J., Klowden, M., Lazarus, J. A., Miller, B. F., & Cohen, D. J. (2019). Clinical workflows and the associated tasks and behaviors to support delivery of integrated behavioral health and primary care. *The Journal of Ambulatory Care Management, 42*(1), 51–65. https://doi.org/10.1097/JAC.0000000000000257

Davis, M. M., Gunn, R., Gowen, L. K., Miller, B. F., Green, L. A., & Cohen, D. J. (2018). A qualitative study of patient experiences of care in integrated behavioral health and primary care settings: More similar than different. *Translational Behavioral Medicine, 8*(5), 649–659. https://doi.org/10.1093/tbm/ibx001

Davy, C., Bleasel, J., Liu, H., Tchan, M., Ponniah, S., & Brown, A. (2015). Effectiveness of chronic care models: Opportunities for improving healthcare practice and health outcomes: A systematic review. *BMC Health Services Research, 15*, Article 194. https://doi.org/10.1186/s12913-015-0854-8

De Maria, M., Tagliabue, S., Ausili, D., Vellone, E., & Matarese, M. (2020). Perceived social support and health-related quality of life in older adults who have multiple chronic conditions and their caregivers: A dyadic analysis. *Social Science & Medicine, 262*, Article 113193. https://doi.org/10.1016/j.socscimed.2020.113193

Deault, L. C. (2010). A systematic review of parenting in relation to the development of comorbidities and functional impairments in children with attention-deficit/hyperactivity disorder (ADHD). *Child Psychiatry and Human Development, 41*(2), 168–192. https://doi.org/10.1007/s10578-009-0159-4

deGruy, F. V., III. (2015). Integrated care: Tools, maps, and leadership. *Journal of the American Board of Family Medicine, 28*(Suppl. 1), S107–S110. https://doi.org/10.3122/jabfm.2015.S1.150106

deGruy, F. V., & Khatri, P. (2019). Everyone leads. In S. B. Gold & L. A. Green (Eds.), *Integrated behavioral health in primary care: Your patients are waiting* (pp. 103–129). Springer Cham. https://doi.org/10.1007/978-3-319-98587-9_5

deGruy, F. V., & McDaniel, S. H. (2021). Proposed requirements for behavioral health in family medicine residencies. *Family Medicine, 53*(7), 516–520. https://doi.org/10.22454/FamMed.2021.380617

DeLago, C., Dickens, B., Phipps, E., Paoletti, A., Kazmierczak, M., & Irigoyen, M. (2018). Qualitative evaluation of individual and group well-child care. *Academic Pediatrics, 18*(5), 516–524. https://doi.org/10.1016/j.acap.2018.01.005

Delamater, A. M., de Wit, M., McDarby, V., Malik, J. A., Hilliard, M. E., Northam, E., & Acerini, C. L. (2018). ISPAD Clinical Practice Consensus Guidelines 2018: Psychological care of children and adolescents with type 1 diabetes. *Pediatric Diabetes, 19*(Suppl. 27), 237–249. https://doi.org/10.1111/pedi.12736

Delbridge, E., Taylor, J., & Hanson, C. (2014). Honoring the "spiritual" in biopsychosocial-spiritual health care: Medical family therapists on the front lines of graduate education, clinical practice, and research. In J. Hodgson, A. Lamson, T. Mendenhall, & D. R. Crane (Eds.), *Medical family therapy:*

Advanced applications (pp. 197–216). Springer International Publishing/ Springer Nature. https://doi.org/10.1007/978-3-319-03482-9_11

Derose, K. P., Gresenz, C. R., & Ringel, J. S. (2011). Understanding disparities in health care access—and reducing them—through a focus on public health. *Health Affairs (Project Hope)*, *30*(10), 1844–1851. https://doi.org/10.1377/ hlthaff.2011.0644

Dhand, A., Luke, D. A., Carothers, B. J., & Evanoff, B. A. (2016). Academic cross-pollination: The role of disciplinary affiliation in research collabora- tion. *PLOS ONE*, *11*(1), Article e0145916. https://doi.org/10.1371/journal. pone.0145916

Dickinson, W. P. (2015). Strategies to support the integration of behavioral health and primary care: What have we learned thus far? *Journal of the Amer- ican Board of Family Medicine*, *28*(Suppl. 1), S102–S106. https://doi.org/ 10.3122/jabfm.2015.S1.150112

Dieleman, J. L., Cao, J., Chapin, A., Chen, C., Li, Z., Liu, A., Horst, C., Kaldjian, A., Matyasz, T., Scott, K. W., Bui, A. L., Campbell, M., Duber, H. C., Dunn, A. C., Flaxman, A. D., Fitzmaurice, C., Naghavi, M., Sadat, N., Shieh, P., . . . Murray, C. J. L. (2020). US health care spending by payer and health condition, 1996–2016. *JAMA*, *323*(9), 863–884. https://doi.org/10.1001/jama.2020.0734

Dobmeyer, A. C., Hunter, C. L., Corso, M. L., Nielsen, M. K., Corso, K. A., Polizzi, N. C., & Earles, J. E. (2016). Primary care behavioral health provider train- ing: Systematic development and implementation in a large medical system. *Journal of Clinical Psychology in Medical Settings*, *23*(3), 207–224. https:// doi.org/10.1007/s10880-016-9464-9

Doherty, W. J., & Baird, M. A. (1983). *Family therapy and family medicine: Toward the primary care of families*. Guilford Press.

Doherty, W. J., McDaniel, S. H., & Baird, M. A. (1996). Five levels of primary care/behavioral healthcare collaboration. *Behavioral Healthcare Tomorrow*, *5*(5), 25–27.

Domar, A. D., Smith, K., Conboy, L., Iannone, M., & Alper, M. (2010). A prospec- tive investigation into the reasons why insured United States patients drop out of in vitro fertilization treatment. *Fertility and Sterility*, *94*(4), 1457–1459. https://doi.org/10.1016/j.fertnstert.2009.06.020

Donarelli, Z., Salerno, L., Lo Coco, G., Allegra, A., Marino, A., & Kivlighan, D. M. (2019). From telescope to binoculars. Dyadic outcome resulting from psycho- logical counselling for infertile couples undergoing ART. *Journal of Reproduc- tive and Infant Psychology*, *37*(1), 13–25. https://doi.org/10.1080/02646838. 2018.1548757

Donnelly, P., & Kirk, P. (2015). Use the PDSA model for effective change manage- ment. *Education for Primary Care*, *26*(4), 279–281. https://doi.org/10.1080/ 14739879.2015.11494356

Dooley, K. (1997). A complex adaptive systems model of organization change. *Nonlinear Dynamics, Psychology, and Life Sciences*, *1*, 69–97. https://doi.org/ 10.1023/A:1022375910940

Druss, B. G., & Mauer, B. J. (2010). Health care reform and care at the behavioral health—Primary care interface. *Psychiatric Services, 61*(11), 1087–1092. https://doi.org/10.1176/ps.2010.61.11.1087

Duke, D. C., Guion, K., Freeman, K. A., Wilson, A. C., & Harris, M. A. (2012). Commentary: Health & behavior codes: Great idea, questionable outcome. *Journal of Pediatric Psychology, 37*(5), 491–495. https://doi.org/10.1093/jpepsy/jsr126

Dunkel Schetter, C., & Tanner, L. (2012). Anxiety, depression and stress in pregnancy: Implications for mothers, children, research, and practice. *Current Opinion in Psychiatry, 25*(2), 141–148. https://doi.org/10.1097/YCO.0b013e3283503680

Durbin, J., Barnsley, J., Finlayson, B., Jaakkimainen, L., Lin, E., Berta, W., & McMurray, J. (2012). Quality of communication between primary health care and mental health care: An examination of referral and discharge letters. *The Journal of Behavioral Health Services & Research, 39*(4), 445–461. https://doi.org/10.1007/s11414-012-9288-9

Dyck, E., & Russell, G. (2020). Challenging psychiatric classification: Healthy autistic diversity and the neurodiversity movement. In S. J. Taylor & A. Brumby (Eds.), *Healthy minds in the twentieth century: In and beyond the asylum* (pp. 167–187). Springer.

Dykens, E. M., Fisher, M. H., Taylor, J. L., Lambert, W., & Miodrag, N. (2014). Reducing distress in mothers of children with autism and other disabilities: A randomized trial. *Pediatrics, 134*(2), e454–e463. https://doi.org/10.1542/peds.2013-3164

Dym, B., & Berman, S. (1986). The primary health care team: Family physician and family therapist in joint practice. *Family Systems Medicine, 4*(1), 9–21. https://doi.org/10.1037/h0089687

Ede, V., Okafor, M., Kinuthia, R., Belay, Z., Tewolde, T., Alema-Mensah, E., & Satcher, D. (2015). An examination of perceptions in integrated care practice. *Community Mental Health Journal, 51*(8), 949–961. https://doi.org/10.1007/s10597-015-9837-9

Egede, L. E., Ruggiero, K. J., & Frueh, B. C. (2020). Ensuring mental health access for vulnerable populations in COVID era. *Journal of Psychiatric Research, 129*, 147–148. https://doi.org/10.1016/j.jpsychires.2020.07.011

Ek, K., Ternestedt, B. M., Andershed, B., & Sahlberg-Blom, E. (2011). Shifting life rhythms: Couples' stories about living together when one spouse has advanced chronic obstructive pulmonary disease. *Journal of Palliative Care, 27*(3), 189–197. https://doi.org/10.1177/082585971102700302

Eklund, H., Findon, J., Cadman, T., Hayward, H., Murphy, D., Asherson, P., Glaser, K., & Xenitidis, K. (2018). Needs of adolescents and young adults with neurodevelopmental disorders: Comparisons of young people and parent perspectives. *Journal of Autism and Developmental Disorders, 48*(1), 83–91. https://doi.org/10.1007/s10803-017-3295-x

Ellis, A., Chebsey, C., Storey, C., Bradley, S., Jackson, S., Flenady, V., Heazell, A., & Siassakos, D. (2016). Systematic review to understand and improve care after stillbirth: A review of parents' and healthcare professionals' experiences. *BMC Pregnancy and Childbirth, 16*, Article 16. https://doi.org/10.1186/s12884-016-0806-2

Ellis, D. A., Frey, M. A., Naar-King, S., Templin, T., Cunningham, P., & Cakan, N. (2005a). Use of multisystemic therapy to improve regimen adherence among adolescents with type 1 diabetes in chronic poor metabolic control: A randomized controlled trial. *Diabetes Care, 28*(7), 1604–1610. https://doi.org/10.2337/diacare.28.7.1604

Ellis, D. A., Frey, M. A., Naar-King, S., Templin, T., Cunningham, P. B., & Cakan, N. (2005b). The effects of multisystemic therapy on diabetes stress among adolescents with chronically poorly controlled Type 1 diabetes: Findings from a randomized, controlled trial. *Pediatrics, 116*(6), e826–e832. https://doi.org/10.1542/peds.2005-0638

Ellis, D. A., Naar-King, S., Chen, X., Moltz, K., Cunningham, P. B., & Idalski-Carcone, A. (2012). Multisystemic therapy compared to telephone support for youth with poorly controlled diabetes: Findings from a randomized controlled trial. *Annals of Behavioral Medicine, 44*(2), 207–215. https://doi.org/10.1007/s12160-012-9378-1

Ellis, D. A., Templin, T., Naar-King, S., Frey, M. A., Cunningham, P. B., Podolski, C. L., & Cakan, N. (2007). Multisystemic therapy for adolescents with poorly controlled Type I diabetes: Stability of treatment effects in a randomized controlled trial. *Journal of Consulting and Clinical Psychology, 75*(1), 168–174. https://doi.org/10.1037/0022-006X.75.1.168

Engel, C. C., Oxman, T., Yamamoto, C., Gould, D., Barry, S., Stewart, P., Kroenke, K., Williams, J. W., Jr., & Dietrich, A. J. (2008). RESPECT-Mil: Feasibility of a systems-level collaborative care approach to depression and post-traumatic stress disorder in military primary care. *Military Medicine, 173*(10), 935–940. https://doi.org/10.7205/MILMED.173.10.935

Engel, G. L. (1977). The need for a new medical model: A challenge for biomedicine. *Science, 196*(4286), 129–136. https://doi.org/10.1126/science.847460

Engel, G. L. (1980). The clinical application of the biopsychosocial model. *The American Journal of Psychiatry, 137*(5), 535–544. https://doi.org/10.1176/ajp.137.5.535

Engler, A. J., & Lasker, J. N. (2000). Predictors of maternal grief in the year after a newborn death. *Illness, Crisis & Loss, 8*(3), 227–243. https://doi.org/10.1177/105413730000800302

Epstein, R. M., Marshall, F., Sanders, M., & Krasner, M. S. (2022). Effect of an intensive mindful practice workshop on patient-centered compassionate care, clinician well-being, work engagement, and teamwork. *Journal of Continuing Education in the Health Professions, 42*(1), 19–27.

Etz, R. S., Zyzanski, S. J., Gonzalez, M. M., Reves, S. R., O'Neal, J. P., & Stange, K. C. (2019). A new comprehensive measure of high-value aspects of primary care. *Annals of Family Medicine, 17*(3), 221–230. https://doi.org/10.1370/afm.2393

Everett, B. G., Higgins, J. A., Haider, S., & Carpenter, E. (2019). Do sexual minorities receive appropriate sexual and reproductive health care and counseling? *Journal of Women's Health, 28*(1), 53–62. https://doi.org/10.1089/jwh.2017.6866

Fairbrother, N., Young, A. H., Janssen, P., Antony, M. M., & Tucker, E. (2015). Depression and anxiety during the perinatal period. *BMC Psychiatry, 15*, Article 206. https://doi.org/10.1186/s12888-015-0526-6

Falconier, M. K., & Kuhn, R. (2019). Dyadic coping in couples: A conceptual integration and a review of the empirical literature. *Frontiers in Psychology, 10*, Article 571. https://doi.org/10.3389/fpsyg.2019.00571

Farrales, L. L., Cacciatore, J., Jonas-Simpson, C., Dharamsi, S., Ascher, J., & Klein, M. C. (2020). What bereaved parents want health care providers to know when their babies are stillborn: A community-based participatory study. *BMC Psychology, 8*, Article 18. https://doi.org/10.1186/s40359-020-0385-x

Fekete, E., Geaghan, T. R., & Druley, J. A. (2009). Affective and behavioural reactions to positive and negative health-related social control in HIV+ men. *Psychology & Health, 24*(5), 501–515. https://doi.org/10.1080/08870440801894674

Feldman, M. A., Anderson, L. M., Shapiro, J. B., Jedraszko, A. M., Evans, M., Weil, L. E. G., Garza, K. P., & Weissberg-Benchell, J. (2018). Family-based interventions targeting improvements in health and family outcomes of children and adolescents with type 1 diabetes: A systematic review. *Current Diabetes Reports, 18*, Article 15. https://doi.org/10.1007/s11892-018-0981-9

Fenton, A. T. H. R., Keating, N. L., Ornstein, K. A., Kent, E. E., Litzelman, K., Rowland, J. H., & Wright, A. A. (2022). Comparing adult-child and spousal caregiver burden and potential contributors. *Cancer, 128*(10), 2015–2024. https://doi.org/10.1002/cncr.34164

Ferrell, B., & Wittenberg, E. (2017). A review of family caregiving intervention trials in oncology. *CA: A Cancer Journal for Clinicians, 67*(4), 318–325. https://doi.org/10.3322/caac.21396

Figueiredo, D., Cruz, J., Jácome, C., & Marques, A. (2016). Exploring the benefits to caregivers of a family-oriented pulmonary rehabilitation program. *Respiratory Care, 61*(8), 1081–1089. https://doi.org/10.4187/respcare.04624

Fiscella, K., & McDaniel, S. H. (2018). The complexity, diversity, and science of primary care teams. *American Psychologist, 73*(4), 451–467. https://doi.org/10.1037/amp0000244

Fischer, M. S., Baucom, D. H., & Cohen, M. J. (2016). Cognitive-behavioral couple therapies: Review of the evidence for the treatment of relationship distress, psychopathology, and chronic health conditions. *Family Process, 55*(3), 423–442. https://doi.org/10.1111/famp.12227

Fixsen, D. L., Naoom, S. F., Blase, K. A., Friedman, R. M., & Wallace, F. (2005). *Implementation research: A synthesis of the literature* (Florida Mental Health Institute Publication #231). University of South Florida, Louis de la Parte

Florida Mental Health Institute, National Implementation Research Network. https://nirn.fpg.unc.edu/resources/implementation-research-synthesis-literature

Flentje, A., Heck, N. C., Brennan, J. M., & Meyer, I. H. (2020). The relationship between minority stress and biological outcomes: A systematic review. *Journal of Behavioral Medicine, 43*(5), 673–694. https://doi.org/10.1007/s10865-019-00120-6

Flores, G., & Committee on Pediatric Research. (2010). Racial and ethnic disparities in the health and health care of children. *Pediatrics, 125*(4), e979–e1020. https://doi.org/10.1542/peds.2010-0188

Flynn, A., Gonzalez, V., Mata, M., Salinas, L. A., & Atkins, A. (2020). Integrated care improves mental health in a medically underserved U.S.-Mexico border population. *Families, Systems & Health, 38*(2), 105–115. https://doi.org/10.1037/fsh0000490

Fockler, M. E., Ladhani, N. N. N., Watson, J., & Barrett, J. F. R. (2017). Pregnancy subsequent to stillbirth: Medical and psychosocial aspects of care. *Seminars in Fetal & Neonatal Medicine, 22*(3), 186–192. https://doi.org/10.1016/j.siny.2017.02.004

Fortney, J. C., Pyne, J. M., Edlund, M. J., Williams, D. K., Robinson, D. E., Mittal, D., & Henderson, K. L. (2007). A randomized trial of telemedicine-based collaborative care for depression. *Journal of General Internal Medicine, 22*(8), 1086–1093. https://doi.org/10.1007/s11606-007-0201-9

Fox, M. A., Hodgson, J. L., & Lamson, A. L. (2012). Integration: Opportunities and challenges for family therapists in primary care. *Contemporary Family Therapy, 34*(2), 228–243. https://doi.org/10.1007/s10591-012-9189-3

Frankel, R. M., Quill, T. E., & McDaniel, S. H. (2003). *The biopsychosocial approach: Past, present, and future.* University of Rochester Press.

Franklin, C., Bolton, K. W., & Guz, S. (2019). Solution-focused brief family therapy. In B. H. Fiese (Ed.), *APA handbook of contemporary family psychology: Family therapy and training* (3rd ed., pp. 139–153). American Psychological Association.

Frazier, M. L., Fainshmidt, S., Klinger, R. L., Pezeshkan, A., & Vracheva, V. (2017). Psychological safety: A meta-analytic review and extension. *Personnel Psychology, 70*(1), 113–165. https://doi.org/10.1111/peps.12183

Fredriksen-Goldsen, K. I., Simoni, J. M., Kim, H. J., Lehavot, K., Walters, K. L., Yang, J., Hoy-Ellis, C. P., & Muraco, A. (2014). The health equity promotion model: Reconceptualization of lesbian, gay, bisexual, and transgender (LGBT) health disparities. *American Journal of Orthopsychiatry, 84*(6), 653–663. https://doi.org/10.1037/ort0000030

Freeman, D. (2011). The behavioral health medical home. In N. A. Cummings & W. T. O'Donohue (Eds.), *Understanding the behavioral healthcare crisis: The promise of integrated care and diagnostic reform* (pp. 250–265). Routledge.

Freeman, D. S., Hudgins, C., & Hornberger, J. (2018). Legislative and policy developments and imperatives for advancing the primary care behavioral health (PCBH) model. *Journal of Clinical Psychology in Medical Settings,* 25(2), 210–223. https://doi.org/10.1007/s10880-018-9557-8

Freeman, D. S., Manson, L., Howard, J., & Hornberger, J. (2018). Financing the primary care behavioral health model. *Journal of Clinical Psychology in Medical Settings,* 25(2), 197–209. https://doi.org/10.1007/s10880-017-9529-4

Friedemann, M. L., & Buckwalter, K. C. (2014). Family caregiver role and burden related to gender and family relationships. *Journal of Family Nursing,* 20(3), 313–336. https://doi.org/10.1177/1074840714532715

Frieden, T. R. (2017). Evidence for health decision making—Beyond randomized, controlled trials. *The New England Journal of Medicine,* 377(5), 465–475. https://doi.org/10.1056/NEJMra1614394

Fu, F., Zhao, H., Tong, F., & Chi, I. (2017). A systematic review of psychosocial interventions to cancer caregivers. *Frontiers in Psychology,* 8, Article 834. https://doi.org/10.3389/fpsyg.2017.00834

Funderburk, J. S., Fielder, R. L., DeMartini, K. S., & Flynn, C. A. (2012). Integrating behavioral health services into a university health center: Patient and provider satisfaction. *Families, Systems & Health,* 30(2), 130–140. https://doi.org/10.1037/a0028378

Funderburk, J. S., Polaha, J., & Beehler, G. P. (2021). What is the recipe for PCBH? Proposed resources, processes, and expected outcomes. *Families, Systems & Health,* 39(4), 551–562. https://doi.org/10.1037/fsh0000669

Funderburk, J. S., & Shepardson, R. L. (2017). Real-world program evaluation of integrated behavioral health care: Improving scientific rigor. *Families, Systems & Health,* 35(2), 114–124. https://doi.org/10.1037/fsh0000253

Gabbay, J., & le May, A. (2004). Evidence based guidelines or collectively constructed "mindlines?" Ethnographic study of knowledge management in primary care. *BMJ,* 329, 1013–1025. https://doi.org/10.1136/bmj.329.7473.1013

Gallant, S. J., Coons, H. L., & Morokoff, P. J. (1994). Psychology and women's health: Some reflections and future directions. In V. J. Adesso (Ed.), *Psychological perspectives on women's health* (pp. 315–346). Taylor & Francis.

Galvão, G. M. M., Morsch, D. S., Tavares, E. C., Bouzada, M. C. F., & Byrd, S. E. (2020). An unrecognizable pain: Neonatal loss and the needs of fathers. *American International Journal of Humanities, Arts and Social Sciences,* 2(3), 1–8.

Gameiro, S., Boivin, J., Peronace, L., & Verhaak, C. M. (2012). Why do patients discontinue fertility treatment? A systematic review of reasons and predictors of discontinuation in fertility treatment. *Human Reproduction Update,* 18(6), 652–669. https://doi.org/10.1093/humupd/dms031

Gance-Cleveland, B. (2005). Motivational interviewing as a strategy to increase families' adherence to treatment regimens. *Journal for Specialists in Pediatric Nursing,* 10(3), 151–155. https://doi.org/10.1111/j.1744-6155.2005.00028.x

García-Huidobro, D., & Mendenhall, T. (2015). Family oriented care: Opportunities for health promotion and disease prevention. *Journal of Family Medicine and Disease Prevention,* 1(2). https://doi.org/10.23937/2469-5793/1510009

García-Huidobro, D., Puschel, K., & Soto, G. (2012). Family functioning style and health: Opportunities for health prevention in primary care. *The British Journal of General Practice, 62*(596), e198–e203. https://doi.org/10.3399/bjgp12X630098

Gardiner, E., Miller, A. R., & Lach, L. M. (2018). Family impact of childhood neurodevelopmental disability: Considering adaptive and maladaptive behaviour. *Journal of Intellectual Disability Research, 62*(10), 888–899. https://doi.org/10.1111/jir.12547

Garland, A. F., Bickman, L., & Chorpita, B. F. (2010). Change what? Identifying quality improvement targets by investigating usual mental health care. *Administration and Policy in Mental Health, 37*(1–2), 15–26. https://doi.org/10.1007/s10488-010-0279-y

Garrison, G. M., Angstman, K. B., O'Connor, S. S., Williams, M. D., & Lineberry, T. W. (2016). Time to remission for depression with collaborative care management (CCM) in primary care. *Journal of the American Board of Family Medicine, 29*(1), 10–17. https://doi.org/10.3122/jabfm.2016.01.150128

Gehlert, S., Murray, A., Sohmer, D., McClintock, M., Conzen, S., & Olopade, O. (2010). The importance of transdisciplinary collaborations for understanding and resolving health disparities. *Social Work in Public Health, 25*(3–4), 408–422. https://doi.org/10.1080/19371910903241124

Gerber, M. R. (2019). Trauma-informed adult primary care. In M. R. Gerber (Ed.), *Trauma-informed healthcare approaches: A guide for primary care* (pp. 125–143). Springer. https://doi.org/10.1007/978-3-030-04342-1_7

Gerhardt, C. (2019). *Families in motion: Dynamics in diverse contexts.* Sage.

Ghabrial, M. A., Classen, C. C., & Maggi, J. D. (2019). Professionally moderated, psychoeducational, web-based support for women living with HIV: An exploratory study. *Journal of HIV/AIDS & Social Services, 18*(1), 1–25. https://doi.org/10.1080/15381501.2018.1530628

Ghorob, A., & Bodenheimer, T. (2015). Building teams in primary care: A practical guide. *Families, Systems & Health, 33*(3), 182–192. https://doi.org/10.1037/fsh0000120

Gibson, C., Arya, N., Ponka, D., Rouleau, K., & Woollard, R. (2016). Approaching a global definition of family medicine: The Besrour Papers: A series on the state of family medicine in the world. *Canadian Family Physician, 62*(11), 891–896.

Giese, A., & Waugh, M. (2017). Conceptual framework for integrated care. In R. E. Feinstein, J. V. Connelly, & M. S. Feinstein (Eds.), *Integrating behavioral health and primary care* (pp. 3–16). Oxford University Press.

Gilliss, C. L. (1991). Family nursing research, theory and practice. *Image: The Journal of Nursing Scholarship, 23*(1), 19–22. https://doi.org/10.1111/j.1547-5069.1991.tb00629.x

Gilliss, C. L. (2002). There is science, and there is life. *Families, Systems & Health, 20*(1), 47–49. https://doi.org/10.1037/h0089565

Gilliss, C. L., Pan, W., & Davis, L. L. (2019). Family involvement in adult chronic disease care: Reviewing the systematic reviews. *Journal of Family Nursing, 25*(1), 3–27. https://doi.org/10.1177/1074840718822365

Glasgow, R. E., Emont, S., & Miller, D. C. (2006). Assessing delivery of the five 'As' for patient-centered counseling. *Health Promotion International, 21*(3), 245–255. https://doi.org/10.1093/heapro/dal017

Glasgow, R. E., Goldstein, M. G., Ockene, J. K., & Pronk, N. P. (2004). Translating what we have learned into practice. Principles and hypotheses for interventions addressing multiple behaviors in primary care. *American Journal of Preventive Medicine, 27*(2, Suppl.), 88–101. https://doi.org/10.1016/j.amepre.2004.04.019

Glueck, B. (2015). Roles, attitudes, and training needs of behavioral health clinicians in integrated primary care. *Journal of Mental Health Counseling, 37*(2), 175–188. https://doi.org/10.17744/mehc.37.2.p84818638n07447r

Goetter, E. M., Frumkin, M. R., Palitz, S. A., Swee, M. B., Baker, A. W., Bui, E., & Simon, N. M. (2020). Barriers to mental health treatment among individuals with social anxiety disorder and generalized anxiety disorder. *Psychological Services, 17*(1), 5–12. https://doi.org/10.1037/ser0000254

Gold, K. J., Sen, A., & Hayward, R. A. (2010). Marriage and cohabitation outcomes after pregnancy loss. *Pediatrics, 125*(5), e1202–e1207. https://doi.org/10.1542/peds.2009-3081

Gold, S. B., & Green, L. A. (Eds.). (2018). *Integrated behavioral health in primary care: Your patients are waiting.* Springer Cham.

Goldberg, D. G., Soylu, T. G., Kitsantas, P., Grady, V. M., Elward, K., & Nichols, L. M. (2021). Burnout among primary care providers and staff: Evaluating the association with practice adaptive reserve and individual behaviors. *Journal of General Internal Medicine, 36*(5), 1222–1228. https://doi.org/10.1007/s11606-020-06367-z

Goldenberg, I., Stanton, M., & Goldenberg, H. (2017). *Family therapy: An overview* (9th ed.). Cengage Learning.

Gonzalez, S., Steinglass, P., & Reiss, D. (1989). Putting the illness in its place: Discussion groups for families with chronic medical illnesses. *Family Process, 28*(1), 69–87. https://doi.org/10.1111/j.1545-5300.1989.00069.x

Goodman, J. H., & Tyer-Viola, L. (2010). Detection, treatment, and referral of perinatal depression and anxiety by obstetrical providers. *Journal of Women's Health, 19*(3), 477–490. https://doi.org/10.1089/jwh.2008.1352

Goodwin, G. F., Blacksmith, N., & Coats, M. R. (2018). The science of teams in the military: Contributions from over 60 years of research. *American Psychologist, 73*(4), 322–333. https://doi.org/10.1037/amp0000259

Goroll, A. H. (2019). Does primary care add sufficient value to deserve better funding? *JAMA Internal Medicine, 179*(3), 372–373. https://doi.org/10.1001/jamainternmed.2018.6707

Gotham, H. J. (2004). Diffusion of mental health and substance abuse treatments: Development, dissemination, and implementation. *Clinical Psychology: Science and Practice, 11*(2), 160–176. https://doi.org/10.1093/clipsy.bph067

Graetz, F., & Smith, A. C. T. (2010). Managing organizational change: A philosophies of change approach. *Journal of Change Management, 10*(2), 135–154. https://doi.org/10.1080/14697011003795602

Gravensteen, I. K., Jacobsen, E. M., Sandset, P. M., Helgadottir, L. B., Rådestad, I., Sandvik, L., & Ekeberg, Ø. (2018). Anxiety, depression and relationship satisfaction in the pregnancy following stillbirth and after the birth of a liveborn baby: A prospective study. *BMC Pregnancy and Childbirth, 18*, Article 41. https://doi.org/10.1186/s12884-018-1666-8

Greaves, C. J., Sheppard, K. E., Abraham, C., Hardeman, W., Roden, M., Evans, P. H., Schwarz, P., & the IMAGE Study Group. (2011). Systematic review of reviews of intervention components associated with increased effectiveness in dietary and physical activity interventions. *BMC Public Health, 11*, Article 119. https://doi.org/10.1186/1471-2458-11-119

Green, L. A., Miller, W. L., Frey, J. J., III, Jason, H., Westberg, J., Cohen, D., Gotler, R. S., & deGruy, F. V. (2022). The time is now: A plan to redesign family medicine residency education. *Family Medicine, 54*(1), 7–15. https://doi.org/10.22454/FamMed.2022.197486

Green, L. A., Wyszewianski, L., Lowery, J. C., Kowalski, C. P., & Krein, S. L. (2007). An observational study of the effectiveness of practice guideline implementation strategies examined according to physicians' cognitive styles. *Implementation Science, 2*, Article 41. https://doi.org/10.1186/1748-5908-2-41

Green, L. W. (2008). Making research relevant: If it is an evidence-based practice, where's the practice-based evidence? *Family Practice, 25*(Suppl. 1), i20–i24. https://doi.org/10.1093/fampra/cmn055

Green, S. M., Donegan, E., Frey, B. N., Fedorkow, D. M., Key, B. L., Streiner, D. L., & McCabe, R. E. (2019). Cognitive behavior therapy for menopausal symptoms (CBT-Meno): A randomized controlled trial. *Menopause, 26*(9), 972–980. https://doi.org/10.1097/GME.0000000000001363

Greene, C. A., Ford, J. D., Ward-Zimmerman, B., Honigfeld, L., & Pidano, A. E. (2016). Strengthening the coordination of pediatric mental health and medical care: Piloting a collaborative model for freestanding practices. *Child & Youth Care Forum, 45*(5), 729–744. https://doi.org/10.1097/GME.0000000000001363

Gregory, E. C. W., MacDorman, M. F., & Martin, J. A. (2014, November). *Trends in fetal and perinatal mortality in the United States, 2006–2012* (NCHS Data Brief No. 169). https://www.cdc.gov/nchs/data/databriefs/db169.pdf

Greil, A. L., Slauson-Blevins, K., & McQuillan, J. (2010). The experience of infertility: A review of recent literature. *Sociology of Health & Illness, 32*(1), 140–162. https://doi.org/10.1111/j.1467-9566.2009.01213.x

Griffen, A., McIntyre, L., Belsito, J. Z., Burkhard, J., Davis, W., Kimmel, M., Stuebe, A., Clark, C., & Meltzer-Brody, S. (2021). Perinatal mental health care in the United States: An overview of policies and programs. *Health Affairs (Project Hope), 40*(10), 1543–1550. https://doi.org/10.1377/hlthaff.2021.00796

Gunn, R., Davis, M. M., Hall, J., Heintzman, J., Muench, J., Smeds, B., Miller, B. F., Miller, W. L., Gilchrist, E., Brown Levey, S., Brown, J., Wise Romero, P.,

& Cohen, D. J. (2015). Designing clinical space for the delivery of integrated behavioral health and primary care. *Journal of the American Board of Family Medicine, 28*(Suppl. 1), S52–S62. https://doi.org/10.3122/jabfm.2015.S1. 150053

Guo, H., Pavek, M., & Loth, K. (2017). Management of childhood obesity and over-weight in primary care visits: Gaps between recommended care and typical practice. *Current Nutrition Reports, 6*(4), 307–314. https://doi.org/10.1007/s13668-017-0221-y

Ha, T., & Granger, D. A. (2016). Family relations, stress, and vulnerability: Biobehavioral implications for prevention and practice. *Family Relations, 65*(1), 9–23. https://doi.org/10.1111/fare.12173

Haack, S., Erickson, J. M., Iles-Shih, M., & Ratzliff, A. (2020). Integration of primary care and behavioral health. In B. L. Levin & A. Hanson (Eds.), *Foundations of behavioral health* (pp. 273–300). https://doi.org/10.1007/978-3-030-18435-3_13

Hagan, J. F., Shaw, J. S., & Duncan, P. M. (Eds.). (2017). *Bright futures: Guidelines for health supervision of infants, children, and adolescents* (4th ed.). Bright Futures/American Academy of Pediatrics. https://www.aap.org/en/practice-management/bright-futures

Halding, A. G., Heggdal, K., & Wahl, A. (2011). Experiences of self-blame and stigmatisation for self-infliction among individuals living with COPD. *Scandinavian Journal of Caring Sciences, 25*(1), 100–107. https://doi.org/10.1111/j.1471-6712.2010.00796.x

Hall, J., Cohen, D. J., Davis, M., Gunn, R., Blount, A., Pollack, D. A., Miller, W. L., Smith, C., Valentine, N., & Miller, B. F. (2015). Preparing the workforce for behavioral health and primary care integration. *Journal of the American Board of Family Medicine, 28*(Suppl. 1), S41–S51. https://doi.org/10.3122/jabfm.2015.S1.150054

Hall, J. E., & Weaver, B. R. (1977). *Distributive nursing practice: A systems approach to community health*. Lippincott Williams & Wilkins.

Hammer, L. B., & Neal, M. B. (2008). Working sandwiched-generation caregivers: Prevalence, characteristics, and outcomes. *The Psychologist Manager Journal, 11*(1), 93–112. https://doi.org/10.1080/10887150801967324

Hammond, D. (2002). Exploring the genealogy of systems thinking. *Systems Research and Behavioral Science, 19*(5), 429–439. https://doi.org/10.1002/sres.499

Haque, S. N. (2021). Telehealth beyond COVID-19. *Psychiatric Services, 72*(1), 100–103. https://doi.org/10.1176/appi.ps.202000368

Hargraves, D., White, C., Frederick, R., Cinibulk, M., Peters, M., Young, A., & Elder, N. (2017). Implementing SBIRT (Screening, Brief Intervention and Referral to Treatment) in primary care: Lessons learned from a multi-practice evaluation portfolio. *Public Health Reviews, 38*, Article 31. https://doi.org/10.1186/s40985-017-0077-0

Harper, A., Taylor Dyches, T., Harper, J., Olsen Roper, S., & South, M. (2013). Respite care, marital quality, and stress in parents of children with autism spectrum disorders. *Journal of Autism and Developmental Disorders, 43*(11), 2604–2616. https://doi.org/10.1007/s10803-013-1812-0

Hashemi, L., Weinreb, J., Weimer, A. K., & Weiss, R. L. (2018). Transgender care in the primary care setting: A review of guidelines and literature. *Federal Practitioner, 35*(7), 30–37.

Health Insurance Portability and Accountability Act (HIPAA), Pub. L. No. 104-191, § 264, 110 Stat. 1936 (1996).

Heazell, A. E. P. (2016). Stillbirth—A challenge for the 21st century. *BMC Pregnancy and Childbirth, 16*, Article 388. https://doi.org/10.1186/s12884-016-1181-8

Heckman, B. W., Mathew, A. R., & Carpenter, M. J. (2015). Treatment burden and treatment fatigue as barriers to health. *Current Opinion in Psychology, 5*, 31–36. https://doi.org/10.1016/j.copsyc.2015.03.004

Helgeson, V. S. (1994). Relation of agency and communion to well-being: Evidence and potential explanations. *Psychological Bulletin, 116*(3), 412–428. https://doi.org/10.1037/0033-2909.116.3.412

Helgeson, V. S., & Palladino, D. K. (2012). Implications of psychosocial factors for diabetes outcomes among children with Type-1 diabetes: A review. *Social and Personality Psychology Compass, 6*(3), 228–242. https://doi.org/10.1111/j.1751-9004.2011.00421.x

Henggeler, S. W., & Schaeffer, C. M. (2016). Multisystemic therapy®: Clinical overview, outcomes and implementation research. *Family Process, 55*(3), 514–528. https://doi.org/10.1111/famp.12232

Hepp, S. L., Suter, E., Jackson, K., Deutschlander, S., Makwarimba, E., Jennings, J., & Birmingham, L. (2015). Using an interprofessional competency framework to examine collaborative practice. *Journal of Interprofessional Care, 29*(2), 131–137. https://doi.org/10.3109/13561820.2014.955910

Heredia, D., Jr., Pankey, T. L., & Gonzalez, C. A. (2021). LGBTQ-affirmative behavioral health services in primary care. *Primary Care: Clinics in Office Practice, 48*(2), 243–257. https://doi.org/10.1016/j.pop.2021.02.005

Higgs, M., & Rowland, D. (2005). All changes great and small: Exploring approaches to change and its leadership. *Journal of Change Management, 5*(2), 121–151. https://doi.org/10.1080/14697010500082902

Hill, J. M. (2015). Behavioral health integration: Transforming patient care, medical resident education, and physician effectiveness. *International Journal of Psychiatry in Medicine, 50*(1), 36–49. https://doi.org/10.1177/0091217415592357

Hills, W., & Hills, K. (2019). Virtual treatments in an integrated primary care-behavioral health practice: An overview of synchronous telehealth services to address rural-urban disparities in mental health care. *Medical Science Pulse, 13*(3), 54–59. https://doi.org/10.5604/01.3001.0013.5239

Hinde, J. M., Bray, J. W., & Cowell, A. J. (2020). Implementation science on the margins: How do we demonstrate the value of implementation strategies? *Families, Systems & Health, 38*(3), 225–231. https://doi.org/10.1037/fsh0000535

Hing, E., Kurtzman, E., Lau, D. T., Taplin, C., & Bindman, A. B. (2017). Characteristics of primary care physicians in patient-centered medical home practices: United States, 2013. *National Health Statistics Reports, 101,* 1–9.

Hodgson, J., Lamson, A., Mendenhall, T., & Crane, D. R. (Eds.). (2014). *Medical family therapy: Advanced applications.* Springer. https://doi.org/10.1007/978-3-319-03482-9

Hodgson, J., Mendenhall, T., & Lamson, A. (2013). Patient and provider relationships: Consent, confidentiality, and mistakes in integrated primary care settings. *Families, Systems, & Health, 31,* 28–40. doi:10.1037/a0031771

Hodgson, J., Trump, L., Wilson, G., & García-Huidobro, D. (2018). Medical family therapy in family medicine. In T. Mendenhall, A. Lamson, J. Hodgson, & M. Baird (Eds.), *Clinical methods in medical family therapy* (pp. 17–59). Springer. https://doi.org/10.1007/978-3-319-68834-3_2

Hoffman, L., Benedetto, E., Huang, H., Grossman, E., Kaluma, D., Mann, Z., & Torous, J. (2019). Augmenting mental health in primary care: A 1-year study of deploying smartphone apps in a multi-site primary care/behavioral health integration program. *Frontiers in Psychiatry, 10,* Article 94. https://doi.org/10.3389/fpsyt.2019.00094

Hoge, M. A., Morris, J. A., Laraia, M., Pomerantz, A., & Farley, T. (2014). *Core competencies for integrated behavioral health and primary care.* SAMHSA-HRSA Center for Integrated Health Solutions.

Hoge, M. A., Paris, M., Jr., Adger, H., Jr., Collins, F. L., Jr., Finn, C. V., Fricks, L., Gill, K. J., Haber, J., Hansen, M., Ida, D. J., Kaplan, L., Northey, W. F., Jr., O'Connell, M. J., Rosen, A. L., Taintor, Z., Tondora, J., & Young, A. S. (2005). Workforce competencies in behavioral health: An overview. *Administration and Policy in Mental Health, 32*(5–6), 593–631. https://doi.org/10.1007/s10488-005-3259-x

Holderle, K. E., Poleshuck, E., Rosenberg, T., & Pulcino, T. (2022). Integrated behavioral health in primary care for adults with complex childhood onset medical and developmental diagnoses. *Journal of Clinical Psychology in Medical Settings, 29*(3), 586–595. https://doi.org/10.1007/s10880-021-09798-w

Holmes, A., & Chang, Y. P. (2022). Effect of mental health collaborative care models on primary care provider outcomes: An integrative review. *Family Practice, 39*(5), 964–970. https://doi.org/10.1093/fampra/cmac026

Holt-Lunstad, J., & Uchino, B. N. (2015). Social support and health. In K. Glanz, B. K. Rimer, & K. V. Viswanath (Eds.), *Health behavior: Theory, research and practice* (pp. 183–204). Jossey-Bass/Wiley.

Hoover, M., & Andazola, J. (2012). Integrated behavioral care training in family practice residency: Opportunities and challenges. *Journal of Clinical Psychology in Medical Settings, 19*(4), 446–450. https://doi.org/10.1007/s10880-012-9353-9

Horevitz, E., Lawson, J., & Chow, J. C. C. (2013). Examining cultural competence in health care: Implications for social workers. *Health & Social Work, 38*(3), 135–145. https://doi.org/10.1093/hsw/hlt015

Horevitz, E., & Manoleas, P. (2013). Professional competencies and training needs of professional social workers in integrated behavioral health in primary care. *Social Work in Health Care, 52*(8), 752–787. https://doi.org/10.1080/00981389.2013.791362

Hornberger, J., & Freeman, D. (2015). Blending behaviorists into the patient-centered medical home. In W. O'Donohue & A. Maragakis (Eds.), *Integrated primary and behavioral care* (pp. 39–59). Springer. https://doi.org/10.1007/978-3-319-19036-5_3

Horton-Deutsch, S., & Sherwood, G. D. (2017). *Reflective practice: Transforming education and improving outcomes* (2nd ed.). Sigma Theta Tau International. https://hsrc.himmelfarb.gwu.edu/books/140

Houben, C. H. M., Spruit, M. A., Groenen, M. T. J., Wouters, E. F. M., & Janssen, D. J. A. (2014). Efficacy of advance care planning: A systematic review and meta-analysis. *Journal of the American Medical Directors Association, 15*(7), 477–489. https://doi.org/10.1016/j.jamda.2014.01.008

Hoyt, M. A., & Stanton, A. L. (2018). Adjustment to chronic illness. In T. A. Revenson & R. A. Gurung (Eds.), *Handbook of health psychology* (pp. 179–194). Routledge. https://doi.org/10.4324/9781315167534-13

Hsieh, W. J., Sbrilli, M. D., Huang, W. D., Hoang, T. M., Meline, B., Laurent, H. K., & Tabb, K. M. (2021). Patients' perceptions of perinatal depression screening: A qualitative study. *Health Affairs (Project Hope), 40*(10), 1612–1617. https://doi.org/10.1377/hlthaff.2021.00804

Hubbard, G., Gorely, T., Ozakinci, G., Polson, R., & Forbat, L. (2016). A systematic review and narrative summary of family-based smoking cessation interventions to help adults quit smoking. *BMC Family Practice, 17*, 73. https://doi.org/10.1186/s12875-016-0457-4

Hunter, C. L., Funderburk, J. S., Polaha, J., Bauman, D., Goodie, J. L., & Hunter, C. M. (2018). Primary care behavioral health (PCBH) model research: Current state of the science and a call to action. *Journal of Clinical Psychology in Medical Settings, 25*(2), 127–156. https://doi.org/10.1007/s10880-017-9512-0

Hunter, C. L., & Goodie, J. L. (2012). Behavioral health in the Department of Defense Patient-Centered Medical Home: History, finance, policy, work force development, and evaluation. *Translational Behavioral Medicine, 2*(3), 355–363. https://doi.org/10.1007/s13142-012-0142-7

Hunter, C. L., Goodie, J. L., Dobmeyer, A. C., & Dorrance, K. A. (2014). Tipping points in the Department of Defense's experience with psychologists in primary care. *American Psychologist, 69*(4), 388–398. https://doi.org/10.1037/a0035806

Hunter, C. L., Goodie, J. L., Oordt, M. S., & Dobmeyer, A. C. (2009). *Integrated behavioral health in primary care: Step-by-step guidance for assessment and intervention.* American Psychological Association.

Hunter, C. L., Goodie, J. L., Oordt, M. S., & Dobmeyer, A. C. (2017). *Integrated behavioral health in primary care: Step-by-step guidance for assessment and intervention* (2nd ed.). American Psychological Association.

Hunter, M. S., & Chilcot, J. (2021). Is cognitive behaviour therapy an effective option for women who have troublesome menopausal symptoms? *British Journal of Health Psychology, 26*(3), 697–708. https://doi.org/10.1111/bjhp.12543

Hunter, M. S., Nuttall, J., & Fenlon, D. (2019). A comparison of three outcome measures of the impact of vasomotor symptoms on women's lives. *Climacteric, 22*(4), 419–423. https://doi.org/10.1080/13697137.2019.1580258

Hutchinson, T. A. (2017). *Whole-person care: Transforming healthcare.* Springer. https://doi.org/10.1007/978-3-319-59005-9

Hymmen, P., Stalker, C. A., & Cait, C. A. (2013). The case for single-session therapy: Does the empirical evidence support the increased prevalence of this service delivery model? *Journal of Mental Health, 22*(1), 60–71. https://doi.org/10.3109/09638237.2012.670880

Ilgen, D. R., Hollenbeck, J. R., Johnson, M., & Jundt, D. (2005). Teams in organizations: From input-process-output models to IMOI models. *Annual Review of Psychology, 56*(1), 517–543. https://doi.org/10.1146/annurev.psych.56.091103.070250

Institute of Medicine Committee on Quality of Health Care in America. (2001). *Crossing the quality chasm: A new health system for the 21st century.* National Academies Press. https://doi.org/10.17226/10027

Institute for Patient- and Family-Centered Care. (2021). *Core concepts of patient and family centered care.* https://www.ipfcc.org/about/pfcc.html

Interprofessional Education Collaborative Expert Panel. (2011). *Core competencies for interprofessional collaborative practice: Report of an expert panel.* Interprofessional Education Collaborative. https://www.ipecollaborative.org/ipec-core-competencies

Jackson, S. E., Steptoe, A., & Wardle, J. (2015). The influence of partner's behavior on health behavior change: The English Longitudinal Study of Ageing. *JAMA Internal Medicine, 175*(3), 385–392. https://doi.org/10.1001/jamainternmed.2014.7554

Jacobi, J. V., Ragone, T. A., & Greenwood, K. (2016). *Integration of behavioral and physical health care: Licensing and reimbursement barriers and opportunities in New Jersey.* Seton Hall University School of Law. https://thenicholsonfoundation.org/sites/default/files/Integration_Healthcare_Seton_Hall_report.pdf

Jacobs, J. C., Blonigen, D. M., Kimerling, R., Slightam, C., Gregory, A. J., Gurmessa, T., & Zulman, D. M. (2019). Increasing mental health care access, continuity, and efficiency for veterans through telehealth with video tablets. *Psychiatric Services, 70*(11), 976–982. https://doi.org/10.1176/appi.ps.201900104

Jaén, C. R., Crabtree, B. F., Palmer, R. F., Ferrer, R. L., Nutting, P. A., Miller, W. L., Stewart, E. E., Wood, R., Davila, M., & Stange, K. C. (2010). Methods for evaluating practice change toward a patient-centered medical home. *Annals of Family Medicine, 8*(Suppl. 1), S9–S20, S92. https://doi.org/10.1370/afm.1108

Jaiswal, J., & Halkitis, P. N. (2019). Towards a more inclusive and dynamic understanding of medical mistrust informed by science. *Behavioral Medicine, 45*(2), 79–85. https://doi.org/10.1080/08964289.2019.1619511

James, C. V., Moonesinghe, R., Wilson-Frederick, S. M., Hall, J. E., Penman-Aguilar, A., & Bouye, K. (2017). Racial/ethnic health disparities among rural adults—United States, 2012–2015. *MMWR Surveillance Summaries, 66*(23), 1–9. https://doi.org/10.15585/mmwr.ss6623a1

Janicke, D. M., Steele, R. G., Gayes, L. A., Lim, C. S., Clifford, L. M., Schneider, E. M., Carmody, J. K., & Westen, S. (2014). Systematic review and meta-analysis of comprehensive behavioral family lifestyle interventions addressing pediatric obesity. *Journal of Pediatric Psychology, 39*(8), 809–825. https://doi.org/10.1093/jpepsy/jsu023

Jannini, E. A., & Nappi, R. E. (2018). Couplepause: A new paradigm in treating sexual dysfunction during menopause and andropause. *Sexual Medicine Reviews, 6*(3), 384–395. https://doi.org/10.1016/j.sxmr.2017.11.002

Jeong, S., & Cho, S. I. (2018). Concordance in the health behaviors of couples by age: A cross-sectional study. *Journal of Preventive Medicine and Public Health, 51*(1), 6–14. https://doi.org/10.3961/jpmph.17.137

Johannsen, M., Damholdt, M. F., Zachariae, R., Lundorff, M., Farver-Vestergaard, I., & O'Connor, M. (2019). Psychological interventions for grief in adults: A systematic review and meta-analysis of randomized controlled trials. *Journal of Affective Disorders, 253*, 69–86. https://doi.org/10.1016/j.jad.2019.04.065

Johnson, K. F., & Freeman, K. L. (2014). Integrating interprofessional education and collaboration competencies (IPEC) into mental health counselor education. *Journal of Mental Health Counseling, 36*(4), 328–344. https://doi.org/10.17744/mehc.36.4.g47567602327j510

Johnson, M. J., & May, C. R. (2015). Promoting professional behaviour change in healthcare: What interventions work, and why? A theory-led overview of systematic reviews. *BMJ Open, 5*(9), Article e008592. https://doi.org/10.1136/bmjopen-2015-008592

Jones, K. M., Carter, M. M., Bianchi, A. L., Zeglin, R. J., & Schulkin, J. (2020). Obstetrician-gynecologist and patient factors associated with intimate partner violence screening in a clinical setting. *Women & Health, 60*(9), 1000–1013. https://doi.org/10.1080/03630242.2020.1784368

Jovicic, A., & McPherson, S. (2020). To support and not to cure: General practitioner management of loneliness. *Health & Social Care in the Community, 28*(2), 376–384. https://doi.org/10.1111/hsc.12869

Kaplan-Sanoff, M., & Briggs, R. D. (2016). Healthy steps for young children: Integrating behavioral health into primary care for young children and their families. In R. D. Briggs (Ed.), *Integrated early childhood behavioral health in primary care* (pp. 71–83). Springer International Publishing. https://doi.org/10.1007/978-3-319-31815-8_5

Karekla, M., Höfer, S., Plantade-Gipch, A., Neto, D. D., Schjødt, B., David, D., Schütz, C., Eleftheriou, A., Pappová, P. K., Lowet, K., McCracken, L., Sargautytė, R., Scharnhorst, J., & Hart, J. (2021). The role of psychologists in healthcare during the COVID-19 pandemic: Lessons learned and recommendations for the future. *European Journal of Psychology Open, 80*(1–2), 5–17. https://doi.org/10.1024/2673-8627/a000003

Kastner, M., Cardoso, R., Lai, Y., Treister, V., Hamid, J. S., Hayden, L., Wong, G., Ivers, N. M., Liu, B., Marr, S., Holroyd-Leduc, J., & Straus, S. E. (2018). Effectiveness of interventions for managing multiple high-burden chronic diseases in older adults: A systematic review and meta-analysis. *CMAJ*, *190*(34), E1004–E1012. https://doi.org/10.1503/cmaj.171391

Kathol, R. G., Butler, M., McAlpine, D. D., & Kane, R. L. (2010). Barriers to physical and mental condition integrated service delivery. *Psychosomatic Medicine*, *72*(6), 511–518. https://doi.org/10.1097/PSY.0b013e3181e2c4a0

Kathol, R. G., deGruy, F., & Rollman, B. L. (2014). Value-based financially sustainable behavioral health components in patient-centered medical homes. *Annals of Family Medicine*, *12*(2), 172–175. https://doi.org/10.1370/afm.1619

Katon, W. (1995). Collaborative care: Patient satisfaction, outcomes, and medical cost-offset. *Family Systems Medicine*, *13*(3–4), 351.

Katon, W. (2012). Collaborative depression care models: From development to dissemination. *American Journal of Preventive Medicine*, *42*(5), 550–552. https://doi.org/10.1016/j.amepre.2012.01.017

Katon, W. J., Lin, E. H., Von Korff, M., Ciechanowski, P., Ludman, E. J., Young, B., Peterson, D., Rutter, C. M., McGregor, M., & McCulloch, D. (2010). Collaborative care for patients with depression and chronic illnesses. *The New England Journal of Medicine*, *363*(27), 2611–2620. https://doi.org/10.1056/NEJMoa1003955

Katon, W., Von Korff, M., Lin, E., Walker, E., Simon, G. E., Bush, T., Robinson, P., & Russo, J. (1995). Collaborative management to achieve treatment guidelines. Impact on depression in primary care. *JAMA*, *273*(13), 1026–1031. https://doi.org/10.1001/jama.1995.03520370068039

Kautz, C., Mauch, D., & Smith, S. A. (2008). *Reimbursement of mental health services in primary care settings* (HHS Pub. No. SMA-08-4324). Center for Mental Health Services, Substance Abuse and Mental Health Services Administration.

Kazak, A. E., Schneider, S., Didonato, S., & Pai, A. L. (2015). Family psychosocial risk screening guided by the pediatric psychosocial preventative health model (PPPHM) using the Psychosocial Assessment Tool (PAT). *Acta Oncologica*, *54*(5), 574–580.

Kearney, L. K., Dollar, K. M., Beehler, G. P., Goldstein, W. R., Grasso, J. R., Wray, L. O., & Pomerantz, A. S. (2020). Creation and implementation of a national interprofessional integrated primary care competency training program: Preliminary findings and lessons learned. *Training and Education in Professional Psychology*, *14*(3), 219–227. https://doi.org/10.1037/tep0000263

Kearney, L. K., Post, E. P., Pomerantz, A. S., & Zeiss, A. M. (2014). Applying the interprofessional patient aligned care team in the Department of Veterans Affairs: Transforming primary care. *American Psychologist*, *69*(4), 399–408. https://doi.org/10.1037/a0035909

Keith, P., & Rogers, M. (2017). Spirituality in the primary care setting. In J. Wattis, S. Curran, & M. Rogers (Eds.), *Spiritually competent practice in health care* (pp. 129–144). CRC Press. https://doi.org/10.1201/9781315188638-9

Keller, M. B., Klerman, G. L., Lavori, P. W., Fawcett, J. A., Coryell, W., & Endicott, J. (1982). Treatment received by depressed patients. *JAMA, 248*(15), 1848–1855. https://doi.org/10.1001/jama.1982.03330150034019

Kellerman, R., & Kirk, L. (2007). Principles of the patient-centered medical home. *American Family Physician, 76*(6), 774–775.

Kepley, H. O., & Streeter, R. A. (2018). Closing behavioral health workforce gaps: A HRSA program expanding direct mental health service access in underserved areas. *American Journal of Preventive Medicine, 54*(6, Suppl. 3), S190–S191. https://doi.org/10.1016/j.amepre.2018.03.006

Kersting, A., & Wagner, B. (2012). Complicated grief after perinatal loss. *Dialogues in Clinical Neuroscience, 14*(2), 187–194. https://doi.org/10.31887/DCNS.2012.14.2/akersting

Kessler, R., & Glasgow, R. E. (2011). A proposal to speed translation of healthcare research into practice: Dramatic change is needed. *American Journal of Preventive Medicine, 40*(6), 637–644. https://doi.org/10.1016/j.amepre.2011.02.023

Kessler, R., & Hitt, J. R. (2016). Re: Electronic health record challenges, workarounds, and solutions observed in practices integrating behavioral health and primary care. *Journal of the American Board of Family Medicine, 29*(2), 289–290. https://doi.org/10.3122/jabfm.2016.02.150355

Kessler, R., & Stafford, D. (2008). Primary care is the de facto mental health system. In R. Kessler & D. Stafford (Eds.). *Collaborative medicine case studies: Evidence in practice* (pp. 9–21). Springer. https://doi.org/10.1007/978-0-387-76894-6_2

Khatri, P., Perry, G., & deGruy, F. V. (2017). Integrated health care at Cherokee Health Systems. In R. E. Feinstein, J. V. Connelly, & M. S. Feinstein (Eds.), *Integrating behavioral health and primary care* (pp. 17–30). Oxford University Press.

Kiesler, C. A. (1992). US mental health policy: Doomed to fail. *American Psychologist, 47*(9), 1077.

Kilo, C. M., & Wasson, J. H. (2010). Practice redesign and the patient-centered medical home: History, promises, and challenges. *Health Affairs (Project Hope), 29*(5), 773–778. https://doi.org/10.1377/hlthaff.2010.0012

Kiran, T., Kopp, A., Moineddin, R., & Glazier, R. H. (2015). Longitudinal evaluation of physician payment reform and team-based care for chronic disease management and prevention. *CMAJ, 187*(17), E494–E502. https://doi.org/10.1503/cmaj.150579

Kirchner, S. R., Gold, S. B., & Miller, B. F. (2019). Where practice meets policy. In S. B. Gold & L. A. Green (Eds.), *Integrated behavioral health in primary care: Your patients are waiting* (pp. 177–202). Springer Cham. https://doi.org/10.1007/978-3-319-98587-9_8

Kirkinis, K., Pieterse, A. L., Martin, C., Agiliga, A., & Brownell, A. (2021). Racism, racial discrimination, and trauma: A systematic review of the social science literature. *Ethnicity & Health, 26*(3), 392–412. https://doi.org/10.1080/13557858.2018.1514453

Kirsh, S. R., Aron, D. C., Johnson, K. D., Santurri, L. E., Stevenson, L. D., Jones, K. R., & Jagosh, J. (2017). A realist review of shared medical appointments: How, for whom, and under what circumstances do they work? *BMC Health Services Research, 17*, Article 113. https://doi.org/10.1186/s12913-017-2064-z

Kissane, D. W., Zaider, T. I., Li, Y., Hichenberg, S., Schuler, T., Lederberg, M., & Del Gaudio, F. (2016). Randomized controlled trial of family therapy in advanced cancer continued into bereavement. *Journal of Clinical Oncology, 34*(16), 1921–1927. https://doi.org/10.1200/JCO.2015.63.0582

Klein, J. T., & Falk-Krzesinski, H. J. (2017). Interdisciplinary and collaborative work: Framing promotion and tenure practices and policies. *Research Policy, 46*(6), 1055–1061. https://doi.org/10.1016/j.respol.2017.03.001

Knafl, K. A., Havill, N. L., Leeman, J., Fleming, L., Crandell, J. L., & Sandelowski, M. (2017). The nature of family engagement in interventions for children with chronic conditions. *Western Journal of Nursing Research, 39*(5), 690–723.

Kohn, L. T., Corrigan, J. M., & Donaldson, M. S. (Eds.). (1999). *To err is human: Building a safer health system*. National Academies Press.

Kolko, D. J., Torres, E., Rumbarger, K., James, E., Turchi, R., Bumgardner, C., & O'Brien, C. (2019). Integrated pediatric health care in Pennsylvania: A survey of primary care and behavioral health providers. *Clinical Pediatrics, 58*(2), 213–225. https://doi.org/10.1177/0009922818810881

Konzen, J., Lambert, J., Miller, M., & Negash, S. (2018). The EIS model: A pilot investigation of a multidisciplinary sex therapy treatment. *Journal of Sex & Marital Therapy, 44*(6), 552–565. https://doi.org/10.1080/0092623X.2018.1436626

Kothandan, S. K. (2014). School based interventions versus family based interventions in the treatment of childhood obesity—A systematic review. *Archives of Public Health, 72*, Article 3. https://doi.org/10.1186/2049-3258-72-3

Kotter, J. P. (1996). *Leading change*. Harvard Business School Press.

Kotter, J. P. (2017). What leaders really do. In A. Hooper (Ed.), *Leadership perspectives* (pp. 7–15). Routledge. https://doi.org/10.4324/9781315250601-2

Kovacs Burns, K., Nicolucci, A., Holt, R. I., Willaing, I., Hermanns, N., Kalra, S., Wens, J., Pouwer, F., Skovlund, S. E., Peyrot, M., & the DAWN2 Study Group. (2013). Diabetes Attitudes, Wishes and Needs second study (DAWN2™): Cross-national benchmarking indicators for family members living with people with diabetes. *Diabetic Medicine, 30*(7), 778–788. https://doi.org/10.1111/dme.12239

Kringos, D. S., Boerma, W. G., Hutchinson, A., van der Zee, J., & Groenewegen, P. P. (2010). The breadth of primary care: A systematic literature review of its core dimensions. *BMC Health Services Research, 10*, Article 65. https://doi.org/10.1186/1472-6963-10-65

Kroenke, K., Spitzer, R. L., & Williams, J. B. (2001). The PHQ-9: Validity of a brief depression severity measure. *Journal of General Internal Medicine, 16*(9), 606–613. https://doi.org/10.1046/j.1525-1497.2001.016009606.x

Kuhn, T. S. (2012). *The structure of scientific revolutions*. University of Chicago Press. https://doi.org/10.7208/chicago/9780226458144.001.0001

Kuo, D. Z., Houtrow, A. J., Arango, P., Kuhlthau, K. A., Simmons, J. M., & Neff, J. M. (2012). Family-centered care: Current applications and future directions in pediatric health care. *Maternal and Child Health Journal, 16*(2), 297–305. https://doi.org/10.1007/s10995-011-0751-7

Kyle, M. A., Aveling, E. L., & Singer, S. (2021). A mixed methods study of change processes enabling effective transition to team-based care. *Medical Care Research and Review, 78*(4), 326–337. https://doi.org/10.1177/1077558719881854

Lambie, G. W., & Milsom, A. (2010). A narrative approach to supporting students diagnosed with learning disabilities. *Journal of Counseling and Development, 88*(2), 196–203. https://doi.org/10.1002/j.1556-6678.2010.tb00009.x

Lamson, A., Phelps, K., Jones, A., & Bagley, R. (2018). Medical family therapy in obstetrics and gynecology. In J. Hodgson, A. Lamson, T. Mendenhall, & D. R. Crane (Eds.), *Medical family therapy* (pp. 147–180). Springer.

Lamson, A. L., Hodgson, J. L., Pratt, K. J., Mendenhall, T. J., Wong, A. G., Sesemann, E. M., Brown, B. J., Taylor, E. S., Williams-Reade, J. M., Blocker, D. J., Harsh Caspari, J., Zubatsky, M., & Martin, M. P. (2022). Couple and family interventions for high mortality health conditions: A strategic review (2010–2019). *Journal of Marital and Family Therapy, 48*(1), 307–345. https://doi.org/10.1111/jmft.12564

Lane, R. D. (2014). Is it possible to bridge the biopsychosocial and biomedical models? *BioPsychoSocial Medicine, 8*, Article 3. https://doi.org/10.1186/1751-0759-8-3

Lanham, H. J., Palmer, R. F., Leykum, L. K., McDaniel, R. R., Jr., Nutting, P. A., Stange, K. C., Crabtree, B. F., Miller, W. L., & Jaén, C. R. (2016). Trust and reflection in primary care practice redesign. *Health Services Research, 51*(4), 1489–1514. https://doi.org/10.1111/1475-6773.12415

Lanoye, A., Stewart, K. E., Rybarczyk, B. D., Auerbach, S. M., Sadock, E., Aggarwal, A., Waller, R., Wolver, S., & Austin, K. (2017). The impact of integrated psychological services in a safety net primary care clinic on medical utilization. *Journal of Clinical Psychology, 73*(6), 681–692. https://doi.org/10.1002/jclp.22367

Lardieri, M. R., Lasky, G. B., & Raney, L. (2014). *Essential elements of effective integrated primary care and behavioral health teams.* SAMHSA-HRSA Center for Integrated Health Solutions.

Larry A. Green Center. (2021). *Quick COVID-19 survey.* https://www.green-center.org/covid-survey

Lau, R., Stevenson, F., Ong, B. N., Dziedzic, K., Treweek, S., Eldridge, S., Everitt, H., Kennedy, A., Qureshi, N., Rogers, A., Peacock, R., & Murray, E. (2016). Achieving change in primary care—Causes of the evidence to practice gap: Systematic reviews of reviews. *Implementation Science, 11*, Article 40. https://doi.org/10.1186/s13012-016-0396-4

Launer, J. (2015). Guidelines and mindlines. *Postgraduate Medical Journal, 91*(1081), 663–664. https://doi.org/10.1136/postgradmedj-2015-133766

Lavallee, D. C., Chenok, K. E., Love, R. M., Petersen, C., Holve, E., Segal, C. D., & Franklin, P. D. (2016). Incorporating patient-reported outcomes into health care to engage patients and enhance care. *Health Affairs (Project Hope)*, *35*(4), 575–582. https://doi.org/10.1377/hlthaff.2015.1362

Law, E. F., Fisher, E., Fales, J., Noel, M., & Eccleston, C. (2014). Systematic review and meta-analysis of parent and family-based interventions for children and adolescents with chronic medical conditions. *Journal of Pediatric Psychology*, *39*(8), 866–886. https://doi.org/10.1093/jpepsy/jsu032

Lebow, J. L. (Ed.). (2016). Empirically supported treatments in couple and family therapy [Special issue]. *Family Process*, *55*(3).

Lekas, H. M., Pahl, K., & Fuller Lewis, C. (2020). Rethinking cultural competence: Shifting to cultural humility. *Health Services Insights*, *13*, Article 1178632920970580. https://doi.org/10.1177/1178632920970580

Leone, E., Dorstyn, D., & Ward, L. (2016). Defining resilience in families living with neurodevelopmental disorder: A preliminary examination of Walsh's framework. *Journal of Developmental and Physical Disabilities*, *28*(4), 595–608. https://doi.org/10.1007/s10882-016-9497-x

Levitt, H. M., Pomerville, A., & Surace, F. I. (2016). A qualitative meta-analysis examining clients' experiences of psychotherapy: A new agenda. *Psychological Bulletin*, *142*(8), 801–830. https://doi.org/10.1037/bul0000057

Lewis, V. A., Colla, C. H., Tierney, K., Van Citters, A. D., Fisher, E. S., & Meara, E. (2014). Few ACOs pursue innovative models that integrate care for mental illness and substance abuse with primary care. *Health Affairs (Project Hope)*, *33*(10), 1808–1816. https://doi.org/10.1377/hlthaff.2014.0353

Lewis Johnson, T. E., Clare, C. A., Johnson, J. E., & Simon, M. A. (2020). Preventing perinatal depression now: A call to action. *Journal of Women's Health*, *29*(9), 1143–1147. https://doi.org/10.1089/jwh.2020.8646

Li, K., Davison, K. K., & Jurkowski, J. M. (2012). Mental health and family functioning as correlates of a sedentary lifestyle among low-income women with young children. *Women & Health*, *52*(6), 606–619. https://doi.org/10.1080/03630242.2012.705243

Li, K. K., Cardinal, B. J., & Acock, A. C. (2013). Concordance of physical activity trajectories among middle-aged and older married couples: Impact of diseases and functional difficulties. *Journals of Gerontology: Series B*, *68*(5), 794–806. https://doi.org/10.1093/geronb/gbt068

Li, S., & Delva, J. (2012). Social capital and smoking among Asian American men: An exploratory study. *American Journal of Public Health*, *102*(Suppl. 2), S212–S221. https://doi.org/10.2105/AJPH.2011.300442

Liblik, K., Mulvagh, S. L., Hindmarch, C. C., Alavi, N., & Johri, A. M. (2021). Depression and anxiety following acute myocardial infarction in women. *Trends in Cardiovascular Medicine*, *32*(6), 341–347.

Lichstein, J. C., Ghandour, R. M., & Mann, M. Y. (2018). Access to the medical home among children with and without special health care needs. *Pediatrics*, *142*(6), Article e20181795. https://doi.org/10.1542/peds.2018-1795

Lindberg, L. D., VandeVusse, A., Mueller, J., & Kirstein, M. (2020, June). *Early impacts of the COVID-19 pandemic: Findings from the 2020 Guttmacher Survey*

of Reproductive Health Experiences. Guttmacher Institute. https://doi.org/
10.1363/2020.31482

Lipsitz, L. A. (2012). Understanding health care as a complex system: The foundation for unintended consequences. *JAMA, 308*(3), 243–244. https://doi.org/
10.1001/jama.2012.7551

Lister, Z., Fox, C., & Wilson, C. M. (2013). Couples and diabetes: A 30-year narrative review of dyadic relational research. *Contemporary Family Therapy,
35*(4), 613–638. https://doi.org/10.1007/s10591-013-9250-x

Lorig, K. R., Sobel, D. S., Ritter, P. L., Laurent, D., & Hobbs, M. (2001). Effect of a self-management program on patients with chronic disease. *Effective Clinical Practice, 4*(6), 256–262.

Lotti, F., & Maggi, M. (2018). Sexual dysfunction and male infertility. *Nature Reviews Urology, 15*(5), 287–307. https://doi.org/10.1038/nrurol.2018.20

Lu, M. C., Kotelchuck, M., Hogan, V. K., Johnson, K., & Reyes, C. (2010). Innovative strategies to reduce disparities in the quality of prenatal care in underresourced settings. *Medical Care Research and Review, 67*(5, Suppl.), 198S–230S.
https://doi.org/10.1177/1077558710374324

Luo, D., Xu, J. J., Cai, X., Zhu, M., Wang, H., Yan, D., & Li, M. Z. (2019). The effects of family functioning and resilience on self-management and glycaemic control among youth with type 1 diabetes. *Journal of Clinical Nursing, 28*(23–24),
4478–4487. https://doi.org/10.1111/jocn.15033

Lutgendorf, M. A. (2019). Intimate partner violence and women's health.
Obstetrics and Gynecology, 134(3), 470–480. https://doi.org/10.1097/AOG.
0000000000003326

Ly, D. P. (2019). Racial and ethnic disparities in the evaluation and management of pain in the outpatient setting, 2006–2015. *Pain Medicine, 20*(2), 223–232.
https://doi.org/10.1093/pm/pny074

Lynch, K. (2019). The trans man and the warrior women. *Transgender Health,
4*(1), 277–279. https://doi.org/10.1089/trgh.2019.0047

Lyon, M. E., Jacobs, S., Briggs, L., Cheng, Y. I., & Wang, J. (2013). Family-centered advance care planning for teens with cancer. *JAMA Pediatrics, 167*(5), 460–467.
https://doi.org/10.1001/jamapediatrics.2013.943

MacDonald, M. B., Bally, J. M., Ferguson, L. M., Lee Murray, B., Fowler-Kerry,
S. E., & Anonson, J. M. (2010). Knowledge of the professional role of others:
A key interprofessional competency. *Nurse Education in Practice, 10*(4), 238–242.
https://doi.org/10.1016/j.nepr.2009.11.012

MacFarlane, P., Anderson, T., & McClintock, A. S. (2015). The early formation of the working alliance from the client's perspective: A qualitative study. *Psychotherapy, 52*(3), 363–372. https://doi.org/10.1037/a0038733

Mann, K., Gordon, J., & MacLeod, A. (2009). Reflection and reflective practice in health professions education: A systematic review. *Advances in Health Sciences Education: Theory and Practice, 14*(4), 595–621. https://doi.org/10.1007/
s10459-007-9090-2

Manne, S. L., Kashy, D. A., Kissane, D., Zaider, T., Heckman, C. J., Penedo, F. J., & Myers, S. (2019). Relationship intimacy processes during treatment for couple-focused interventions for prostate cancer patients and their spouses. *Journal of Psychosocial Oncology Research and Practice, 1*(2), e7. https://doi.org/10.1097/OR9.0000000000000007

Manne, S. L., Siegel, S., Kashy, D., & Heckman, C. J. (2014). Cancer-specific relationship awareness, relationship communication, and intimacy among couples coping with early-stage breast cancer. *Journal of Social and Personal Relationships, 31*(3), 314–334. https://doi.org/10.1177/0265407513494950

Markin, R. D. (2017). An introduction to the special section on psychotherapy for pregnancy loss: Review of issues, clinical applications, and future research direction. *Psychotherapy, 54*(4), 367–372. https://doi.org/10.1037/pst0000134

Marlowe, D., Capobianco, J., & Greenberg, C. (2014). Getting reimbursed for MedFT: Financial models toward sustainability. In J. Hodgson, A. Lamson, T. Mendenhall, & D. R. Crane (Eds.), *Medical family therapy* (pp. 437–449). Springer. https://doi.org/10.1007/978-3-319-03482-9_23

Marlowe, D., Hodgson, J., Lamson, A., White, M., & Irons, T. (2012). Medical family therapy in a primary care setting: A framework for integration. *Contemporary Family Therapy, 34*(2), 244–258. https://doi.org/10.1007/s10591-012-9195-5

Marques, A., Jácome, C., Cruz, J., Gabriel, R., Brooks, D., & Figueiredo, D. (2015). Family-based psychosocial support and education as part of pulmonary rehabilitation in COPD: A randomized controlled trial. *Chest, 147*(3), 662–672. https://doi.org/10.1378/chest.14-1488

Mårtensson, J., Dracup, K., Canary, C., & Fridlund, B. (2003). Living with heart failure: Depression and quality of life in patients and spouses. *The Journal of Heart and Lung Transplantation, 22*(4), 460–467. https://doi.org/10.1016/S1053-2498(02)00818-5

Martin, M. P., White, M. B., Hodgson, J. L., Lamson, A. L., & Irons, T. G. (2014). Integrated primary care: A systematic review of program characteristics. *Families, Systems & Health, 32*(1), 101–115. https://doi.org/10.1037/fsh0000017

Martire, L. M. (2013). Couple-oriented interventions for chronic illness: Where do we go from here? *Journal of Social and Personal Relationships, 30*(2), 207–214. https://doi.org/10.1177/0265407512453786

Martire, L. M., & Helgeson, V. S. (2017). Close relationships and the management of chronic illness: Associations and interventions. *American Psychologist, 72*(6), 601–612. https://doi.org/10.1037/amp0000066

Martire, L. M., Schulz, R., Helgeson, V. S., Small, B. J., & Saghafi, E. M. (2010). Review and meta-analysis of couple-oriented interventions for chronic illness. *Annals of Behavioral Medicine, 40*(3), 325–342. https://doi.org/10.1007/s12160-010-9216-2

Massachusetts College of Pharmacy and Health Sciences. (2021, July 13). *Interprofessional education funding opportunities.* https://mcphs.libguides.com/c.php?g=883690&p=6350226

Mautone, J. A., Cabello, B., Egan, T. E., Rodrigues, N. P., Davis, M., Figge, C. J., Sass, A. J., & Williamson, A. A. (2020). Exploring predictors of treatment engagement in urban integrated primary care. *Clinical Practice in Pediatric Psychology, 8*(3), 228–240. https://doi.org/10.1037/cpp0000366

Mayberry, L. S., & Osborn, C. Y. (2014). Family involvement is helpful and harmful to patients' self-care and glycemic control. *Patient Education and Counseling, 97*(3), 418–425. https://doi.org/10.1016/j.pec.2014.09.011

Mazzoni, S., Brewer, S., Durfee, J., Pyrzanowski, J., Barnard, J., Dempsey, A. F., & O'Leary, S. T. (2017). Patient perspectives of obstetrician-gynecologists as primary care providers. *The Journal of Reproductive Medicine, 62*(1–2), 3–8.

McColl-Kennedy, J. R., Vargo, S. L., Dagger, T. S., Sweeney, J. C., & Kasteren, Y. V. (2012). Health care customer value cocreation practice styles. *Journal of Service Research, 15*(4), 370–389. https://doi.org/10.1177/1094670512442806

McConnell, K. J. (2019). Investing in primary care and dismantling fee-for-service. *The Milbank Quarterly, 97*(3), 636–640. https://doi.org/10.1111/1468-0009.12399

McCool-Myers, M., Theurich, M., Zuelke, A., Knuettel, H., & Apfelbacher, C. (2018). Predictors of female sexual dysfunction: A systematic review and qualitative analysis through gender inequality paradigms. *BMC Women's Health, 18*, Article 108. https://doi.org/10.1186/s12905-018-0602-4

McCusker, C. G., Doherty, N., Molloy, B., Rooney, N., Mulholland, C., Sands, A., & Casey, F. (2009). A controlled trial of early interventions to promote maternal adjustment and development in infants born with severe congenital heart disease. *Child: Care, Health and Development, 36*, 110–117. https://doi.org/10.1111/j.1365-2214.2009.01026.x

McCusker, C. G., Doherty, N. N., Molloy, B., Rooney, N., Mulholland, C., Sands, A., Craig, B., Stewart, M., & Casey, F. (2012). A randomized controlled trial of interventions to promote adjustment in children with congenital heart disease entering school and their families. *Journal of Pediatric Psychology, 37*(10), 1089–1103. https://doi.org/10.1093/jpepsy/jss092

McDaniel, S. H., Belar, C. D., Schroeder, C., Hargrove, D. S., & Freeman, E. L. (2002). A training curriculum for professional psychologists in primary care. *Professional Psychology, Research and Practice, 33*(1), 65–72. https://doi.org/10.1037/0735-7028.33.1.65

McDaniel, S. H., Campbell, T. L., Hepworth, J., & Lorenz, A. (2005). *Family-oriented primary care* (2nd ed.). Springer.

McDaniel, S. H., Campbell, T. L., Rosenberg, T., Schultz, S., & deGruy, F. (2014). Innovations in teaching about transdisciplinary professionalism and professional norms. In P. Cuff (Ed.), *Establishing transdisciplinary professionalism for improving health outcomes: Workshop Summary* (pp. 101–107). National Academies Press.

McDaniel, S. H., Doherty, W. J., & Hepworth, J. (2014). *Medical family therapy and integrated care* (2nd ed.). American Psychological Association. https://doi.org/10.1037/14256-000

McDaniel, S. H., & Fogerty, C. T. (2009). What primary care psychology has to offer the patient-centered medical home. *Professional Psychology, Research and Practice, 40*(5), 483–492. https://doi.org/10.1037/a0016751

McDaniel, S. H., Grus, C. L., Cubic, B. A., Hunter, C. L., Kearney, L. K., Schuman, C. C., Karel, M. J., Kessler, R. S., Larkin, K. T., McCutcheon, S., Miller, B. F., Nash, J., Qualls, S. H., Connolly, K. S., Stancin, T., Stanton, A. L., Sturm, L. A., & Johnson, S. B. (2014). Competencies for psychology practice in primary care. *American Psychologist, 69*(4), 409–429. https://doi.org/10.1037/a0036072

McDaniel, S. H., Hepworth, J., & Doherty, W. J. (1992). *Medical family therapy: A biopsychosocial approach to families with health problems.* Basic Books.

McDaniel, S. H., Hepworth, J., & Doherty, W. J. (1997). *The shared experience of illness: Stories of patients, families, and their therapists.* Basic Books.

McDaniel, S. H., & Pisani, A. R. (2012). Family dynamics and caregiving for people with disabilities. In R. C. Talley & J. E. Crews (Eds.), *Multiple dimensions of caregiving and disability: Research, practice, and policy* (pp. 11–28). Springer. https://doi.org/10.1007/978-1-4614-3384-2_2

McEvoy, M., McElvaney, R., & Glover, R. (2021). Understanding vaginismus: A biopsychosocial perspective. *Sexual and Relationship Therapy.* https://doi.org/10.1080/14681994.2021.2007233

McEwen, M. M., Pasvogel, A., & Murdaugh, C. (2019). Effects of a family-based diabetes intervention on family social capital outcomes for Mexican American adults. *The Diabetes Educator, 45*(3), 272–286. https://doi.org/10.1177/0145721719837899

McEwen, M. M., Pasvogel, A., Murdaugh, C., & Hepworth, J. (2017). Effects of a family-based diabetes intervention on behavioral and biological outcomes for Mexican American adults. *The Diabetes Educator, 43*(3), 272–285. https://doi.org/10.1177/0145721717706031

McGill, K., Bhullar, N., Pearce, T., Batterham, P. J., Wayland, S., & Maple, M. (2022). Effectiveness of brief contact interventions for bereavement: A systematic review. *OMEGA—Journal of Death and Dying*, Article 00302228221108289. https://doi.org/10.1177/00302228221108289

McGinty, E. E., Presskreischer, R., Breslau, J., Brown, J. D., Domino, M. E., Druss, B. G., Horvitz-Lennon, M., Murphy, K. A., Pincus, H. A., & Daumit, G. L. (2021). Improving physical health among people with serious mental illness: The role of the specialty mental health sector. *Psychiatric Services, 72*(11), 1301–1310. https://doi.org/10.1176/appi.ps.202000768

McGoldrick, M., Gerson, R., & Petry, S. S. (2020). *Genograms: Assessment and treatment* (4th ed.). W. W. Norton & Company.

McGrath, R. E., & O'Donohue, W. (2015). The importance of stepped-care protocols for the redesign of behavioral health care in patient-centered medical homes. In W. O'Donohue & A. Maragakis (Eds.), *Integrated primary and behavioral care* (pp. 97–114). Springer. https://doi.org/10.1007/978-3-319-19036-5_6

McKenney, K. M., Martinez, N. G., & Yee, L. M. (2018). Patient navigation across the spectrum of women's health care in the United States. *American Journal of Obstetrics and Gynecology, 218*(3), 280–286. https://doi.org/10.1016/j.ajog.2017.08.009

Mead, M. (1968). The cybernetics of cybernetics. In H. von Foerster, J. D. White, L. J. Peterson, & J. K. Russel (Eds.), *Purposive systems* (pp. 1–11). Spartan Books.

Meadows, D. H. (2008). *Thinking in systems: A primer.* Chelsea Green Publishers.

Medina-Martínez, J., Saus-Ortega, C., Sánchez-Lorente, M. M., Sosa-Palanca, E. M., García-Martínez, P., & Mármol-López, M. I. (2021). Health inequities in LGBT people and nursing interventions to reduce them: A systematic review. *International Journal of Environmental Research and Public Health, 18*(22), Article 11801. https://doi.org/10.3390/ijerph182211801

Mehta, N. (2011). Mind-body dualism: A critique from a health perspective. *Mens Sana Monographs, 9*(1), 202–209. https://doi.org/10.4103/0973-1229.77436

Mendenhall, T., Lamson, A., Hodgson, J., & Baird, M. (Eds.). (2018). *Clinical methods in medical family therapy.* Springer. https://doi.org/10.1007/978-3-319-68834-3

Mendenhall, T., Lamson, A., Hodgson, J., Tyndall, L., Williams-Reade, J., & Trudea, S. (2018, March 5). Core clinical competencies for family therapists working in healthcare settings. *The AAMFT Blog.* https://blog.aamft.org/2018/03/core-clinical-competencies-for-family-therapists-working-in-healthcare-settings.html

Mihata, K. (1997). The persistence of emergence. In R. A. Eve, S. Horsfall, & M. E. Lee (Eds.), *Chaos, complexity & sociology: Myths, models & theories* (pp. 30–38). Sage.

Miles, A. (2015). From EBM to PCH: Always predictable, now inexorable. Editorial introduction to the 2015 Evidence Based Medicine thematic issue of the *Journal of Evaluation in Clinical Practice. Journal of Evaluation in Clinical Practice, 21*(6), 983–987. https://doi.org/10.1111/jep.12525

Miles, P. V., Conway, P. H., & Pawlson, L. G. (2013). Physician professionalism and accountability: The role of collaborative improvement networks. *Pediatrics, 131*(Suppl. 4), S204–S209. https://doi.org/10.1542/peds.2012-3786G

Miller, B. F., Gilchrist, E. C., Ross, K. M., Wong, S. L., & Green, L. A. (2016). *Creating a culture of whole health: Recommendations for integrating behavioral health and primary care.* Eugene S. Farley, Jr., Health Policy Center.

Miller, B. F., & Hubley, S. H. (2017). The history of fragmentation and the promise of integration: A primer on behavioral health and primary care. In M. E. Maruish (Ed.), *Handbook of psychological assessment in primary care settings* (pp. 55–73). Routledge.

Miller, B. F., Mendenhall, T. J., & Malik, A. D. (2009). Integrated primary care: An inclusive three-world view through process metrics and empirical discrimination. *Journal of Clinical Psychology in Medical Settings, 16,* 21–30. https://doi.org/10.1007/s10880-008-9137-4

Miller, B. F., Petterson, S., Burke, B. T., Phillips, R. L., Jr., & Green, L. A. (2014). Proximity of providers: Colocating behavioral health and primary care and the prospects for an integrated workforce. *American Psychologist, 69*(4), 443–451. https://doi.org/10.1037/a0036093

Miller, B. F., Ross, K. M., Davis, M. M., Melek, S. P., Kathol, R., & Gordon, P. (2017). Payment reform in the patient-centered medical home: Enabling and sustaining integrated behavioral health care. *American Psychologist, 72*(1), 55–68. https://doi.org/10.1037/a0040448

Miller, B. F., Talen, M. R., & Patel, K. K. (2013). Advancing integrated behavioral health and primary care: The critical importance of behavioral health in health care policy. In M. R. Talen & A. Burke Valeras (Eds.), *Integrated behavioral health in primary care* (pp. 53–62). Springer. https://doi.org/10.1007/978-1-4614-6889-9_4

Miller, E. (2020). Torts: Just walk away: How an overbroad foreseeability of harm standard could kill "curbside consultations"—Warren v. Dinter, 926 NW 2d 370 (Minn. 2019). *Mitchell Hamline Law Review, 46*(3), Article 6.

Miller, T. A., & DiMatteo, M. R. (2013). Importance of family/social support and impact on adherence to diabetic therapy. *Diabetes, Metabolic Syndrome and Obesity, 6*, 421–426. https://doi.org/10.2147/DMSO.S36368

Miller, W. L., Crabtree, B. F., Nutting, P. A., Stange, K. C., & Jaén, C. R. (2010). Primary care practice development: A relationship-centered approach. *Annals of Family Medicine, 8*(Suppl. 1), S68–S79, S92. https://doi.org/10.1370/afm.1089

Miller, W. L., Rubinstein, E. B., Howard, J., & Crabtree, B. F. (2019). Shifting implementation science theory to empower primary care practices. *Annals of Family Medicine, 17*(3), 250–256. https://doi.org/10.1370/afm.2353

Miller-Matero, L. R., Dykuis, K. E., Albujoq, K., Martens, K., Fuller, B. S., Robinson, V., & Willens, D. E. (2016). Benefits of integrated behavioral health services: The physician perspective. *Families, Systems & Health, 34*(1), 51–55. https://doi.org/10.1037/fsh0000182

Mills, T. A., Ricklesford, C., Heazell, A. E. P., Cooke, A., & Lavender, T. (2016). Marvellous to mediocre: Findings of national survey of UK practice and provision of care in pregnancies after stillbirth or neonatal death. *BMC Pregnancy and Childbirth, 16*, Article 101. https://doi.org/10.1186/s12884-016-0891-2

Minkoff, K., & Parks, J. (2015). Primary health–behavioral health integration for the population of individuals with serious mental illness. In W. O'Donohue & A. Maragakas (Eds.), *Integrated primary and behavioral healthcare role in medical homes and chronic disease management* (pp. 171–199). Springer. https://doi.org/10.1007/978-3-319-19036-5_10

Moieni, M., & Eisenberger, N. I. (2020). Social isolation and health. In K. Sweeny, M. L. Robbins, & L. M. Cohen (Eds.), *The Wiley encyclopedia of health psychology* (pp. 695–702). John Wiley & Sons. https://doi.org/10.1002/9781119057840.ch121

Mojtabai, R., Olfson, M., Sampson, N. A., Jin, R., Druss, B., Wang, P. S., Wells, K. B., Pincus, H. A., & Kessler, R. C. (2011). Barriers to mental health treatment:

Results from the National Comorbidity Survey Replication. *Psychological Medicine, 41*(8), 1751–1761. https://doi.org/10.1017/S0033291710002291

Mondesire, F. L., White, K., Liese, A. D., & McLain, A. C. (2016). Gender, illness-related diabetes social support and glycemic control among middle-aged and older adults. *Journal of Gerontology: Series B, 71*(6), 1081–1088. https://doi.org/10.1093/geronb/gbv061

Moore, J., Mule, C., & McDaniel, S. H. (2023). Family systems. In H. Feldman, E. Elias, N. Blum, T. Stancin, & M. Jimenez (Eds.), *Developmental behavioral pediatrics* (5th ed.). Elsevier.

Moore Simas, T. A., Flynn, M. P., Kroll-Desrosiers, A. R., Carvalho, S. M., Levin, L. L., Biebel, K., & Byatt, N. (2018). A systematic review of integrated care interventions addressing perinatal depression care in ambulatory obstetric care settings. *Clinical Obstetrics and Gynecology, 61*(3), 573–590. https://doi.org/10.1097/GRF.0000000000000360

Moscato, E., Patronick, J., & Wade, S. L. (2022). Family functioning and adaptation following pediatric brain tumor: A systematic review. *Pediatric Blood & Cancer, 69*(2). https://doi.org/10.1002/pbc.29470

Moseson, H., Zazanis, N., Goldberg, E., Fix, L., Durden, M., Stoeffler, A., Hastings, Cudlitz, L., Lesser-Lee, B., Letcher, L., Reyes, A., & Obedin-Maliver, J. (2020). The imperative for transgender and gender nonbinary inclusion: Beyond women's health. *Obstetrics and Gynecology, 135*(5), 1059–1068.

Moye, J. (2019). Healthcare systems meet family systems: Improving healthcare for older adults and their families. *Clinical Gerontologist, 42*(5), 461–462. https://doi.org/10.1080/07317115.2019.1651485

Moyer, V. A. (2013). Screening and behavioral counseling interventions in primary care to reduce alcohol misuse: U.S. preventive services task force recommendation statement. *Annals of Internal Medicine, 159*(3), 210–218. https://doi.org/10.7326/0003-4819-159-3-201308060-00652

Mueller, K. L., Hudson, T. W., III, Bruns, D., Algire, D. Z., Buchta, W. G., Christian, J. H., Cloeren, M., Das, R., & Eisenhart, M., Frangos, S. A., Gillaspy, S., Hammel, R., Havens, C., Marks, S., Melvin, J., Moses, X. J. E., Persell, S., Pushkin, G., Rodrigues, S., . . . & Wright, C. V. (2020). Recommendations from the 2019 Symposium on Including Functional Status Measurement in Standard Patient Care. *Journal of Occupational and Environmental Medicine, 62*(8), e457–e466.

Mullin, D. J., & Funderburk, J. S. (2013). Implementing clinical interventions in integrated behavioral health settings: Best practices and essential elements. In M. Talen & V. A. Burke (Eds.), *Integrated behavioral health in primary care* (pp. 273–297). Springer. https://doi.org/10.1007/978-1-4614-6889-9_13

Mulvale, G., Embrett, M., & Razavi, S. D. (2016). 'Gearing Up' to improve interprofessional collaboration in primary care: A systematic review and conceptual framework. *BMC Family Practice, 17*, Article 83. https://doi.org/10.1186/s12875-016-0492-1

Mulvaney-Day, N., Marshall, T., Downey Piscopo, K., Korsen, N., Lynch, S., Karnell, L. H., Moran, G. E., Daniels, A. S., & Ghose, S. S. (2018). Screening for behavioral health conditions in primary care settings: A systematic review of the literature. *Journal of General Internal Medicine, 33*(3), 335–346. https://doi.org/10.1007/s11606-017-4181-0

Muntingh, A. D., van der Feltz-Cornelis, C. M., van Marwijk, H. W., Spinhoven, P., & van Balkom, A. J. (2016). Collaborative care for anxiety disorders in primary care: A systematic review and meta-analysis. *BMC Family Practice, 17,* Article 62. https://doi.org/10.1186/s12875-016-0466-3

Muse, A. R., Lamson, A. L., Didericksen, K. W., Hodgson, J. L., & Schoemann, A. M. (2022). Clinical, operational, and financial evaluation practices in integrated behavioral health care. *Families, Systems & Health, 40*(3), 312–321. https://doi.org/10.1037/fsh0000683

Nash, J. M., McKay, K. M., Vogel, M. E., & Masters, K. S. (2012). Functional roles and foundational characteristics of psychologists in integrated primary care. *Journal of Clinical Psychology in Medical Settings, 19*(1), 93–104. https://doi.org/10.1007/s10880-011-9290-z

Natale, R. A., Messiah, S. E., Asfour, L., Uhlhorn, S. B., Delamater, A., & Arheart, K. L. (2014). Role modeling as an early childhood obesity prevention strategy: Effect of parents and teachers on preschool children's healthy lifestyle habits. *Journal of Developmental and Behavioral Pediatrics, 35*(6), 378–387. https://doi.org/10.1097/DBP.0000000000000074

National Academies of Sciences, Engineering, and Medicine. (2020). *Social isolation and loneliness in older adults: Opportunities for the health care system.* National Academies Press. https://nap.nationalacademies.org/catalog/25663/social-isolation-and-loneliness-in-older-adults-opportunities-for-the

National Academies of Sciences, Engineering, and Medicine. (2021). *Implementing high-quality primary care: Rebuilding the foundation of health care.* The National Academies Press. https://nap.nationalacademies.org/catalog/25983/implementing-high-quality-primary-care-rebuilding-the-foundation-of-health

National Center for Health Statistics (U.S.). (2016). *Health, United States, 2015: With special feature on racial and ethnic health disparities* (DHHS publication No. 2016-1232). U.S. Department of Health and Human Services, Centers for Disease Control and Prevention. https://stacks.cdc.gov/view/cdc/39108

Nelson, G., Bakkum-Gamez, J., Kalogera, E., Glaser, G., Altman, A., Meyer, L. A., Taylor, J. S., Iniesta, M., Lasala, J., Mena, G., Scott, M., Gillis, C., Elias, K., Wijk, L., Huang, J., Nygren, J., Ljungqvist, O., Ramirez, P. T., & Dowdy, S. C. (2019). Guidelines for perioperative care in gynecologic/oncology: Enhanced Recovery After Surgery (ERAS) Society recommendations—2019 update. *International Journal of Gynecological Cancer, 29*(4), 651–668. https://doi.org/10.1136/ijgc-2019-000356

Nelson, K. M., Helfrich, C., Sun, H., Hebert, P. L., Liu, C. F., Dolan, E., Taylor, L., Wong, E., Maynard, C., Hernandez, S. E., Sanders, W., Randall, I., Curtis, I., Schectman, G., Stark, R., & Fihn, S. D. (2014). Implementation of the patient-centered medical home in the Veterans Health Administration: Associations with patient satisfaction, quality of care, staff burnout, and hospital and emergency department use. *JAMA Internal Medicine, 174*(8), 1350–1358. https://doi.org/10.1001/jamainternmed.2014.2488

Nemours Childrens Health Center for Healthcare Delivery Services. (2023). *Psychosocial assessment tool (PAT).* https://www.psychosocialassessmenttool.org

Newton, D. C., & McCabe, M. P. (2008). Sexually transmitted infections: Impact on individuals and their relationships. *Journal of Health Psychology, 13*(7), 864–869. https://doi.org/10.1177/1359105308095058

Ng, R. M. K., Chan, T. F., Herrman, H., & Dowrick, C. (2021). What do psychiatrists think about primary mental health competencies among family doctors? A WPA-WONCA global survey. *BJPsych International, 18*(1), 18–22. https://doi.org/10.1192/bji.2020.32

Nieuwboer, M. S., van der Sande, R., van der Marck, M. A., Olde Rikkert, M. G. M., & Perry, M. (2019). Clinical leadership and integrated primary care: A systematic literature review. *The European Journal of General Practice, 25*(1), 7–18. https://doi.org/10.1080/13814788.2018.1515907

Noël, P. H., Lanham, H. J., Palmer, R. F., Leykum, L. K., & Parchman, M. L. (2013). The importance of relational coordination and reciprocal learning for chronic illness care within primary care teams. *Health Care Management Review, 38*(1), 20–28. https://doi.org/10.1097/HMR.0b013e3182497262

Norfleet, K. R., Ratzliff, A. D., Chan, Y. F., Raney, L. E., & Unützer, J. (2016). The role of the integrated care psychiatrist in community settings: A survey of psychiatrists' perspectives. *Psychiatric Services, 67*(3), 346–349. https://doi.org/10.1176/appi.ps.201400592

Northouse, L., Williams, A. L., Given, B., & McCorkle, R. (2012). Psychosocial care for family caregivers of patients with cancer. *Journal of Clinical Oncology, 30*(11), 1227–1234. https://doi.org/10.1200/JCO.2011.39.5798

Norton, S. A., Wittink, M. N., Duberstein, P. R., Prigerson, H. G., Stanek, S., & Epstein, R. M. (2019). Family caregiver descriptions of stopping chemotherapy and end-of-life transitions. *Supportive Care in Cancer, 27*(2), 669–675. https://doi.org/10.1007/s00520-018-4365-0

Nutting, P. A., Crabtree, B. F., Stewart, E. E., Miller, W. L., Palmer, R. F., Stange, K. C., & Jaén, C. R. (2010). Effect of facilitation on practice outcomes in the National Demonstration Project model of the patient-centered medical home. *Annals of Family Medicine, 8*(Suppl. 1), S33–S44, S92. https://doi.org/10.1370/afm.1119

Nuzum, D., Meaney, S., & O'Donoghue, K. (2014). The impact of stillbirth on consultant obstetrician gynaecologists: A qualitative study. *BJOG, 121*(8), 1020–1028. https://doi.org/10.1111/1471-0528.12695

O'Brien, M. (2007). Ambiguous loss in families of children with autism spectrum disorders. *Family Relations, 56*(2), 135–146. https://doi.org/10.1111/j.1741-3729.2007.00447.x

Ofonedu, M. E., Belcher, H. M. E., Budhathoki, C., & Gross, D. A. (2017). Understanding barriers to initial treatment engagement among underserved families seeking mental health services. *Journal of Child and Family Studies*, 26(3), 863–876. https://doi.org/10.1007/s10826-016-0603-6

Ogbeide, S., Buck, D. S., & Reiter, J. (2014, October 16–18). *Mapping new territory: Implementing the primary care behavioral health (PCBH) model in homeless shelter clinics* [Paper presentation]. Collaborative Family Healthcare Association Annual Conference, Washington, DC, United States.

Okafor, M., Ede, V., Kinuthia, R., & Satcher, D. (2018). Explication of a behavioral health-primary care integration learning collaborative and its quality improvement implications. *Community Mental Health Journal*, 54(8), 1109–1115. https://doi.org/10.1007/s10597-017-0230-8

O'Loughlin, K., Donovan, E. K., Radcliff, Z., Ryan, M., & Rybarczyk, B. (2019). Using integrated behavioral healthcare to address behavioral health disparities in underserved populations. *Translational Issues in Psychological Science*, 5(4), 374–389. https://doi.org/10.1037/tps0000213

O'Malley, A. S., Gourevitch, R., Draper, K., Bond, A., & Tirodkar, M. A. (2015). Overcoming challenges to teamwork in patient-centered medical homes: A qualitative study. *Journal of General Internal Medicine*, 30(2), 183–192. https://doi.org/10.1007/s11606-014-3065-9

O'Rourke, H. M., Collins, L., & Sidani, S. (2018). Interventions to address social connectedness and loneliness for older adults: A scoping review. *BMC Geriatrics*, 18, Article 214. https://doi.org/10.1186/s12877-018-0897-x

OpenNotes. (2021). Education and research for healthcare transparency. https://www.opennotes.org/?s=Education+and+research+for+healthcare+transparency.+

Oppenheim, J., Stewart, W., Zoubak, E., Donato, I., Huang, L., & Hudock, W. (2016). Launching forward: The integration of behavioral health in primary care as a key strategy for promoting young child wellness. *American Journal of Orthopsychiatry*, 86(2), 124–131. https://doi.org/10.1037/ort0000149

Östlund, U., & Persson, C. (2014). Examining family responses to family systems nursing interventions: An integrative review. *Journal of Family Nursing*, 20(3), 259–286. https://doi.org/10.1177/1074840714542962

Overbeck, G., Davidsen, A. S., & Kousgaard, M. B. (2016). Enablers and barriers to implementing collaborative care for anxiety and depression: A systematic qualitative review. *Implementation Science*, 11, Article 165. https://doi.org/10.1186/s13012-016-0519-y

Oxman, T. E., Schulberg, H. C., Greenberg, R. L., Dietrich, A. J., Williams, J. W., Jr., Nutting, P. A., & Bruce, M. L. (2006). A fidelity measure for integrated management of depression in primary care. *Medical Care*, 44(11), 1030–1037. https://doi.org/10.1097/01.mlr.0000233683.82254.63

Palacio, G., C., Krikorian, A., Gómez-Romero, M. J., & Limonero, J. T. (2020). Resilience in caregivers: A systematic review. *The American Journal of Hospice & Palliative Care*, 37(8), 648–658. https://doi.org/10.1177/1049909119893977

Pamungkas, R. A., Chamroonsawasdi, K., & Vatanasomboon, P. (2017). A systematic review: Family support integrated with diabetes self-management among uncontrolled type II diabetes mellitus patients. *Behavioral Sciences*, *7*(3), Article 62. https://doi.org/10.3390/bs7030062

Parekh, N., Jarlenski, M., & Kelley, D. (2018). Prenatal and postpartum care disparities in a large Medicaid program. *Maternal and Child Health Journal*, *22*(3), 429–437. https://doi.org/10.1007/s10995-017-2410-0

Park, M. J., Noh, G. O., & Jung, H. S. (2019). Coping with symptoms after education for self-management of chronic diseases. *International Journal of Advanced Culture Technology*, *7*(1), 89–95.

Parmelli, E., Flodgren, G., Beyer, F., Baillie, N., Schaafsma, M. E., & Eccles, M. P. (2011). The effectiveness of strategies to change organisational culture to improve healthcare performance: A systematic review. *Implementation Science*, *6*, Article 33. https://doi.org/10.1186/1748-5908-6-33

Pasch, L. A., & Sullivan, K. T. (2017). Stress and coping in couples facing infertility. *Current Opinion in Psychology*, *13*, 131–135. https://doi.org/10.1016/j.copsyc.2016.07.004

Pascucci, D., Sassano, M., Nurchis, M. C., Cicconi, M., Acampora, A., Park, D., Morano, C., & Damiani, G. (2021). Impact of interprofessional collaboration on chronic disease management: Findings from a systematic review of clinical trial and meta-analysis. *Health Policy*, *125*(2), 191–202. https://doi.org/10.1016/j.healthpol.2020.12.006

Patel, A., Sharma, P. S. V. N., & Kumar, P. (2018). Role of mental health practitioner in infertility clinics: A review on past, present and future directions. *Journal of Human Reproductive Sciences*, *11*(3), 219–228. https://doi.org/10.4103/jhrs.JHRS_41_18

Patient Protection and Affordable Care Act, 42 U.S.C. § 18001 *et seq.* (2010).

Pavli, A., Theodoridou, M., & Maltezou, H. C. (2021). Post-COVID syndrome: Incidence, clinical spectrum, and challenges for primary healthcare professionals. *Archives of Medical Research*, *52*(6), 575–581. https://doi.org/10.1016/j.arcmed.2021.03.010

Pecukonis, E., Doyle, O., & Bliss, D. L. (2008). Reducing barriers to interprofessional training: Promoting interprofessional cultural competence. *Journal of Interprofessional Care*, *22*(4), 417–428. https://doi.org/10.1080/13561820802190442

Peek, C. J. (2006). Appealing to what matters in chronic care. *Biofeedback*, *34*(4), 141–144.

Peek, C. J. (2008). Planning care in the clinical, operational, and financial worlds. In R. Kessler & D. Stafford (Eds.), *Collaborative medicine case studies* (pp. 25–38). Springer. https://doi.org/10.1007/978-0-387-76894-6_3

Peek, C. J. (2010). Building a medical home around the patient: What it means for behavior. *Families, Systems & Health*, *28*(4), 322–333. https://doi.org/10.1037/a0022043

Peek, C. J. (2019). What is integrated behavioral health? In S. B. Gold & L. A. Green (Eds.), *Integrated behavioral health in primary care: Your patients are waiting* (pp. 11–32). Springer Cham. https://doi.org/10.1007/978-3-319-98587-9_2

Peek, C. J., Cohen, D. J., & deGruy, F. V., III. (2014). Research and evaluation in the transformation of primary care. *American Psychologist, 69*(4), 430–442. https://doi.org/10.1037/a0036223

Peek, C. J., & National Integration Academy Council. (2013, April). *Lexicon for behavioral health and primary care integration: Concepts and definitions developed by expert consensus.* Agency for Healthcare Research and Quality. https://integrationacademy.ahrq.gov/sites/default/files/2020-06/Lexicon.pdf

Péloquin, K., Brassard, A., Arpin, V., Sabourin, S., & Wright, J. (2018). Whose fault is it? Blame predicting psychological adjustment and couple satisfaction in couples seeking fertility treatment. *Journal of Psychosomatic Obstetrics and Gynaecology, 39*(1), 64–72. https://doi.org/10.1080/0167482X.2017.1289369

Pence, B. W., O'Donnell, J. K., & Gaynes, B. N. (2012). The depression treatment cascade in primary care: A public health perspective. *Current Psychiatry Reports, 14*(4), 328–335. https://doi.org/10.1007/s11920-012-0274-y

Pennebaker, J. W. (2012). *The psychology of physical symptoms.* Springer Science & Business Media.

Petrie, K. J., & Jones, A. S. K. (2019). Coping with chronic illness. In C. D. Llewellyn, S. Ayers, C. McManus, S. Newman, K. J. Petrie, T. A. Revenson, & J. Weinman (Eds.), *Cambridge handbooks in psychology. The Cambridge handbook of psychology, health and medicine* (pp. 110–114). Cambridge University Press.

Pharr, J. R. (2021). Health disparities among lesbian, gay, bisexual, transgender, and nonbinary adults 50 years old and older in the United States. *LGBT Health, 8*(7), 473–485. https://doi.org/10.1089/lgbt.2021.0009

Phillips, R. L., Jr., McCauley, L. A., & Koller, C. F. (2021). Implementing high-quality primary care: A report from the National Academies of Sciences, Engineering, and Medicine. *JAMA, 325*(24), 2437–2438. https://doi.org/10.1001/jama.2021.7430

Pietromonaco, P. R., & Collins, N. L. (2017). Interpersonal mechanisms linking close relationships to health. *American Psychologist, 72*(6), 531–542. https://doi.org/10.1037/amp0000129

Piland Springer, N., Turns, B., & Masterson, M. (2018). A systemic and contextual lens of disability: Family stress, ambiguous loss, and meaning making. In B. Nelson Goff & N. Piland Springer (Eds.), *Intellectual and developmental disabilities: A roadmap for families and professionals* (pp. 17–31). Routledge, Taylor & Francis Group. https://doi.org/10.4324/9781315562490

Pinquart, M. (2018). Parenting stress in caregivers of children with chronic physical condition—A meta-analysis. *Stress and Health, 34*(2), 197–207. https://doi.org/10.1002/smi.2780

Plaufcan, M. R., Wamboldt, F. S., & Holm, K. E. (2012). Behavioral and characterological self-blame in chronic obstructive pulmonary disease. *Journal of Psychosomatic Research, 72*(1), 78–83. https://doi.org/10.1016/j.jpsychores.2011.10.004

Poleshuck, E. L., & Woods, J. (2014). Psychologists partnering with obstetricians and gynecologists: Meeting the need for patient-centered models of women's health care delivery. *American Psychologist, 69*(4), 344–354. https://doi.org/10.1037/a0036044

Pomerantz, A., Cole, B. H., Watts, B. V., & Weeks, W. B. (2008). Improving efficiency and access to mental health care: Combining integrated care and advanced access. *General Hospital Psychiatry, 30*(6), 546–551. https://doi.org/10.1016/j.genhosppsych.2008.09.004

Pomerantz, A. S., Corson, J. A., & Detzer, M. J. (2009). The challenge of integrated care for mental health: Leaving the 50 minute hour and other sacred things. *Journal of Clinical Psychology in Medical Settings, 16*(1), 40–46. https://doi.org/10.1007/s10880-009-9147-x

Pomerantz, A., & The Primary Mental Health Care Clinic at the White River Junction VA Medical Center. (2005). 2005 APA Gold Award: Improving treatment engagement and integrated care of veterans. *Psychiatric Services, 56*(10), 1306–1308. https://doi.org/10.1176/appi.ps.56.10.1306

Pomerantz, A. S., Shiner, B., Watts, B. V., Detzer, M. J., Kutter, C., Street, B., & Scott, D. (2010). The White River model of colocated collaborative care: A platform for mental and behavioral health care in the medical home. *Families, Systems & Health, 28*(2), 114–129. https://doi.org/10.1037/a0020261

Popp, J. M., Robinson, J. L., Britner, P. A., & Blank, T. O. (2014). Parent adaptation and family functioning in relation to narratives of children with chronic illness. *Journal of Pediatric Nursing, 29*(1), 58–64. https://doi.org/10.1016/j.pedn.2013.07.004

Possemato, K., Johnson, E. M., Beehler, G. P., Shepardson, R. L., King, P., Vair, C. L., Funderburk, J. S., Maisto, S. A., & Wray, L. O. (2018). Patient outcomes associated with primary care behavioral health services: A systematic review. *General Hospital Psychiatry, 53*, 1–11. https://doi.org/10.1016/j.genhosppsych.2018.04.002

Powers, M. A., Bardsley, J. K., Cypress, M., Funnell, M. M., Harms, D., Hess-Fischl, A., Hooks, B., Isaacs, D., Mandel, E. D., Maryniuk, M. D., Norton, A., Rinker, J., Siminerio, L. M., & Uelmen, S. (2020). Diabetes self-management education and support in adults with type 2 diabetes: A consensus report of the American Diabetes Association, the Association of Diabetes Care & Education Specialists, the Academy of Nutrition and Dietetics, the American Academy of Family Physicians, the American Academy of PAs, the American Association of Nurse Practitioners, and the American Pharmacists Association. *Diabetes Care, 43*(7), 1636–1649. https://doi.org/10.2337/dci20-0023

Pratt, K., VanFossen, C., Didericksen, K., Aamar, R., & Berge, J. (2018). Medical family therapy in pediatrics. In T. Mendenhall, A. Lamson, J. Hodgson, & M. Baird. (Eds.), *Clinical methods in medical family therapy* (pp. 61–85). Springer International. https://doi.org/10.1007/978-3-319-68834-3_3

Pratt, K. J., & Sonney, J. T. (2020). Family science and family-based research in integrated and health care contexts: Future considerations for families, systems, & health. *Families, Systems & Health, 38*(1), 1–5. https://doi.org/10.1037/fsh0000477

Pratt, K. J., Van Fossen, C. A., Utržan, D. S., & Berge, J. M. (2020). Family-based prevention and intervention for child physical health conditions. In K. S. Wampler (Series Ed.) & L. M. McWey (Vol. Ed.), *The handbook of systemic family therapy: Vol. 2. Systemic family therapy with children and adolescents* (pp. 217–239). Wiley-Blackwell.

Priest, J. B., Roberson, P. N. E., & Woods, S. B. (2019). In our lives and under our skin: An investigation of specific psychological mediators linking family relationships and health using the biobehavioral family model. *Family Process, 58*(1), 79–99. https://doi.org/10.1111/famp.12357

Primary Care Collaborative. (2015, September). *Patient-centered medical home: What is the patient-centered medical home?* https://www.pcpcc.org/resource/patient-centered-medical-home-what-patient-centered-medical-home-pcmh#:~:text=The%20patient%2Dcentered%20medical%20home,the%20patient%2C%20and%20advocates%20and

Prime, H., Wade, M., & Browne, D. T. (2020). Risk and resilience in family well-being during the COVID-19 pandemic. *American Psychologist, 75*(5), 631–643. https://doi.org/10.1037/amp0000660

Prince, M., Patel, V., Saxena, S., Maj, M., Maselko, J., Phillips, M. R., & Rahman, A. (2007). No health without mental health. *The Lancet, 370*(9590), 859–877. https://doi.org/10.1016/S0140-6736(07)61238-0

Prinz, R. J., Sanders, M. R., Shapiro, C. J., Whitaker, D. J., & Lutzker, J. R. (2009). Population-based prevention of child maltreatment: The U.S. Triple P system population trial. *Prevention Science, 10*(1), 1–12. https://doi.org/10.1007/s11121-009-0123-3

Prochaska, J. O., Norcross, J. C., & DiClemente, C. C. (2013). Applying the stages of change. *Psychotherapy in Australia, 19*(2), 10–15.

Prochaska, J. O., & Velicer, W. F. (1997). The transtheoretical model of health behavior change. *American Journal of Health Promotion, 12*(1), 38–48. https://doi.org/10.4278/0890-1171-12.1.38

Prochaska, J. O., Velicer, W. F., Redding, C., Rossi, J. S., Goldstein, M., DePue, J., Greene, G. W., Rossi, S. R., Sun, X., Fava, J. L., Laforge, R., Rakowski, W., & Plummer, B. A. (2005). Stage-based expert systems to guide a population of primary care patients to quit smoking, eat healthier, prevent skin cancer, and receive regular mammograms. *Preventive Medicine, 41*(2), 406–416. https://doi.org/10.1016/j.ypmed.2004.09.050

Psihogios, A. M., Fellmeth, H., Schwartz, L. A., & Barakat, L. P. (2019). Family functioning and medical adherence across children and adolescents with chronic health conditions: A meta-analysis. *Journal of Pediatric Psychology, 44*(1), 84–97. https://doi.org/10.1093/jpepsy/jsy044

Purkey, E., Patel, R., & Phillips, S. P. (2018). Trauma-informed care: Better care for everyone. *Canadian Family Physician, 64*(3), 170–172.

Quinn, M., & Fujimoto, V. (2016). Racial and ethnic disparities in assisted reproductive technology access and outcomes. *Fertility and Sterility, 105*(5), 1119–1123. https://doi.org/10.1016/j.fertnstert.2016.03.007

Rajaei, A., & Jensen, J. F. (2020). Empowering patients in integrated behavioral health-care settings: A narrative approach to medical family therapy. *The Family Journal, 28*(1), 48–55. https://doi.org/10.1177/1066480719893958

Ramisch, J. L., & Poland, N. (2020). Systemic approaches for children, adolescents and families living with neurodevelopmental disorder. In K. S. Wampler (Series Ed.) & L. M. McWey (Volume Ed.), *The handbook of systemic family therapy: Vol. 2. Systemic family therapy with children and adolescents* (pp. 369–396). Wiley-Blackwell.

Raney, L. (2013). Integrated care: The evolving role of psychiatry in the era of health care reform. *Psychiatric Services, 64*(11), 1076–1078. https://doi.org/10.1176/appi.ps.201300311

Raney, L. E. (2015). Integrating primary care and behavioral health: The role of the psychiatrist in the collaborative care model. *The American Journal of Psychiatry, 172*(8), 721–728. https://doi.org/10.1176/appi.ajp.2015.15010017

Raney, L. E. (2017). *Integrated care: Working at the interface of primary care and behavioral health.* American Psychiatric Publishing.

Raney, L., Bergman, D., Torous, J., & Hasselberg, M. (2017). Digitally driven integrated primary care and behavioral health: How technology can expand access to effective treatment. *Current Psychiatry Reports, 19*, Article 86. https://doi.org/10.1007/s11920-017-0838-y

Raney, L. E., Lasky, G. B., & Scott, C. (Eds.). (2017). *Integrated care: A guide for effective implementation.* American Psychiatric Publishing.

Ransom, D. C. (1984). Random notes: The patient is not a dirty window. *Family Systems Medicine, 2*(2), 230–233. https://doi.org/10.1037/h0091809

Rasin-Waters, D., Abel, V., Kearney, L. K., & Zeiss, A. (2018). The integrated care team approach of the Department of Veterans Affairs (VA): Geriatric primary care. *Archives of Clinical Neuropsychology, 33*(3), 280–289. https://doi.org/10.1093/arclin/acx129

Ratzliff, A., Unützer, J., & Pascualy, M. (2014). Training psychiatrists for integrated care. In L. E. Raney (Ed.), *Integrated care: Working at the interface of primary care and behavioral health* (pp. 113–138). American Psychiatric Publishing.

Ravaldi, C., Levi, M., Angeli, E., Romeo, G., Biffino, M., Bonaiuti, R., & Vannacci, A. (2018). Stillbirth and perinatal care: Are professionals trained to address parents' needs? *Midwifery, 64*, 53–59. https://doi.org/10.1016/j.midw.2018.05.008

Rawson, J. V., & Moretz, J. (2016). Patient- and family-centered care: A primer. *Journal of the American College of Radiology, 13*(12), P1544–P1549. https://doi.org/10.1016/j.jacr.2016.09.003

Read, S. C., Carrier, M. E., Boucher, M. E., Whitley, R., Bond, S., & Zelkowitz, P. (2014). Psychosocial services for couples in infertility treatment: What do couples really want? *Patient Education and Counseling, 94*(3), 390–395. https://doi.org/10.1016/j.pec.2013.10.025

Reardon, D. C. (2018). The abortion and mental health controversy: A comprehensive literature review of common ground agreements, disagreements, actionable recommendations, and research opportunities. *SAGE Open Medicine*, *6*, Article 2050312118807624. https://doi.org/10.1177/2050312118807624

Rees, S. N., Crowe, M., & Harris, S. (2021). The lesbian, gay, bisexual and transgender communities' mental health care needs and experiences of mental health services: An integrative review of qualitative studies. *Journal of Psychiatric and Mental Health Nursing*, *28*(4), 578–589. https://doi.org/10.1111/jpm.12720

Regan, T. W., Lambert, S. D., Girgis, A., Kelly, B., Kayser, K., & Turner, J. (2012). Do couple-based interventions make a difference for couples affected by cancer?: A systematic review. *BMC Cancer*, *12*, 1–14.

Regier, D. A., Goldberg, I. D., & Taube, C. A. (1978). The de facto US mental health services system: A public health perspective. *Archives of General Psychiatry*, *35*(6), 685–693. https://doi.org/10.1001/archpsyc.1978.01770300027002

Reising, V., Diegel-Vacek, L., Dadabo, L., Martinez, M., Moore, K., & Corbridge, S. (2022). Closing the gap: Collaborative care addresses social determinants of health. *The Nurse Practitioner*, *47*(4), 41–47. https://doi.org/10.1097/01.NPR.0000822572.45824.3f

Reiter, J. T., Dobmeyer, A. C., & Hunter, C. L. (2018). The primary care behavioral health (PCBH) model: An overview and operational definition. *Journal of Clinical Psychology in Medical Settings*, *25*(2), 109–126. https://doi.org/10.1007/s10880-017-9531-x

Restauri, N., & Sheridan, A. D. (2020). Burnout and posttraumatic stress disorder in the coronavirus disease 2019 (COVID-19) pandemic: Intersection, impact, and interventions. *Journal of the American College of Radiology*, *17*(7), 921–926. https://doi.org/10.1016/j.jacr.2020.05.021

Reuben, D. B., Levy-Storms, L., Yee, M. N., Lee, M., Cole, K., Waite, M., Nichols, L., & Frank, J. C. (2004). Disciplinary split: A threat to geriatrics interdisciplinary team training. *Journal of the American Geriatrics Society*, *52*(6), 1000–1006. https://doi.org/10.1111/j.1532-5415.2004.52272.x

Richardson, L. P., McCarty, C. A., Radovic, A., & Suleiman, A. B. (2017). Research in the integration of behavioral health for adolescents and young adults in primary care settings: A systematic review. *The Journal of Adolescent Health*, *60*(3), 261–269. https://doi.org/10.1016/j.jadohealth.2016.11.013

Richman, E. L., Lombardi, B. M., & Zerden, L. D. (2020). Mapping colocation: Using national provider identified data to assess primary care and behavioral health colocation. *Families, Systems & Health*, *38*(1), 16–23. https://doi.org/10.1037/fsh0000465

Rizq, R., Hewey, M., Salvo, L., Spencer, M., Varnaseri, H., & Whitfield, J. (2010). Reflective voices: Primary care mental health workers' experiences in training and practice. *Primary Health Care Research and Development*, *11*(1), 72–86. https://doi.org/10.1017/S1463423609990375

Roberts, A. L., Gilman, S. E., Breslau, J., Breslau, N., & Koenen, K. C. (2011). Race/ethnic differences in exposure to traumatic events, development of post-traumatic stress disorder, and treatment-seeking for post-traumatic stress disorder in the United States. *Psychological Medicine, 41*(1), 71–83. https://doi.org/10.1017/S0033291710000401

Robertson, L., Akré, E. R., & Gonzales, G. (2021). Mental health disparities at the intersections of gender identity, race, and ethnicity. *LGBT Health, 8*(8), 526–535. https://doi.org/10.1089/lgbt.2020.0429

Robinson, C. A. (2017). Families living well with chronic illness: The healing process of moving on. *Qualitative Health Research, 27*(4), 447–461. https://doi.org/10.1177/1049732316675590

Robinson, P. J., & Reiter, J. T. (2016). *Behavioral consultation and primary care: A guide to integrating services* (2nd ed.). Springer. https://doi.org/10.1007/978-3-319-13954-8

Robinson, W. D., Jones, A. C., Felix, D. S., & McPhee, D. P. (2020). Systemic family therapy in medical settings. In K. S. Wampler & L. M. McWey (Eds.), *The handbook of systemic family therapy* (Vol. 1, pp. 659–681). Wiley-Blackwell.

Robinson-Smith, G., Harmer, C., Sheeran, R., & Bellino Vallo, E. (2016). Couples' coping after stroke—A pilot intervention study. *Rehabilitation Nursing, 41*(4), 218–229. https://doi.org/10.1002/rnj.213

Rocca, C. H., Samari, G., Foster, D. G., Gould, H., & Kimport, K. (2020). Emotions and decision rightness over five years following an abortion: An examination of decision difficulty and abortion stigma. *Social Science & Medicine, 248*, 112704. https://doi.org/10.1016/j.socscimed.2019.112704

Roderick, S. S., Burdette, N., Hurwitz, D., & Yeracaris, P. (2017). Integrated behavioral health practice facilitation in patient centered medical homes: A promising application. *Families, Systems & Health, 35*(2), 227–237. https://doi.org/10.1037/fsh0000273

Rodriguez, H. P., Meredith, L. S., Hamilton, A. B., Yano, E. M., & Rubenstein, L. V. (2015). Huddle up!: The adoption and use of structured team communication for VA medical home implementation. *Health Care Management Review, 40*(4), 286–299. https://doi.org/10.1097/HMR.0000000000000036

Rodríguez, V. M., Corona, R., Bodurtha, J. N., & Quillin, J. M. (2016). Family ties: The role of family context in family health history communication about cancer. *Journal of Health Communication, 21*(3), 346–355. https://doi.org/10.1080/10810730.2015.1080328

Rogers, E. M. (1995). *Diffusion of innovations* (4th ed.). Free Press.

Rogers, E. M., Medina, U. E., Rivera, M. A., & Wiley, C. J. (2005). Complex adaptive systems and the diffusion of innovations. *The Innovation Journal, 10*(3), 1–26.

Rolland, J. (1994). *Families, illness, and disability: An integrative treatment model.* Basic Books.

Rolland, J. S. (2018). *Helping couples and families navigate illness and disability: An integrated approach.* Guilford Press.

Rook, L. (2013). Mental models: A robust definition. *The Learning Organization, 20*(1), 38–47. https://doi.org/10.1108/09696471311288519

Rosenberg, T., Fogarty, C. T., Privitera, M., & McDaniel, S. H. (2017). Team-based integrated primary care. In R. E. Feinstein, J. V. Connelly, & M. S. Feinstein

(Eds.), *Integrating behavioral health and primary care* (pp. 46–64). Oxford University Press.

Rosland, A. M., Heisler, M., & Piette, J. D. (2012). The impact of family behaviors and communication patterns on chronic illness outcomes: A systematic review. *Journal of Behavioral Medicine, 35*(2), 221–239. https://doi.org/10.1007/s10865-011-9354-4

Rosland, A. M., & Piette, J. D. (2010). Emerging models for mobilizing family support for chronic disease management: A structured review. *Chronic Illness, 6*(1), 7–21. https://doi.org/10.1177/1742395309352254

Rossen, L. M., Ahrens, K. A., & Branum, A. M. (2018). Trends in risk of pregnancy loss among US women, 1990–2011. *Paediatric and Perinatal Epidemiology, 32*(1), 19–29. https://doi.org/10.1111/ppe.12417

Rossom, R. C., Solberg, L. I., Magnan, S., Crain, A. L., Beck, A., Coleman, K. J., Katzelnick, D., Williams, M. D., Neely, C., Ohnsorg, K., Whitebird, R., Brandenfels, E., Pollock, B., Ferguson, R., Williams, S., & Unützer, J. (2017). Impact of a national collaborative care initiative for patients with depression and diabetes or cardiovascular disease. *Focus—American Psychiatric Publishing, 15*(3), 324–332. https://doi.org/10.1176/appi.focus.150304

Rozemond, M. (1998). *Descartes's dualism.* Harvard University Press. https://doi.org/10.4159/9780674042926

Rozensky, R. H. (2012). Psychology in academic health centers: A true healthcare home. *Journal of Clinical Psychology in Medical Settings, 19*(4), 353–363. https://doi.org/10.1007/s10880-012-9312-5

Rozensky, R. H., Grus, C. L., Goodie, J. L., Bonin, L., Carpenter, B. D., Miller, B. F., Ross, K. M., Rybarczyk, B. D., Stewart, A., & McDaniel, S. H. (2018). A curriculum for an interprofessional seminar on integrated primary care: Developing competencies for interprofessional collaborative practice. *Journal of Allied Health, 47*(3), e61–e66.

Ruddy, N. B., Borresen, D. A., & Gunn, W. B., Jr. (2008). *The collaborative psychotherapist: Creating reciprocal relationships with medical professionals.* American Psychological Association. https://doi.org/10.1037/11754-000

Rugkåsa, J., Tveit, O. G., Berteig, J., Hussain, A., & Ruud, T. (2020). Collaborative care for mental health: A qualitative study of the experiences of patients and health professionals. *BMC Health Services Research, 20,* Article 844. https://doi.org/10.1186/s12913-020-05691-8

Runyan, C. N., Carter-Henry, S., & Ogbeide, S. (2018). Ethical challenges unique to the primary care behavioral health (PCBH) model. *Journal of Clinical Psychology in Medical Settings, 25,* 224–236.

Russell, L. B., Ibuka, Y., & Carr, D. (2008). How much time do patients spend on outpatient visits?: The American time use survey. *Patient, 1*(3), 211–222. https://doi.org/10.2165/1312067-200801030-00008

Ryan, J., Doty, M. M., Hamel, L., Norton, M., Abrams, M. K., & Brodie, M. (2015, August 15). *Primary care providers' views of recent trends in health care delivery and payment: Findings from the Commonwealth Fund/Kaiser Family*

Foundation 2015 National Survey of Primary Care Providers. https://doi.org/ 10.26099/3qrf-gb06

Ryan, P., & Sawin, K. J. (2009). The individual and family self-management theory: Background and perspectives on context, process, and outcomes. *Nursing Outlook, 57*(4), 217–225.e6. https://doi.org/10.1016/j.outlook.2008.10.004

Salas, E., Reyes, D. L., & McDaniel, S. H. (2018). The science of teamwork: Progress, reflections, and the road ahead. *American Psychologist, 73*(4), 593–600. https://doi.org/10.1037/amp0000334

Salas, E., Shuffler, M. L., Thayer, A. L., Bedwell, W. L., & Lazzara, E. H. (2015). Understanding and improving teamwork in organizations: A scientifically based practical guide. *Human Resource Management, 54*(4), 599–622. https:// doi.org/10.1002/hrm.21628

Salas, E., Sims, D. E., & Burke, C. S. (2005). Is there a "big five" in teamwork? *Small Group Research, 36*(5), 555–599. https://doi.org/10.1177/1046496405277134

Salmi, L., Blease, C., Hägglund, M., Walker, J., & DesRoches, C. M. (2021). US policy requires immediate release of records to patients. *BMJ, 372*, n426. https://doi.org/10.1136/bmj.n426

Samsel, C., Ribeiro, M., Ibeziako, P., & DeMaso, D. R. (2017). Integrated behavioral health care in pediatric subspecialty clinics. *Child and Adolescent Psychiatric Clinics, 26*(4), 785–794. https://doi.org/10.1016/j.chc.2017.06.004

Sanchez, K. (2017). Collaborative care in real-world settings: Barriers and opportunities for sustainability. *Patient Preference and Adherence, 11*, 71–74. https://doi.org/10.2147/PPA.S120070

Sanders, J., & Blaylock, R. (2021). "Anxious and traumatised": Users' experiences of maternity care in the UK during the COVID-19 pandemic. *Midwifery, 102*, 103069. https://doi.org/10.1016/j.midw.2021.103069

Sandoval, B. E., Bell, J., Khatri, P., & Robinson, P. J. (2018). Toward a unified integration approach: Uniting diverse primary care strategies under the primary care behavioral health (PCBH) model. *Journal of Clinical Psychology in Medical Settings, 25*(2), 187–196.

Santoro, N., Epperson, C. N., & Mathews, S. B. (2015). Menopausal symptoms and their management. *Endocrinology and Metabolism Clinics, 44*(3), 497–515. https://doi.org/10.1016/j.ecl.2015.05.001

Sav, A., King, M. A., Whitty, J. A., Kendall, E., McMillan, S. S., Kelly, F., Hunter, B., & Wheeler, A. J. (2015). Burden of treatment for chronic illness: A concept analysis and review of the literature. *Health Expectations, 18*(3), 312–324. https:// doi.org/10.1111/hex.12046

Saxon, V., Mukherjee, D., & Thomas, D. (2018). Behavioral health crisis stabilization centers: A new normal. *Journal of Mental Health and Clinical Psychology, 2*(3), 23–26. https://doi.org/10.29245/2578-2959/2018/3.1124

Scharf, D. M., Eberhart, N. K., Hackbarth, N. S., Horvitz-Lennon, M., Beckman, R., Han, B., Lovejoy, S. L., Pincus, H. A., & Burnam, M. A. (2014). *Evaluation of the SAMHSA primary and behavioral health care integration (PBHCI) grant program: Final report (Task 13)*. RAND Corporation. https://www.jstor.org/stable/10.7249/j.ctt6wq97z

Schiebinger, L., & Stefanick, M. L. (2016). Gender matters in biological research and medical practice. *Journal of the American College of Cardiology, 67*(2), 136–138. https://doi.org/10.1016/j.jacc.2015.11.029

Schneider, E. C., Sarnak, D. O., Squires, D., Shah, A., & Doty, M. M. (2017, July 14). *Mirror, mirror 2017: International comparison reflects flaws and opportunities for better U.S. healthcare*. The Commonwealth Fund. http://www.hcfat.org/Mirror_Mirror_2017_International_Comparison.pdf

Schroeder, C. S. (1979). Psychologists in a private pediatric practice. *Journal of Pediatric Psychology, 4*(1), 5–18. https://doi.org/10.1093/jpepsy/4.1.5

Schroeder, C. S. (2004). A collaborative practice in primary care. In B. W. Wildman & T. Stancin (Eds.), *Treating children's psychosocial problems in primary care* (pp. 1–32). Information Age Publishing.

Schulz, R., Beach, S. R., Czaja, S. J., Martire, L. M., & Monin, J. K. (2020). Family caregiving for older adults. *Annual Review of Psychology, 71*(1), 635–659. https://doi.org/10.1146/annurev-psych-010419-050754

Scott, V. C., Kenworthy, T., Godly-Reynolds, E., Bastien, G., Scaccia, J., McMickens, C., Rachel, S., Cooper, S., Wrenn, G., & Wandersman, A. (2017). The Readiness for Integrated Care Questionnaire (RICQ): An instrument to assess readiness to integrate behavioral health and primary care. *American Journal of Orthopsychiatry, 87*(5), 520–530. https://doi.org/10.1037/ort0000270

Sederer, L. I. (2009). Science to practice: Making what we know what we actually do. *Schizophrenia Bulletin, 35*(4), 714–718. https://doi.org/10.1093/schbul/sbp040

Sekoni, A. O., Gale, N. K., Manga-Atangana, B., Bhadhuri, A., & Jolly, K. (2017). The effects of educational curricula and training on LGBT-specific health issues for healthcare students and professionals: A mixed-method systematic review. *Journal of the International AIDS Society, 20*(1), Article 21624. https://doi.org/10.7448/IAS.20.1.21624

Selladurai, R., Hobson, C., Selladurai, R. I., & Greer, A. (Eds.). (2020). *Evaluating challenges and opportunities for healthcare reform*. IGI Global. https://doi.org/10.4018/978-1-7998-2949-2

Serrano, N., Cordes, C., Cubic, B., & Daub, S. (2018). The state and future of the primary care behavioral health model of service delivery workforce. *Journal of Clinical Psychology in Medical Settings, 25*(2), 157–168. https://doi.org/10.1007/s10880-017-9491-1

Shanafelt, T. D., West, C. P., Sinsky, C., Trockel, M., Tutty, M., Satele, D. V., Carlasare, L. E., & Dyrbye, L. N. (2019). Changes in burnout and satisfaction with work-life integration in physicians and the general US working population between 2011 and 2017. *Mayo Clinic Proceedings, 94*(9), 1681–1694. https://doi.org/10.1016/j.mayocp.2018.10.023

Shaw, E. K., Howard, J., Etz, R. S., Hudson, S. V., & Crabtree, B. F. (2012). How team-based reflection affects quality improvement implementation:

A qualitative study. *Quality Management in Health Care, 21*(2), 104–113. https://doi.org/10.1097/QMH.0b013e31824d4984

Shekelle, P. G., & Begashaw, M. (2021). *What are the effects of different team-based primary care structures on the quadruple aim of care? A rapid review.* U.S. Department of Veterans Affairs, Veterans Health Administration, Health Services Research & Development.

Sher, T., Braun, L., Domas, A., Bellg, A., Baucom, D. H., & Houle, T. T. (2014). The partners for life program: A couples approach to cardiac risk reduction. *Family Process, 53*(1), 131–149. https://doi.org/10.1111/famp.12061

Sheridan, B., Chien, A. T., Peters, A. S., Rosenthal, M. B., Brooks, J. V., & Singer, S. J. (2018). Team-based primary care: The medical assistant perspective. *Health Care Management Review, 43*(2), 115–125. https://doi.org/10.1097/HMR.0000000000000136

Shields, C. G., Finley, M. A., Chawla, N., & Meadors, W. P. (2012). Couple and family interventions in health problems. *Journal of Marital and Family Therapy, 38*(1), 265–280. https://doi.org/10.1111/j.1752-0606.2011.00269.x

Shin, D. W., Shin, J., Kim, S. Y., Yang, H. K., Cho, J., Youm, J. H., Choi, G. S., Hong, N. S., Cho, B., & Park, J. H. (2016). Family avoidance of communication about cancer: A dyadic examination. *Cancer Research and Treatment, 48*(1), 384–392. https://doi.org/10.4143/crt.2014.280

Sia, C., Tonniges, T. F., Osterhus, E., & Taba, S. (2004). History of the medical home concept. *Pediatrics, 113*(Suppl. 4), 1473–1478. https://doi.org/10.1542/peds.113.S4.1473

Siantz, E., Redline, B., & Henwood, B. (2021). Practice facilitation in integrated behavioral health and primary care settings: A scoping review. *The Journal of Behavioral Health Services & Research, 48*(1), 133–155. https://doi.org/10.1007/s11414-020-09709-1

Sikka, R., Morath, J. M., & Leape, L. (2015). The Quadruple Aim: Care, health, cost and meaning in work. *BMJ Quality & Safety, 24*(10), 608–610. https://doi.org/10.1136/bmjqs-2015-004160

Simmons, M. M., Gabrielian, S., Byrne, T., McCullough, M. B., Smith, J. L., Taylor, T. J., O'Toole, T. P., Kane, V., Yakovchenko, V., McInnes, D. K., & Smelson, D. A. (2017). A Hybrid III stepped wedge cluster randomized trial testing and implementation strategy to facilitate the use of an evidence-based practice in VA Homeless Primary Care Treatment Programs. *Implementation Science, 12*, Article 46. https://doi.org/10.1186/s13012-017-0563-2

Simon, N. M. (2013). Treating complicated grief. *JAMA, 310*(4), 416–423. https://doi.org/10.1001/jama.2013.8614

Simonovich, S. D., Nidey, N. L., Gavin, A. R., Piñeros-Leaño, M., Hsieh, W. J., Sbrilli, M. D., Ables-Torres, L. A., Huang, H., Ryckman, K., & Tabb, K. M. (2021). Meta-analysis of antenatal depression and adverse birth outcomes in US populations, 2010–20: Study is a meta-analysis of antenatal depression and adverse birth outcomes in the US, 2010–20. *Health Affairs (Project Hope)*, *40*(10), 1560–1565. https://doi.org/10.1377/hlthaff.2021.00801

Sinsky, C. A., Jerzak, J. T., & Hopkins, K. D. (2021). Telemedicine and team-based care: The perils and the promise. *Mayo Clinic Proceedings*, *96*(2), 429–437. https://doi.org/10.1016/j.mayocp.2020.11.020

Sinsky, C. A., Willard-Grace, R., Schutzbank, A. M., Sinsky, T. A., Margolius, D., & Bodenheimer, T. (2013). In search of joy in practice: A report of 23 high-functioning primary care practices. *Annals of Family Medicine*, *11*(3), 272–278. https://doi.org/10.1370/afm.1531

Smith, E. E., Rome, L. P., & Freedheim, D. K. (1967). The clinical psychologist in the pediatric office. *The Journal of Pediatrics*, *71*(1), 48–51. https://doi.org/10.1016/S0022-3476(67)80229-4

Smith, J. D., Berkel, C., Jordan, N., Atkins, D. C., Narayanan, S. S., Gallo, C., Grimm, K. J., Dishion, T. J., Mauricio, A. M., Rudo-Stern, J., Meachum, M. K., Winslow, E., & Bruening, M. M. (2018). An individually tailored family-centered intervention for pediatric obesity in primary care: Study protocol of a randomized type II hybrid effectiveness-implementation trial (Raising Healthy Children study). *Implementation Science*, *13*, Article 11. https://doi.org/10.1186/s13012-017-0697-2

Smith, J. D., Fu, E., & Kobayashi, M. A. (2020). Prevention and management of child-hood obesity and its psychological and health comorbidities. *Annual Review of Clinical Psychology*, *16*(1), 351–378. https://doi.org/10.1146/annurev-clinpsy-100219-060201

Smith, J. D., & Polaha, J. (2017). Using implementation science to guide the integration of evidence-based family interventions into primary care. *Families, Systems & Health*, *35*(2), 125–135. https://doi.org/10.1037/fsh0000252

Sockalingam, S., Arena, A., Serhal, E., Mohri, L., Alloo, J., & Crawford, A. (2018). Building provincial mental health capacity in primary care: An evaluation of a Project ECHO mental health program. *Academic Psychiatry*, *42*(4), 451–457. https://doi.org/10.1007/s40596-017-0735-z

Sockalingam, S., Clarkin, C., Serhal, E., Pereira, C., & Crawford, A. (2020). Responding to health care professionals' mental health needs during COVID-19 through the rapid implementation of Project ECHO. *The Journal of Continuing Education in the Health Professions*, *40*(3), 211–214. https://doi.org/10.1097/CEH.0000000000000311

Solberg, L. I., Crain, A. L., Jaeckels, N., Ohnsorg, K. A., Margolis, K. L., Beck, A., Whitebird, R. R., Rossom, R. C., Crabtree, B. F., & Van de Ven, A. H. (2013). The DIAMOND initiative: Implementing collaborative care for depression in 75 primary care clinics. *Implementation Science*, *8*, Article 135. https://doi.org/10.1186/1748-5908-8-135

Sommers, B. D., Gawande, A. A., & Baicker, K. (2017). Health insurance cover-age and health—What the recent evidence tells us. *The New England Journal of Medicine*, *377*(6), 586–593. https://doi.org/10.1056/NEJMsb1706645

Southam-Gerow, M. A., & Prinstein, M. J. (2014). Evidence base updates: The evolution of the evaluation of psychological treatments for children and adolescents. *Journal of Clinical Child and Adolescent Psychology, 43*(1), 1–6. https://doi.org/10.1080/15374416.2013.855128

Spain, D., Sin, J., Paliokosta, E., Furuta, M., Prunty, J. E., Chalder, T., Murphy, D. G., & Happé Francesca, G. (2017). Family therapy for autism spectrum disorders. *Cochrane Database of Systematic Reviews, 2017*(5), Article CD011894. https://doi.org/10.1002/14651858.CD011894.pub2

Speice, J., & McDaniel, S. H. (2015). Training the medical family therapist in an integrated care setting. In K. Jordan (Ed.), *Couple, marriage, and family therapy supervision* (pp. 371–390). Springer.

Springer, N. P., Turns, B., & Masterson, M. (2017). A systemic and contextual lens of disability: Family stress, ambiguous loss, and meaning making. In B. Nelson Goff & N. Piland Springer (Eds.), *Intellectual and developmental disabilities: A roadmap for families and professionals* (pp. 17–31). Routledge.

Stancin, T., & Perrin, E. C. (2014). Psychologists and pediatricians: Opportunities for collaboration in primary care. *American Psychologist, 69*(4), 332–343. https://doi.org/10.1037/a0036046

Stange, K. C., Nutting, P. A., Miller, W. L., Jaén, C. R., Crabtree, B. F., Flocke, S. A., & Gill, J. M. (2010). Defining and measuring the patient-centered medical home. *Journal of General Internal Medicine, 25*(6), 601–612. https://doi.org/10.1007/s11606-010-1291-3

Steinbrecher, N., Koerber, S., Frieser, D., & Hiller, W. (2011). The prevalence of medically unexplained symptoms in primary care. *Psychosomatics, 52*(3), 263–271. https://doi.org/10.1016/j.psym.2011.01.007

Stephens, K. A., Van Eeghen, C., Mollis, B., Au, M., Brennhofer, S. A., Martin, M., & Kessler, R. (2020). Defining and measuring core processes and structures in integrated behavioral health in primary care: A cross-model framework. *Translational behavioral medicine, 10*(3), 527–538.

Stevens, G. W. (2013). Toward a process-based approach of conceptualizing change readiness. *The Journal of Applied Behavioral Science, 49*(3), 333–360. https://doi.org/10.1177/0021886313475479

Stewart, D. E., & Yuen, T. (2011). A systematic review of resilience in the physically ill. *Psychosomatics, 52*(3), 199–209. https://doi.org/10.1016/j.psym.2011.01.036

St. George, S. M. S., Kobayashi, M. A., Noriega Esquives, B. S., Ocasio, M. A., Wagstaff, R. G., & Dorcius, D. P. (2022). Pediatric obesity prevention and treatment among Hispanics: A systematic review and meta-analysis. *American Journal of Preventive Medicine, 62*(3), 438–449. https://doi.org/10.1016/j.amepre.2021.10.003

Striepe, M. I., & Coons, H. L. (2002). Women's health in primary care: Interdisciplinary interventions. *Families, Systems & Health, 20*(3), 237–251. https://doi.org/10.1037/h0089578

Stroh, D. P. (2015). *Systems thinking for social change: A practical guide to solving complex problems, avoiding unintended consequences, and achieving lasting results*. Chelsea Green Publishing.

Sturhahn, J. S., Buck, K., & Heru, A. M. (2017). Best practice for family-centered health care: A three step model. In R. E. Feinstein, J. V. Connelly, & M. S. Feinstein (Eds.), *Integrating behavioral health and primary care* (pp. 514–526). Oxford University Press.

Sturmberg, J. P. (2018). Health system redesign. *How to make health care person-centered, equitable, and sustainable*. Springer. https://doi.org/10.1007/978-3-319-64605-3

Suleman, A., Mootz, J. J., Feliciano, P., Nicholson, T., O'Grady, M. A., Wall, M., Mandell, D. S., Stockton, M., Teodoro, E., Anube, A., Novela, A., Mocumbi, A. O., Gouveia, L., & Wainberg, M. L. (2021). Scale-up study protocol of the implementation of a mobile health SBIRT approach for alcohol use reduction in Mozambique. *Psychiatric Services, 72*(10), 1199–1208. https://doi.org/10.1176/appi.ps.202000086

Sulmasy, D. P. (2009). Spirituality, religion, and clinical care. *Chest, 135*(6), 1634–1642. https://doi.org/10.1378/chest.08-2241

Sunderji, N., Waddell, A., Gupta, M., Soklaridis, S., & Steinberg, R. (2016). An expert consensus on core competencies in integrated care for psychiatrists. *General Hospital Psychiatry, 41*, 45–52. https://doi.org/10.1016/j.genhosppsych.2016.05.003

Sundquist, J., Li, X., Johansson, S. E., & Sundquist, K. (2005). Depression as a predictor of hospitalization due to coronary heart disease. *American Journal of Preventive Medicine, 29*(5), 428–433. https://doi.org/10.1016/j.amepre.2005.08.002

Sung-Chen, P., Sung, Y. W., Zhao, X., & Brownson, R. C. (2013). Family-based models for childhood-obesity intervention: A systematic review of randomized controlled trials. *Obesity Reviews, 14*(4), 265–278. https://doi.org/10.1111/obr.12000

Swartz, K., & Collins, L. G. (2019). Caregiver care. *American Family Physician, 99*(11), 699–706.

Swavely, D., O'Gurek, D. T., Whyte, V., Schieber, A., Yu, D., Tien, A. Y., & Freeman, S. L. (2020). Primary care practice redesign: Challenges in improving behavioral health care for a vulnerable patient population. *American Journal of Medical Quality, 35*(2), 101–109. https://doi.org/10.1177/1062860619855136

Sweeney, J. C., Danaher, T. S., & McColl-Kennedy, J. R. (2015). Customer effort in value cocreation activities: Improving quality of life and behavioral intentions of health care customers. *Journal of Service Research, 18*(3), 318–335. https://doi.org/10.1177/1094670515572128

Sycz, L., Kreher, D., & Garroway, A. (2021). *Caring for patients with a sexual trauma history: A mixed methods preliminary needs assessment of OB/GYN clinicians* [Unpublished manuscript]. Department of Obstetrics and Gynecology and Psychiatry, University of Rochester School of Medicine and Dentistry.

Szafran, O., Torti, J. M. I., Kennett, S. L., & Bell, N. R. (2018). Family physicians' perspectives on interprofessional teamwork: Findings from a qualitative study. *Journal of Interprofessional Care, 32*(2), 169–177. https://doi.org/10.1080/13561820.2017.1395828

Tai, D. B. G., Shah, A., Doubeni, C. A., Sia, I. G., & Wieland, M. L. (2021). The disproportionate impact of COVID-19 on racial and ethnic minorities in the United States. *Clinical Infectious Diseases, 72*(4), 703–706. https://doi.org/10.1093/cid/ciaa815

Talmon, M. (2012). When less is more: Lessons from 25 years of attempting to maximize the effect of each (and often only) therapeutic encounter. *Australian and New Zealand Journal of Family Therapy, 33*(1), 6–14. https://doi.org/10.1017/aft.2012.2

Tannenbaum, S. I., & Cerasoli, C. P. (2013). Do team and individual debriefs enhance performance? A meta-analysis. *Human Factors, 55*(1), 231–245. https://doi.org/10.1177/0018720812448394

Tannenbaum, S., & Salas, E. (2020). *Teams that work: The seven drivers of team effectiveness.* Oxford University Press. https://doi.org/10.1093/oso/9780190056964.001.0001

Tatz, S. (2019). Should we minister to the lonely? *Australian Medicine, 31*(2), 16–17.

Tedstone Doherty, D., & Kartalova-O'Doherty, Y. (2010). Gender and self-reported mental health problems: Predictors of help seeking from a general practitioner. *British Journal of Health Psychology, 15*(1), 213–228. https://doi.org/10.1348/135910709X457423

Thompson, M., & McCracken, L. M. (2011). Acceptance and related processes in adjustment to chronic pain. *Current Pain and Headache Reports, 15*(2), 144–151. https://doi.org/10.1007/s11916-010-0170-2

Thota, A. B., Sipe, T. A., Byard, G. J., Zometa, C. S., Hahn, R. A., McKnight-Eily, L. R., Chapman, D. P., Abraido-Lanza, A. F., Pearson, J. L., Anderson, C. W., Gelenberg, A. J., Hennessy, K. D., Duffy, F. F., Vernon-Smiley, M. E., Nease, D. E. J., Jr., Williams, S. P., & the Community Preventive Services Task Force. (2012). Collaborative care to improve the management of depressive disorders: A community guide systematic review and meta-analysis. *American Journal of Preventive Medicine, 42*(5), 525–538. https://doi.org/10.1016/j.amepre.2012.01.019

Toledano-Toledano, F., & Domínguez-Guedea, M. T. (2019). Psychosocial factors related with caregiver burden among families of children with chronic conditions. *BioPsychoSocial Medicine, 13*, Article 6. https://doi.org/10.1186/s13030-019-0147-2

Torrence, N. D., Mueller, A. E., Ilem, A. A., Renn, B. N., DeSantis, B., & Segal, D. L. (2014). Medical provider attitudes about behavioral health consultants in integrated primary care: A preliminary study. *Families, Systems & Health, 32*(4), 426–432. https://doi.org/10.1037/fsh0000078

Tosone, C. (Ed.). (2020). *Shared trauma, shared resilience during a pandemic: Social work in the time of COVID-19*. Springer Nature.

Traa, M. J., De Vries, J., Bodenmann, G., & Den Oudsten, B. L. (2015). Dyadic coping and relationship functioning in couples coping with cancer: A systematic review. *British Journal of Health Psychology, 20*(1), 85–114. https://doi.org/10.1111/bjhp.12094

Trad, N. K., Wharam, J. F., & Druss, B. (2020). Addressing loneliness in the era of COVID-19. *JAMA Health Forum, 1*(6), e200631. https://doi.org/10.1001/jamahealthforum.2020.0631

Tramonti, F., Bonfiglio, L., Bongioanni, P., Belviso, C., Fanciullacci, C., Rossi, B., Chisari, C., & Carboncini, M. C. (2019). Caregiver burden and family functioning in different neurological diseases. *Psychology, Health and Medicine, 24*(1), 27–34. https://doi.org/10.1080/13548506.2018.1510131

Treanor, C. J., Santin, O., Prue, G., Coleman, H., Cardwell, C. R., O'Halloran, P., & Donnelly, M. (2019). Psychosocial interventions for informal caregivers of people living with cancer. *Cochrane Database of Systematic Reviews, 2019*(6), Article CD009912. https://doi.org/10.1002/14651858.CD009912.pub2

Turgoose, D., Ashwick, R., & Murphy, D. (2018). Systematic review of lessons learned from delivering tele-therapy to veterans with post-traumatic stress disorder. *Journal of Telemedicine and Telecare, 24*(9), 575–585. https://doi.org/10.1177/1357633X17730443

Twomey, C., O'Reilly, G., & Byrne, M. (2015). Effectiveness of cognitive behavioural therapy for anxiety and depression in primary care: A meta-analysis. *Family Practice, 32*(1), 3–15. https://doi.org/10.1093/fampra/cmu060

Tyler, E. T., Hulkower, R. L., & Kaminski, J. W. (2017, March). *Behavioral health integration in pediatric primary care*. Milbank Memorial Fund.

Unützer, J. (2014). Which flavor of integrated care? *Psychiatric News, 45*(20), 8.

Unützer, J. (2016). All hands on deck. *Psychiatric News, 51*(5), 22–23. https://doi.org/10.1176/appi.pn.2016.3a28

Unützer, J., Katon, W., Callahan, C. M., Williams, J. W., Jr., Hunkeler, E., Harpole, L., Hoffing, M., Della Penna, R. D., Noël, P. H., Lin, E. H. B., Areán, P. A., Hegel, M. T., Tang, L., Belin, T. R., Oishi, S., & Langston, C. (2002). Collaborative care management of late-life depression in the primary care setting: A randomized controlled trial. *JAMA, 288*(22), 2836–2845. https://doi.org/10.1001/jama.288.22.2836

U.S. Senate Committee on Finance. (2022). *Mental health care in the United States: The case for government action*. https://www.finance.senate.gov/imo/media/doc/SFC%20Mental%20Health%20Report%20March%202022.pdf

Ussher, J. M. (2013). Diagnosing difficult women and pathologising femininity: Gender bias in psychiatric nosology. *Feminism & Psychology, 23*(1), 63–69. https://doi.org/10.1177/0959353512467968

Usuba, K., Li, A. K. C., & Nowrouzi-Kia, B. (2019). Trend of the burden of chronic illnesses: Using the Canadian Community Health Survey. *Public Health, 177*, 10–18. https://doi.org/10.1016/j.puhe.2019.07.019

Van Fossen, C. A., Wexler, R., Purtell, K. McMaster Family Assessment Tool M., Slesnick, N., Taylor, C., & Pratt, K. J. (2022). Family functioning screening, referral, and behavioral health utilization in a family medicine setting. *Families, Systems & Health, 40*(1), 21–34. https://doi.org/10.1037/fsh0000652

Van Hoof, T. J., Harrison, L. G., Miller, N. E., Pappas, M. S., & Fischer, M. A. (2015). Characteristics of academic detailing: Results of a literature review. *American Health & Drug Benefits, 8*(8), 414–422.

Van Houtven, C. H., Hastings, S. N., & Colón-Emeric, C. (2019). A path to high-quality team-based care for people with serious illness. *Health Affairs (Project Hope), 38*(6), 934–940. https://doi.org/10.1377/hlthaff.2018.05486

Van Schoors, M., Caes, L., Knoble, N. B., Goubert, L., Verhofstadt, L. L., & Alderfer, M. A. (2017). Systematic review: Associations between family functioning and child adjustment after pediatric cancer diagnosis: A meta-analysis. *Journal of Pediatric Psychology, 42*(1), 6–18.

Varker, T., Brand, R. M., Ward, J., Terhaag, S., & Phelps, A. (2019). Efficacy of synchronous telepsychology interventions for people with anxiety, depression, posttraumatic stress disorder, and adjustment disorder: A rapid evidence assessment. *Psychological Services, 16*(4), 621–635. https://doi.org/10.1037/ser0000239

Varkey, P., Horne, A., & Bennet, K. E. (2008). Innovation in health care: A primer. *American Journal of Medical Quality, 23*(5), 382–388. https://doi.org/10.1177/1062860608317695

Vickers, K. S., Ridgeway, J. L., Hathaway, J. C., Egginton, J. S., Kaderlik, A. B., & Katzelnick, D. J. (2013). Integration of mental health resources in a primary care setting leads to increased provider satisfaction and patient access. *General Hospital Psychiatry, 35*(5), 461–467. https://doi.org/10.1016/j.genhosppsych.2013.06.011

Vogel, M. E., Kirkpatrick, H. A., Collings, A. S., Cederna-Meko, C. L., & Grey, M. J. (2012). Integrated care: Maturing the relationship between psychology and primary care. *Professional Psychology, Research and Practice, 43*(4), 271–280. https://doi.org/10.1037/a0029204

Volgsten, H., Jansson, C., Svanberg, A. S., Darj, E., & Stavreus-Evers, A. (2018). Longitudinal study of emotional experiences, grief and depressive symptoms in women and men after miscarriage. *Midwifery, 64*, 23–28. https://doi.org/10.1016/j.midw.2018.05.003

Volk, J., Palaker, D., O'Brien, M., & Goe, C. L. (2021, June 23). *States' actions to expand telemedicine access during COVID-19 and future policy considerations.* The Commonwealth Fund. https://www.commonwealthfund.org/publications/issue-briefs/2021/jun/states-actions-expand-telemedicine-access-covid-19

von Foerster, H. (2003). *Understanding understanding: Essays on cybernetics and cognition.* Springer-Verlag.

Wade, D. T., & Halligan, P. W. (2017). The biopsychosocial model of illness: A model whose time has come. *Clinical Rehabilitation, 31*(8), 995–1004. https://doi.org/10.1177/0269215517709890

Wagner, E. H., Austin, B. T., & Von Korff, M. (1996). Organizing care for patients with chronic illness. *The Milbank Quarterly, 74*(4), 511–544. https://doi.org/10.2307/3350391

Waldstein, S. R., Neumann, S. A., Drossman, D. A., & Novack, D. H. (2001). Teaching psychosomatic (biopsychosocial) medicine in United States medical schools: Survey findings. *Psychosomatic Medicine, 63*(3), 335–343. https://doi.org/10.1097/00006842-200105000-00001

Walsh, F. (2015). *Strengthening family resilience* (3rd ed.). Guilford Press.

Walter, H. J., Vernacchio, L., Trudrell, E. K., Bromberg, J., Goodman, E., Barton, J., Young, G. J., DeMaso, D. R., & Focht, G. (2019). Five-year outcomes of behavioral health integration in pediatric primary care. *Pediatrics, 144*(1), Article e20183243. https://doi.org/10.1542/peds.2018-3243

Wang, P. S., Lane, M., Olfson, M., Pincus, H. A., Wells, K. B., & Kessler, R. C. (2005). Twelve-month use of mental health services in the United States: Results from the National Comorbidity Survey Replication. *Archives of General Psychiatry, 62*(6), 629–640. https://doi.org/10.1001/archpsyc.62.6.629

Ward, B. W., Schiller, J. S., & Goodman, R. A. (2014). Multiple chronic conditions among U.S. adults: A 2012 update. *Preventing Chronic Disease, 11*, E62.

Ward, W., Zagoloff, A., Rieck, C., & Robiner, W. (2018). Interprofessional education: Opportunities and challenges for psychology. *Journal of Clinical Psychology in Medical Settings, 25*(3), 250–266. https://doi.org/10.1007/s10880-017-9538-3

Ward-Zimmerman, B., Gunn, W. B., Ruddy, N. B., Vogel, M. E., Cubic, B. A., Kearney, L. A., Neumann, C., Stillman, M. A., & Wells, S. (Eds.). (2021). *Integrated primary care psychology: An introductory curriculum.* Society for Health Psychology.

Warren, J. C., Smalley, K. B., & Barefoot, K. N. (2016). Psychological well-being among transgender and genderqueer individuals. *International Journal of Transgenderism, 17*(3–4), 114–123. https://doi.org/10.1080/15532739.2016.1216344

Waters, H., & Graf, M. (2018). *The costs of chronic disease in the U.S.* Milken Institute. https://milkeninstitute.org/sites/default/files/reports-pdf/ChronicDiseases-HighRes-FINAL.pdf

Watson, W. H., & McDaniel, S. H. (2005). Managing emotional reactivity in couples facing illness: Smoothing out the emotional roller coaster. In M. Harway (Ed.), *Handbook of couples therapy* (pp. 253–271). Wiley.

Waugh, M., Calderone, J., Brown Levey, S., Lyon, C., Thomas, M., deGruy, F., & Shore, J. H. (2019). Using telepsychiatry to enrich existing integrated primary care. *Telemedicine Journal and e-Health, 25*(8), 762–768. https://doi.org/10.1089/tmj.2018.0132

Weller, J., Boyd, M., & Cumin, D. (2014). Teams, tribes and patient safety: Overcoming barriers to effective teamwork in healthcare. *Postgraduate Medical Journal, 90*(1061), 149–154. https://doi.org/10.1136/postgradmedj-2012-131168

Wells, H., Crowe, M., & Inder, M. (2020). Why people choose to participate in psychotherapy for depression: A qualitative study. *Journal of Psychiatric and Mental Health Nursing, 27*(4), 417–424. https://doi.org/10.1111/jpm.12597

White, N., & Newman, E. (2016). Shared recovery: Couples' experiences after treatment for colorectal cancer. *European Journal of Oncology Nursing, 21,* 223–231. https://doi.org/10.1016/j.ejon.2015.10.008

Whitebird, R. R., Solberg, L. I., Jaeckels, N. A., Pietruszewski, P. B., Hadzic, S., Unützer, J., Ohnsorg, K. A., Rossom, R. C., Beck, A., Joslyn, K. E., & Rubenstein, L. V. (2014). Effective implementation of collaborative care for depression: What is needed? *The American Journal of Managed Care, 20*(9), 699–707.

Whitfield, J., LePoire, E., Stanczyk, B., Ratzliff, A., & Cerimele, J. M. (2022). Remote collaborative care with off-site behavioral health care managers: A systematic review of clinical trials. *Journal of the Academy of Consultation-Liaison Psychiatry, 63*(1), 71–85. https://doi.org/10.1016/j.jaclp.2021.07.012

Widmer, E. D., Girardin, M., & Ludwig, C. (2018). Conflict structures in family networks of older adults and their relationship with health-related quality of life. *Journal of Family Issues, 39*(6), 1573–1597. https://doi.org/10.1177/0192513X17714507

Wiebe, S. A., & Johnson, S. M. (2016). A review of the research in emotionally focused therapy for couples. *Family Process, 55*(3), 390–407.

Wielen, L. M., Gilchrist, E. C., Nowels, M. A., Petterson, S. M., Rust, G., & Miller, B. F. (2015). Not near enough: Racial and ethnic disparities in access to nearby behavioral health care and primary care. *Journal of Health Care for the Poor and Underserved, 26*(3), 1032–1047. https://doi.org/10.1353/hpu.2015.0083

Wiener, L., Kazak, A. E., Noll, R. B., Patenaude, A. F., & Kupst, M. J. (2015). Standards for the psychosocial care of children with cancer and their families: An introduction to the special issue. *Pediatric Blood & Cancer, 62*(Suppl. 5), S419–S424. https://doi.org/10.1002/pbc.25675

Wilbur, K., Snyder, C., Essary, A. C., Reddy, S., Will, K. K., & Saxon, M. (2020). Developing workforce diversity in the health professions: A social justice perspective. *Health Profession Education, 6*(2), 222–229. https://doi.org/10.1016/j.hpe.2020.01.002

Wilfong, K. M., Goodie, J. L., Curry, J. C., Hunter, C. L., & Kroke, P. C. (2019). The impact of brief interventions on functioning among those demonstrating anxiety, depressive, and adjustment disorder symptoms in primary care: The effectiveness of the Primary Care Behavioral Health (PCBH) model. *Journal of Clinical Psychology in Medical Settings, 29*(2), 318–331.

Willard-Grace, R., Hessler, D., Rogers, E., Dubé, K., Bodenheimer, T., & Grumbach, K. (2014). Team structure and culture are associated with lower burnout in primary care. *Journal of the American Board of Family Medicine, 27*(2), 229–238. https://doi.org/10.3122/jabfm.2014.02.130215

Williams, D., Eckstrom, J., Avery, M., & Unützer, J. (2015). Perspectives of behavioral health clinicians in a rural integrated primary care/mental health program. *The Journal of Rural Health, 31*(4), 346–353. https://doi.org/10.1111/jrh.12114

Williams-Reade, J., Freitas, C., & Lawson, L. (2014). Narrative-informed medical family therapy: Using narrative therapy practices in brief medical encounters. *Families, Systems & Health, 32*(4), 416–425. https://doi.org/10.1037/fsh0000082

Willis, B., & O'Donohue, W. T. (2018). The neglected constructs of health literacy, shared decision-making, and patient-centered care in behavioral health: An integrated model. In M. P. Duckworth & W. T. O'Donohue (Eds.), *Behavioral medicine and integrated care* (pp. 147–174). Springer.

Wilson, J. L. (1964). Growth and development of pediatrics: Presidential address—1964. *The Journal of Pediatrics, 65*(6), 984–991. https://doi.org/10.1016/S0022-3476(64)80031-7

Wilson, P. G. (2004). The Air Force experience: Integrating behavioral health providers into primary care. In R. G. Frank, S. H. McDaniel, J. H. Bray, & M. Heldring (Eds.), *Primary care psychology* (pp. 169–185). American Psychological Association. https://doi.org/10.1037/10651-009

Wolff, J. L., & Jacobs, B. J. (2015). Chronic illness trends and the challenges to family caregivers: Organization and system health barriers. In J. E. Gaugler & R. L. Kane (Eds.), *Family caregiving in the new normal* (pp. 79–103). Elsevier. https://doi.org/10.1016/B978-0-12-417046-9.00007-6

Wolff, J. L., & Roter, D. L. (2011). Family presence in routine medical visits: A meta-analytical review. *Social Science & Medicine, 72*(6), 823–831. https://doi.org/10.1016/j.socscimed.2011.01.015

Wolk, C. B., Alter, C. L., Kishton, R., Rado, J., Atlas, J. A., Press, M. J., Jordan, N., Grant, M., Livesey, C., Rosenthal, L. J., & Smith, J. D. (2021). Improving payment for collaborative mental health care in primary care. *Medical Care, 59*(4), 324–326. https://doi.org/10.1097/MLR.0000000000001485

Wong, E. C., Jaycox, L. H., Ayer, L., Batka, C., Harris, R., Naftel, S., & Paddock, S. M. (2015). Evaluating the implementation of the re-engineering systems of primary care treatment in the military (RESPECT-Mil). *Rand Health Quarterly, 5*(2), 13.

Wood, E., Ohlsen, S., & Ricketts, T. (2017). What are the barriers and facilitators to implementing collaborative care for depression? A systematic review. *Journal of Affective Disorders, 214*, 26–43. https://doi.org/10.1016/j.jad.2017.02.028

Woods, S. B., Bridges, K., & Carpenter, E. N. (2020). The critical need to recognize that families matter for adult health: A systematic review of the literature. *Family Process, 59*(4), 1608–1626. https://doi.org/10.1111/famp.12505

World Health Organization. (2010). *Framework for action on interprofessional education & collaborative practice.* http://apps.who.int/iris/bitstream/10665/70185/1/WHO_HRH_HPN_10.3_eng.pdf

Wranik, W. D., Price, S., Haydt, S. M., Edwards, J., Hatfield, K., Weir, J., & Doria, N. (2019). Implications of interprofessional primary care team characteristics for health services and patient health outcomes: A systematic review with narrative synthesis. *Health Policy, 123*(6), 550–563. https://doi.org/10.1016/j.healthpol.2019.03.015

Wright, A. A., Keating, N. L., Ayanian, J. Z., Chrischilles, E. A., Kahn, K. L., Ritchie, C. S., Weeks, J. C., Earle, C. C., & Landrum, M. B. (2016). Family perspectives on aggressive cancer care near the end of life. *JAMA, 315*(3), 284–292. https://doi.org/10.1001/jama.2015.18604

Wynne, L. C., Shields, C. G., & Sirkin, M. I. (1992). Illness, family theory, and family therapy: I. Conceptual issues. *Family Process, 31*(1), 3–18. https://doi.org/10.1111/j.1545-5300.1992.00003.x

Wysocki, T., Harris, M. A., Buckloh, L. M., Mertlich, D., Lochrie, A. S., Mauras, N., & White, N. H. (2007). Randomized trial of behavioral family systems therapy for diabetes: Maintenance of effects on diabetes outcomes in adolescents. *Diabetes Care, 30*(3), 555–560. https://doi.org/10.2337/dc06-1613

Wysocki, T., Harris, M. A., Buckloh, L. M., Mertlich, D., Lochrie, A. S., Taylor, A., Sadler, M., Mauras, N., & White, N. H. (2006). Effects of behavioral family systems therapy for diabetes on adolescents' family relationships, treatment adherence, and metabolic control. *Journal of Pediatric Psychology, 31*(9), 928–938. https://doi.org/10.1093/jpepsy/jsj098

Wysocki, T., Harris, M. A., Buckloh, L. M., Mertlich, D., Lochrie, A. S., Taylor, A., Sadler, M., & White, N. H. (2008). Randomized, controlled trial of behavioral family systems therapy for diabetes: Maintenance and generalization of effects on parent-adolescent communication. *Behavior Therapy, 39*(1), 33–46. https://doi.org/10.1016/j.beth.2007.04.001

Yang, Q., Chen, Y., & Wendorf Muhamad, J. (2017). Social support, trust in health information, and health information seeking behaviors (HISBs): A study using the 2012 Annenberg National Health Communication Survey (ANHCS). *Health Communication, 32*(9), 1142–1150. https://doi.org/10.1080/10410236.2016.1214220

Yim, I. S., Tanner Stapleton, L. R., Guardino, C. M., Hahn-Holbrook, J., & Dunkel Schetter, C. (2015). Biological and psychosocial predictors of postpartum depression: Systematic review and call for integration. *Annual Review of Clinical Psychology, 11*(1), 99–137. https://doi.org/10.1146/annurev-clinpsy-101414-020426

Young, N. S., Ioannidis, J. P. A., & Al-Ubaydli, O. (2008). Why current publication practices may distort science. *PLOS Medicine, 5*(10), e201. https://doi.org/10.1371/journal.pmed.0050201

Young-Hyman, D., de Groot, M., Hill-Briggs, F., Gonzalez, J. S., Hood, K., & Peyrot, M. (2016). Psychosocial care for people with diabetes: A position statement of the American Diabetes Association. *Diabetes Care, 39*(12), 2126–2140. https://doi.org/10.2337/dc16-2053

Yu, L., Mo, L., Tang, Y., Huang, X., & Tan, J. (2014). Effects of nursing intervention models on social adaption capability development in preschool children with malignant tumors: A randomized control trial. *Psycho-Oncology, 23*(6), 708–712. https://doi.org/10.1002/pon.3572

Zallman, L., Joseph, R., O'Brien, C., Benedetto, E., Grossman, E., Arsenault, L., & Sayah, A. (2017). Does behavioral health integration improve primary care providers' perceptions of health-care system functioning and their own knowledge? *General Hospital Psychiatry, 46,* 88–93. https://doi.org/10.1016/j.genhosppsych.2017.03.005

Zeckhauser, R. (2021). Strategic sorting: The role of ordeals in health care. *Economics and Philosophy, 37*(1), 64–81. https://doi.org/10.1017/S0266267120000139

Zhang, X., Wang, G., Wang, H., Wang, X., Ji, T., Hou, D., Wu, J., Sun, J., & Zhu, B. (2020). Spouses' perceptions of and attitudes toward female menopause: A mixed-methods systematic review. *Climacteric, 23*(2), 148–157. https://doi.org/10.1080/13697137.2019.1703937

Zhang, Y. (2018). Family functioning in the context of an adult family member with illness: A concept analysis. *Journal of Clinical Nursing, 27*(15–16), 3205–3224. https://doi.org/10.1111/jocn.14500

Zimmer, Z., Jagger, C., Chiu, C. T., Ofstedal, M. B., Rojo, F., & Saito, Y. (2016). Spirituality, religiosity, aging and health in global perspective: A review. *SSM—Population Health, 2,* 373–381. https://doi.org/10.1016/j.ssmph.2016.04.009

Zimmermann, M., O'Donohue, W., & Vechiu, C. (2020). A primary care prevention system for behavioral health: The behavioral health annual wellness checkup. *Journal of Clinical Psychology in Medical Settings, 27*(2), 268–284. https://doi.org/10.1007/s10880-019-09658-8

Zubatsky, M., & Mendenhall, T. (2018). Medical family therapy in endocrinology. In T. Mendenhall, A. Lamson, J. Hodgson, & M. Baird (Eds.), *Clinical methods in medical family therapy* (pp. 293–319). Springer. https://doi.org/10.1007/978-3-319-68834-3_11

Zuckerman, B. (2016). Two-generation pediatric care: A modest proposal. *Pediatrics, 137*(1), Article e20153447. https://doi.org/10.1542/peds.2015-3447

Index

About the Authors

Nancy Breen Ruddy, PhD, is a professor of clinical psychology at Antioch University New England in Keene, New Hampshire. She directs the health psychology curriculum, which centers on primary care psychology. Prior to joining Antioch in 2020, she spent 3 decades training both medical and mental health professionals to provide integrated behavioral health. Her roles spanned multiple disciplines and training levels, including medical residency faculty, psychology postdoctoral fellowship director, postgraduate training program faculty, and curriculum design expert. Dr. Ruddy is a licensed psychologist and medical family therapist, having obtained both Clinical Member and Approved Supervisor status in the American Association for Marriage and Family Therapy. She has served as the chair of the Integrated Primary Care Interest Group in the Society for Health Psychology and is a past-president of the Society. Dr. Ruddy was recognized for her contributions to the field of health psychology with the Timothy B. Jeffrey Memorial Award for Outstanding Contributions to Clinical Health Psychology in 2013. In addition, she has consulted to dozens of healthcare systems to facilitate the integration of behavioral health services into medical settings. Dr. Ruddy has published numerous book chapters and articles on integrated healthcare, as well as the 2008 American Psychological Association book, *The Collaborative Psychotherapist: Creating Reciprocal Relationships With Medical Professionals.*

Susan H. McDaniel, PhD, ABPP, is the Dr. Laurie Sands Distinguished Professor of Families & Health at the University of Rochester Medical Center (URMC), where she has multiple roles. She is the director of the URMC Physician Communication Coaching and Leadership Development Program. She is the vice chair of the Department of Family Medicine and, in the Department of Psychiatry, she is chief psychologist and the director of the Institute for the

Family. Dr. McDaniel's career is dedicated to integrating psychological and relational science and practice into healthcare. She has won many awards and authored well over 100 journal articles and authored and/or edited 17 books; translations of some of these works represent 10 languages. The American Psychological Association (APA) published five of these books— *Medical Family Therapy and Integrated Care, Family Therapy, Primary Care Psychology, Integrating Family Therapy,* and *Casebook for Integrating Family Therapy*—as well as special issues of the *American Psychologist*, one on psychology and primary care and other on the science of teamwork. Dr. McDaniel served as coeditor, with Thomas Campbell, MD, of *Families, Systems, & Health,* for 12 years and as associate editor for the *American Psychologist* for 10 years. She is a frequent speaker at national and international medical and mental health meetings. Dr. McDaniel has held many leadership positions in mental health and primary care, including serving as the 2016 president of the APA.